MOOD DISORDERS

Edited by **Neşe Kocabaşoğlu**

Mood Disorders
http://dx.doi.org/10.5772/55930
Edited by Neşe Kocabaşoğlu

Contributors

Ana Polona Mivšek, Tita Stanek Zidaric, Jana Hroudova, Zdenek Fisar, Jiri Raboch, Alfonso Valenzuela, Rodrigo Valenzuela Baez, Aleksandra Suwalska, Dorota Łojko, Dagmar Breznoscakova, Andreea Letitia Arsene, Niculina Mitrea, Cristina Manuela Dragoi, Alina Crenguta Nicolae, Doina Draganescu, Dumitru Lupuliasa, Ion-Bogdan Dumitrescu, Dragos Florian Ciolan, Nasser Haddjeri, Ouissame Mnie-Filali, Erika Abrial, Laura Lambás-Señas, Yong-Ku Kim, Bertalan Dudas, Irene Lehner-Adam, Toshihiko Yanagita, Wendy Cross

Published by InTech

Janeza Trdine 9, 51000 Rijeka, Croatia

Publishing Process Manager Danijela Duric
Technical Editor InTech DTP team
Cover InTech Design team

Additional hard copies can be obtained from orders@intechopen.com

Mood Disorders, Edited by Neşe Kocabaşoğlu
p. cm.
ISBN 978-953-51-0959-4

For EU product safety concerns:
IN TECH d.o.o., Prolaz Marije Krucifikse Kozulić 3, 51000 Rijeka, Croatia,
info@intechopen.com or visit our website at intechopen.com.

Meet the editor

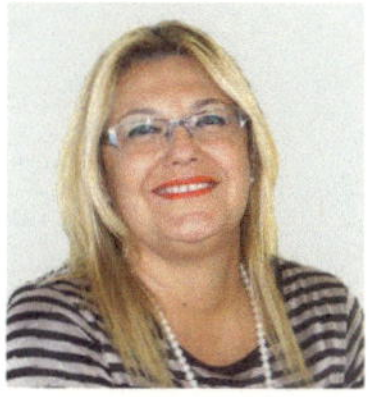

Professor Doctor Neşe Kocabaşoğlu has been born in 1960 in Istanbul, Turkey. She graduated from Besiktas Ataturk Deneme High School in 1997 and from Istanbul University Cerrahpasa Medical Faculty in 1983. She completed her mandatory medical service in Mersin, Turkey from 1984 to 1986. In 1986, she got back to Cerrahpasa Medical Faculty and started as an assistant doctor in Psychiaty Department. When she became psychiatry specialist in 1991, she started to work as teaching assistant in the same department. In 1995 she got the title of associate professor. She became a professor in 2001 and is still a professor lecturer in Cerrahpasa Medical Faculty.
She is a founder member of Turkish Psychiatry Association, founded in 1995 and has its headquarters in Ankara. She is also a member of Sexual Health Institute (CİSED) in Turkey and an international member of American Psychiatry Association. She works as the publishing secretary of the regularly published magazines New Symposium Psychiatry and Neurological Sciences Magazine as well as the publishing advisory committee member of the Okmeydani Medical Journal and Clinical Psychopharmalogical Journal. She has done much research about social psychiatry and anxiety disorders. Parallel to her work, she founded Cerrahpasa Medical Faculty Psychiatry Department's Anxiety Disorders Unit.

Contents

Preface

If we look at the history of development of the science of psychiatry in the world we will see that the important change and developments have occurred in the last 50 years.

Mood disorders are thought to be a group of diseases which are mainly a result of disturbance of mood and it is also characterized by cognitive, psychomotor and interpersonal psycho-physiological disorders. These people lose self control and they have an extremely distressed life.

Mood disorders are emotional tone disorders that affect perception of patients and their interest to themselves, others and environment profoundly.

In this book, we touched on different subjects, such as relationship of mood disorders with mother-infant, mitochondrial functions, Omega 3 (DHA) and glycid metabolism. Also, we paid attention to cognitive factors in euthymic BD with Lithium treatment. You will find the topics interested which are focused on murine models for developing an individualized neuropsychopharmacotherapy based on the behavior typology; relationships of mood disorders with biological markers; genetic factors; cognitive behavioral therapy; 5-HT system; depression-culture relationship; and neuronal insulin receptor signaling.

It can be said that the owners of different topics cooperate sincerely and prepared their own issues with great precision in preparation of this book. Our common stance here is "what's new on the agenda under the heading of Mood Disorders" and what our friends are doing. However, we know that the reader wants to reach more comprehensive and detailed information, here a feature of the scientist is acceptance of each resource in his hands as a new starting point.

I thank to all of those who have contributed during the publication of this book, to all my colleagues named on this book, to Publishing Process Manager Silvia Vlase and Head of Production Ms. Danijela Duric. They facilitated the duty of the editor with their careful work.

This book is dedicated to people who have psychiatric problems and people who care for them.

Prof. Dr. Neşe Kocabaşoğlu
Istanbul University,
Faculty of Medicine,
Department of Psychiatry
Istanbul / Turkey

Chapter 1

Murine Models for Developping an Individualized Neuropsychopharmacotherapy Based on the Behaviour Typology

Andreea Letitia Arsene, Niculina Mitrea,
Dumitru Lupuliasa, Cristina Manuela Dragoi,
Alina Crenguta Nicolae, Ion-Bogdan Dumitrescu,
Dragos Florian Ciolan and Doina Draganescu

Additional information is available at the end of the chapter

http://dx.doi.org/10.5772/53323

1. Introduction

A drug administered in the same dosage, under similar conditions, to adult individuals from a population homogeneous in race, gender and age, triggers different pharmacological effects. This phenomenon represents the pharmacological variability in a relatively homogeneous population, as a natural expression of the biological variability of the response to any stimulus. The cause of the pharmacological variability to a drug is often considerably different between the individuals of the same population. The pharmacology variability (pharmacokinetics, pharmaco-dynamics and pharmaco-toxicological) is therefore of two types: inter-individual (on population level) and, respectively, intra-individual (on individual level).

General mechanisms of the pharmacological variability

They can be grouped into: pharmacokinetic mechanisms (variations in the drug concentrations in the plasma and in the substrate receptor) and pharmaco-dynamic mechanisms (variations regarding the drug-receptor substrate complex).

Pharmacokinetic mechanisms of the pharmacological variability

The variations in the drug concentrations in plasma and on the level of the receptor substrate represent the pharmacokinetic variability which contributes to the pharmaco-dynamic, pharmaco-therapeutic and pharmaco-toxicological variability. The cases are represented by inter and intra-individual differences, in the rate of the physiological processes: absorption; distribution (transport, diffusion, storage); epuration (biotransformation, excretion).

The most extensive and complex pharmacokinetic variability is manifested in the biotransformation process, being caused by the following phenomena: enzyme induction or inhibition, induced by various factors including by the inducing drugs or enzyme inhibitors; enzymopathies genetically determined.

Pharmaco-dynamic mechanisms of the pharmacological variability

The variations regarding the complex drug- receptor substrate induce the pharmaco-toxicological and pharmaco-dynamic variability. The causes are represented by inter-intra-individual differences, in the functional state of the receptor system (R) - the effect on the number and the binding capacity of R, the state of intermediate links in the chain of the receptor-effector system and to the physiological agonist concentrations (chemical mediator) and certain ions in the R level.

The biological variability in the functional state of the receptor-effector system is determined by the following phenomena: desensitization of R ("down" - adjustment) or sensitization of R ("up" - adjustment), caused by various factors, including the agonist drugs and the antagonists drugs or of illnesses of the receptors (autoimmune diseases, genetic diseases, aberrations induced by mutagens and oncogenes drugs, diseases of the link of coupling R – effector, represented by Gs protein).

The types of pharmacological variability

In accordance with these multiple mechanism generating individual reactivity on the drug effect, the pharmacological variability can be classified into several types:

- By the criterion of the area of expansion of the population: inter-individual and intra-individual variability.
- By the criterion of the appearance time: congenital and acquired variability;
- By the criterion of the statistical classification: normal, uni-modal variability (Gaussian type) and abnormal (bimodal or multimodal).

From a statistical viewpoint (reported on the average response of most individuals), the pharmacological variability is manifested either uni-modal (Gaussian) or polimodal.

- *The normalvariability* depends on the physiological type (CNS type, endocrine, metabolic, etc.) and on the ability to physiological control the enzyme functions (induction and enzyme inhibition) and the receptors ("up" and "down" adjustment). The normal relationship between the intensity of the pharmaco-dynamic effect (the response) and the number of the individuals from a community which respond with the same intensity, on the same dose of medication, it is represented in Cartesian graph by the frequency-distribution curve.
- *The abnormal variability* is the consequence of the genetic diseases (receptoropaties and enzymopathies) or the immunological mechanisms (allergic and autoimmune). In this case, the normal frequency-distribution curve with the allure of a bell looks bimodal, trimodal or even multimodal.

Psychoneuroendocrine behavior typology, factor of the biological and pharmacological variability

The psychoneuroendocrine typology should be considered within the factors generating biological and pharmacological variability. We refer to the following two types of psychoneuroendocrine behaviours, described in literature:

- the adrenergic type "A". The differentiation of the adrenergic typology was first realized in 1978 by RH Rosenman, by describing some specific behavioral characteristics that predispose it to the emergence and the development of cardiovascular diseases: competitiveness, sharp ambition, continuous involvement in multiple and diverse activities, with a sense of haste and time urgency, irritability, impulsivity, reduced ability to disconnect and relaxation.

- the opioid type "O". The "non-A" type, opposite to the adrenergic type from the behavior point of view, with the psychoneuroendocrine predominance of the endogenous opioid system. It has the following characteristics: defensive, calm, relaxed, non-aggressive, introverted, resistant to pain, but with predisposition to the hiperalgia post-stress syndrome.

Based on the studies performed and published by Rosenman RH on the adrenergic psychoneuroendocrine type (A) [30], numerous experimental and clinical studies have been performed to highlight the neuroendocrine grounds of the opposite behavioral type, usually called type B or "non-A". In this regard there was hypothesized that the "non-A" type has, in fact, opioid neuroendocrine bases and was suggested as type "O". This hypothesis was based on the following theoretical and practical considerations:

1. The endogenous opioid system (through a cybernetic mechanism of "feedback" type) operates as a modulator system of the activator, "alarm", adrenergic (operating through a cybernetic mechanism of "feed-before" type) systems. Between these two systems there are highly complex interrelationships, their non-synchronization or physiological alterations resulting in different pathological conditions such as the coronary disease or cardiac ischemia. It was also shown that stress, adrenaline and endogenous opioids act through some very well correlated mechanisms [8].

2. Pharmacological research has shown that the adrenergic system and the endogenous opioid system are closely-correlated and involved in the informational aggression syndrome [7,8]. Thus, it was shown that there are two types of individuals: those who have the *adrenergic type of behavior* associated with *basal pain hypersensitivity,* and others having the *opioidergic type of behavior* associated with *pain hyposensitivity* [8].

Therefore, in order to differentiate the human and murine adrenergic and opioid types, the literature presents the following methods:

- for human subjects: personality questionnaire - personality type O was found to be opposite (complementary) to type A, corresponding to type B ("non-A");

- or humans and animals: the reaction to pain - it should be registered the time for the pain reaction occurrence by using the heat stimuli.

Parameter followed	Type A	Type O
1. Hostility	1.1 Hostile	No
	1.2 Irritable, angry	No
	1.3 Aggressive	Defensive
	1.4 Agitated	Relaxed
	1.5 Randy	Calm
	1.6 Extroverted	Introvert
2. The spirit of competition	2.1 Fighter	No
	2.2 Ambitious	No
	2.3 Dominant	No
	2.4 Confident	No
	2.5 Deep involvement in an activity, failing to distraction	No
	2.6 Hyperactive	Slow
3. The urgency of time	3.1 Hurry	Calm, slow
	3.2 Tense	Relaxed
	3.3 Alert	Fear
	3.4 Strained countenance	Relaxed
4. Appetite	4.1 Great (increases in stress)	Anorexia

Table 1. Personality questionnaire for differentiating typologies A and O [7]

Assessment of the behavioral type of adrenergic type in children [13,16]

The clinical trials have included children of different ages (3-13 years) being included both boys and girls. There were pursued the following parameters:

- the time in which the child likes to play;
- the impatience;
- the competitiveness;
- the anger;
- the aggressiveness;
- the crisis time;
- the cardiovascular response (the systolic blood pressure, the diastolic blood pressure, the heart rate);
- the variation of the urinary catecholamine concentrations in basal and stress state.

These studies highlighted that the characteristic features of A type can be measured from the early childhood (3-6 years). It was also noted that boys obtained higher scores for the A type behavior, compared with the girls. In addition, the cardiovascular responses and the urinary concentrations of catecholamines were much higher in boys than in girls, both in basal state and in stress.

The assessment of the behavioral type of adrenergic type in men and women [13,14]

The specialty literature describes numerous clinical studies that have attempted to differentiate the adrenergic feminine typology by the male typology. In this respect it was found that the sex factor does not significantly influence the personality traits specific to adrenergic, major differences occurring with the installation of stressful situations. Thus, it was found that in stress, the systolic blood pressure, the heart rate and the urinary catecholamine levels are significantly lower in women than men. Basically, the women's physiological reactivity is much less competitive than the men's, in the same stressful situation.

Clinical studies on the impact of A Type behavior on the cardiovascular physiological reactivity.

Numerous clinical studies have been performed [14,16,17,19] to correlate the characteristic features of A type with the cardiovascular responses, in stress. Heart rate, EKG, blood pressure and peripheral vasoconstriction were mesured. Type A individuals revealed increase cardiovascular responsiveness.

Clinical studies for investigating the physiological reactivity of A type with sympathomimetic or sympatholytic drugs [13,27,29].

There were carried out numerous research studies of the cardiovascular responses (systolic and diastolic blood pressure, heart rate), in individuals with personality of type A, treated with beta-adrenolitic. The results showed that these drugs reduced in type A statistically significant cardiovascular physiological parameters investigated, compared with type B.

A number of clinical studies investigated the antagonistic potency in sympathetic/parasympathetic systems in type A, compared with type B. In this purpose were evaluated the specific cardiovascular parameters (e.g. the amplitude of T wave from electrocardiogram) after the administration of sympathomimetic drugs (isoproterenol, norepinephrine, etc). In all cases the return to normal, physiological limits of the studied cardiovascular parameters was achieved much faster (significant) in type B, suggesting a lower parasympathetic antagonism in the adrenergic type.

Murine and clinical studies on the impact of A Type behavior on the CNS physiopathology

Published clinical studies, reported the prevalence of bipolar disorder and the ciclotimic temper within the adrenergic behavioral type [2,3,7].

Experimetal actometry test (for investigation the spontaneous motor activity), the platform test, the inclined plane test and the plate with holes test (to research the evasion-investigation behavior), the cross-maze test (for investigating the anxiety), were performed on animals. Their results revealed a significant predisposition to anxiety of the adrenergic type together with an higher agitation [7].

In our previous studies [2] we evaluated the cerebral monoaminergic status, in mice identified as adrenergic or opioid types, compared with the intermediate N type. We mesured the neuronal levels of noradrenaline, serotonin, dopamine and GABA, both in basal state and after acute stress in order to establish some potential predictive biomarkers for an individualized therapy according to the behaviour typology.

2. Objectives

Individuals variability in regard to their reactivity to thermic stimuli constitutes an accepted predictive factor for establishing the behavioural typology in animals [8] namely the adrenergic and opioid types. Thus, the reported validated murine model is the hot-plate test. Accordingly, the jumping time off the 60°C heated plate characterizes animals' endogenous analgesia: the A type of behaviour is associated with basal pain hypersensitivity, while the O type correlates with pain hyposensitivity.

Therefore, after the endogenous analgesic screening, mice were divided into three working groups: the adrenergic "A" type, the equilibrated, intermediate, "N" type and the "O" type, according to Gauss normal distribution curve.

The murine models described were used for investigating the thymic tonus in scute stress, the circadian cronovariability of the thymic tonus and the variability of the antidepressant effect of imipramine, fluoxetine and lithium.

- Studies regarding the thymic tonus in acute stress to adrenergic and opioid types
- Circadian cronovariability of the thymic tonus, within each psychoneuroendocrin type
- Research of the variability of the antidepressant effect of imipramine, fluoxetine and lithium to adrenergic and opioid psychoneuroendocrine types

3. Matherials and methods

Animals

Five-week-old Albino Swiss male mice were purchased from the Biobase of "Carol Davila" University (Bucharest, Romania). They were housed five per cage at a room temperature of 25 ± 1 ºC and 45-55% relative humidity with free access to food and water. Mice were maintained under standardized 12h light-dark cycle (lights on at 7a.m., lights off at 7p.m.) for 1 week before the experiments. All animals used in this study were maintained in facilities fully accreditated and the experiments described here were performed in compliance with the European Communities Council Directive of 24 November 1986 (86/609/EEC) and Ordinance No. 37 of the Romanian Government from 2nd February 2002.

Identification of the murine behavioral type

For the identification of the murine behavior type the hot plate test (Ugo Basile apparatus) was employed, previously described. Briefly, mice were behaviourally characterized based on their endogenous analgesia expressed as the jumping time off the 60 ºC heated plate. Three murine behavioural working groups were drawn: the adrenergic A type (with low endogenous analgesia, low pain reactivity – including thermic pain stimuli), the opioid O type (high endogenous analgesia, high pain reactivity) and the intermediate N type.

Forced swimming test (FST)

To investigate the acute stress-related activity within the murine behavioural categories described, the forced swimming test (FST) was used as stressor (immobilization stress). The procedure was performed according to a previous report (Porsolt et al., 1977). Briefly, mice were placed individually into plastic cylinders (height, 25cm; diameter, 10cm) containing 10 cm of water maintained at 21-23 ºC, and left there for 5 min. A mouse was considered to be immobile when it floated in an upright position and made only small movements to keep its head above water. The duration of immobility was recorded during the 5-min testing period.

FST was also used to establish, within the three murine behavioural typologies described, a pharmacological response pattern after the administration of some psychotropic drugs.

Drugs and treatment procedure

Imipramin, fluoxetin and lithium carbonate were purchased from Sigma. Other routine reagents were of the highest purity commercially available. The drugs were dissolved in sterilized saline. To investigate the influence of the drugs on mice behaviour (expressed as immobility time during the FST), groups of 10 mice from each behavioural typology were injected intraperitoneally, for 10 days, at 9 a.m., the following doses: saline, imipramin 10mg/kg, fluoxetin 10mg/kg, lithium carbonate 70mg/kg. The animals were subjected to the FST before and after drugs administration.

Statistical analysis

For the statistical analysis of the data there were used one-way ANOVA, Spearman coefficient and Pearson coefficient. (SPSS software).

4. Results and discussion

Identification of the murine behavioral type

Individuals variability in regard to their reactivity to thermic stimuli constitutes an accepted predictive factor for establishing the behavioural typology in animals, namely the adrenergic and opioid types. Thus, the reported validated murine model is the hot plate test. Accordingly, the jumping time off the 60 ºC heated plate characterizes animals' endogenous pain responses (endogenous analgesia): the adrenergic type of behavior was associated with basal pain hypersensitivity, and the opioidergic type of behavior was correlated with pain hyposensitivity.

The average value of the jumping time off the 60 ºC heated plate was 30.8±5.36sec. Mice that possessed a value of the jumping time (Jt) of M ± 1SD were selected as intermediate, N type. Mice that registered Jt< M – SD were selected as adrenergic A type, while Jt>M +1SD marked the non-A type (O type) mice.

The differential physiological effects (endogenous algic response) after exposure to the 60 ºC heated plate resulted in a statistical significant difference between A and O type ($p<0.001$), Spearman correlation=0.9812. (figure 1).

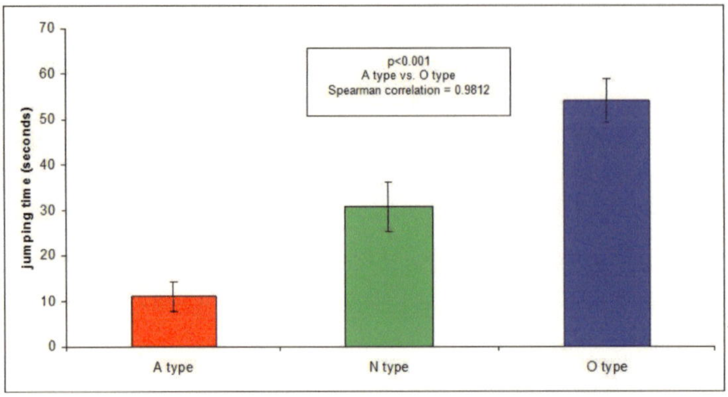

Figure 1. The establishment of the behavioural typology in animals according to the differential physiological effects (endogenous algic response) after the exposure to the 60 °C heated plate (hot plate test)

According to the hot-plate test, the group of animals was distributed as follows (figure 2):

- 30% adrenergic mice;
- 37% normal,intermediate mice;
- 33% opioid animals.

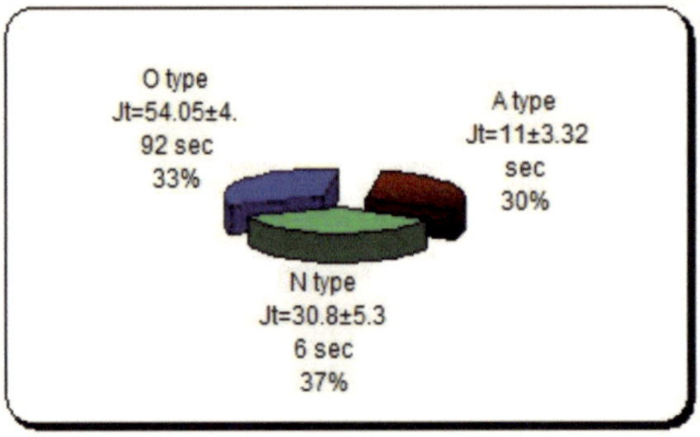

Figure 2. The distribution of the studied animals according to their pain sensitivity

The behavioural screen of the adrenergic and opioid murine typologies after acute stress

The literature shows that, under stress, the clinical manifestations depend on the balance between the adrenergic system and opioid endogenous system [7,8]. For these reasons, under stress, there is great behavioral variability of the psychoneuroendocrine types A and O. This aspect has been shown by means of complex clinical tests, where types A and O have been exposed to the sustained chronic stress. The research results have shown a significant tendency of type A towards the depressive syndrome, in case of the advanced chronic stress. Assuming that the adrenergic, psychoneuroendocrine behavioral type is characterized by competitiveness, combativeness and alertness, we proposed to assess the thymic tonus of adrenergic type, in comparison with the opioid type, under acute stress induced by forced swimming ("desperation") test.

Each individual from each group was submitted to FST and results are depicted in figure 3. As it can be seen the immobilization time is higher in the O type (90.5±23.77 sec), compared with both the A type (37.6±10.64 sec; p<0.001) and N type (81.9±15.54 sec; p<0.05).

	A type	N type	O type
Jt (sec)	11±3.32	30.8 ±5.36	54.05 ± 4.92
Timob(sec)	37.6 ± 10.64	81.9 ± 15.54	90.5 ± 23.77

Table 2. The average values of the jumping time off the heated plate (Jt) and the immobility time (Timob) during FST for the studied behaviour types

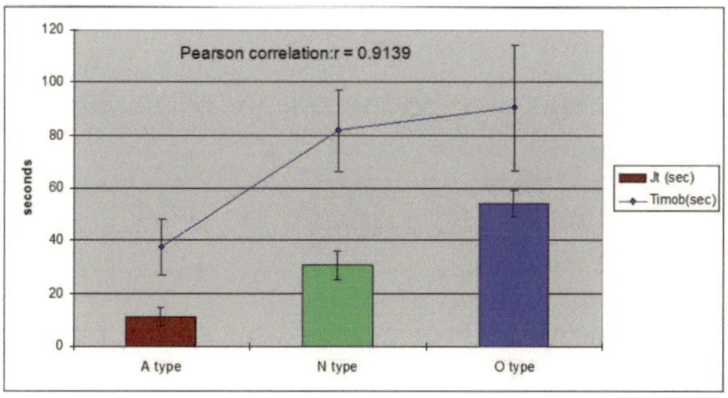

Figure 3. Correlations of the results obtined after submitting the animals to the hot plate test and the forced swimming test

One-way Anova revealed a significant different behavioural reactivity (expressed as immobility time) between the A, N and O groups (F=3.037; p< 0.001). Eventhough the frequency of immobility counts (seconds) is lower for the adrenergics, the A type pattern of the swimming behaviour during FST positively correlates with the O type (Pearson coefficient = 0.9139).

Cronovariability of acute stress-related behavioural patterns

The circadian change of the acute stress responsiveness during FST, related to the adrenergic and opioid behaviour patterns was registered hourly, between 9 and 13 a.m. FST is a consummatory behavioural test in which the homeostatic control of the animal's stress responsiveness and adaptation depends both on the neuronal excitability and neurondocrine reactivity. Previous studies reported an enhanced glucocorticoid and mineralocorticoid responses for the A type of behaviour, together with a high norepinephrine and epinephrine status during specific cognitive tasks, which postulated the basis of psychophyysiological mechanisms of high blood pressue, ischemic cardiopathy, myocardial infarction and sudden death. Recent studies also reported low urinary free cortisol levels togetherwith high urinary norepinephrine excretion in patients with endogenous type depressive disorder, bipolar disorder, paranoid schizophrenia(). All these reports may seem contradictory, but, in fact, many studies reported that the hypothalamic-pituitary-adrenal (HPA) axis plays a pivotal role during organisms adaptation to stress. There was also reported that the activity of HPA axis is influenced by pschychological factors (conflict, the sense of control, etc.) which act through the corticosteroid/catecholamiergic receptor system within the hippocampus.

Neuroendocrine studies have shown that glucocorticoids, mineralocorticoids and catecholamines regulate the stress-activated neural metabolism, modulate the stress response and control the subsequent adaptive behaviour of animals [4,5,10,26]. There was demonstrated that a proper balance between glucocorticoids, mineralocorticoids and catecholamines is of paramount importance for the homeostatic control of organisms' stress and adaptation.

In this regard, we aimed to assess the acute stress behaviour profile of the A type, compared with both the the opioidergic O type and the normal N type, during FST.

In order to assess the chronovariability of the thymic tonus in the three psychoneuroendocrine types, the initial communities of animals corresponding to types A, N and O have been redivided, as follows:

- Group 1A: consisting of adrenergic type animals, for which the immobilization time was monitored between 9-10 am
- Group 2A: consisting of adrenergic type animals, for which the immobilization time was monitored between 10 to 11 am
- Group 3A: consisting of adrenergic type animals, for which the immobilization time was monitored between 11 to 12 am
- Group 4A: consisting of adrenergic type animals, for which the immobilization time was monitored between 12 to 13 pm
- Group 1N: consisting of intermediate, balanced type of animals, for which the immobilization time was monitored between 9-10 am
- Group 2N: consisting of intermediate, normal type of animals, for which the immobilization time was monitored between 10 to 11 am
- Group 3N: consisting of intermediate type of animals, for which the immobilization time was monitored between 11 to 12 am
- Group 4N: consisting of normal type animals, for which the immobilization time was monitored between 12-13 pm
- Group 1O: consisting of opioid type animals for which the immobilization time was monitored between 9-10 am
- Group 2O: consisting of opioid type animals for which the immobilization time was monitored between 10-11 am
- Group3O: consisting of opioid type animals for which the immobilization time was monitored between 11-12 am

- Group 4O: f consisting of opioid type animals for which the immobilization time was monitored between 12 to 13 pm

The murine behavioural type	Group 1 9-10a.m	Group 2 10-11a.m.	Group 3 11-12a.m.	Group 4 12-13p.m.
A type	92.73± 25.03	113 ± 35.19	126.3 ± 36.6	105.55 ± 28.2
N type	69.55 ± 20.55	79.83 ± 27.42	100.1 ± 21.89	56.27 ± 17.33
O type	91.16 ± 25.26	125.5 ± 44.25	134.6 ±46.7	98.92 ± 28.53

Table 3. The average values of the immobility time (Timob) during FST for the studied behaviour types at different daily hours

Considering the assessment of the chronovariability of the thymic tonus in the adrenergic psychoneuroendocrine type, during FST, it was registered a gradual increase of the immobilization time, during morning hours, continued at noon(12-13 pm), by a significant decrease (figure 4).

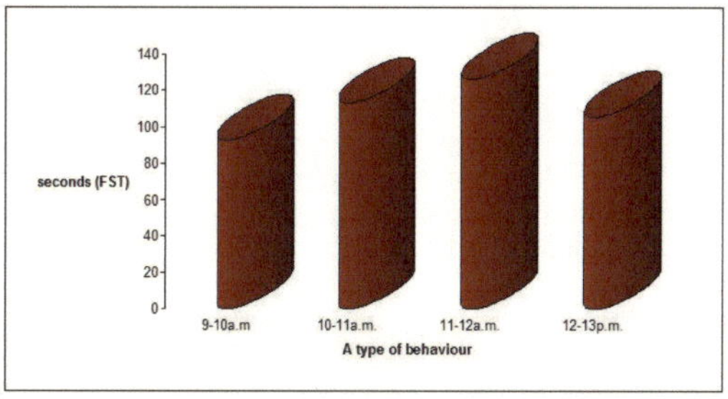

Figure 4. The assessment of the chronovariability of the thymic tonus in the adrenergic psychoneuroendocrine type, during FST

The same pattern was observed for the assessment of the chronovariability of the thymic tonus in the balanced psychoneuroendocrine type, during FST (figure 5).

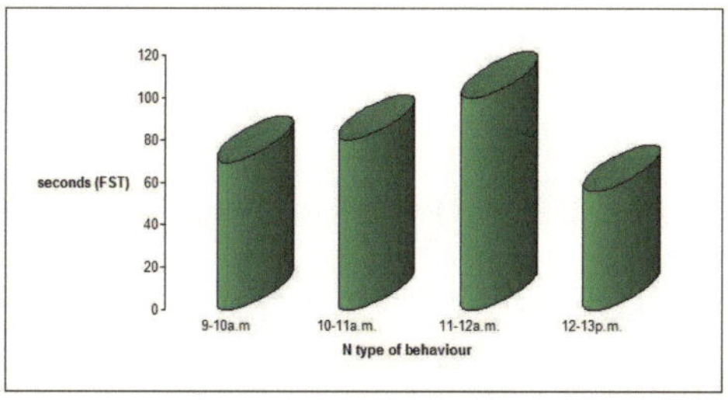

Figure 5. The assessment of the chronovariability of the thymic tonus in the normal psychoneuroendocrine type, during FST

For the opioid psychoneuroendocrine type, it was registered a gradual increase of the immobilization time, at 9-10 am, 10-11 am, 11-12 am, continued at 12-13 pm) by a significant decrease (figure 6).

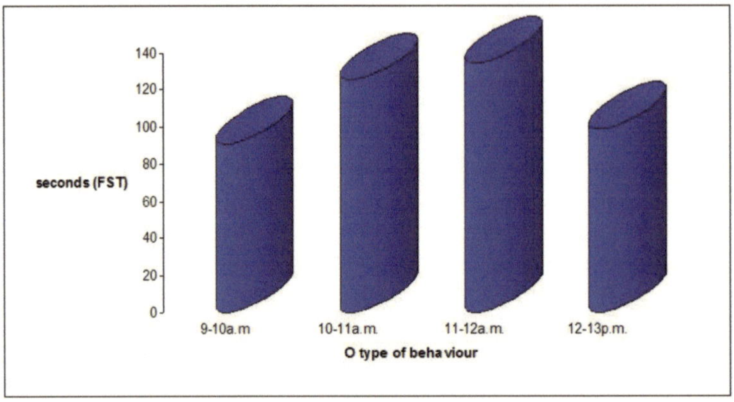

Figure 6. The assessment of the chronovariability of the thymic tonus in the opioid psychoneuroendocrine type, during FST

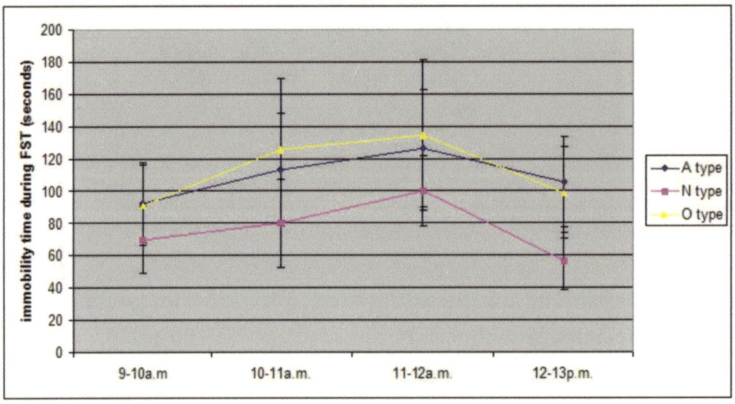

Figure 7. The assessment of the chronovariability of the thymic tonus in the adrenergic, normal and opioid psychoneuroendocrine types, during FST

Analyzing the experimental results obtained, we can highlight some interesting points:

- between 9-10 we have recorded the lowest values of immobilization time (maximum thymic tonus) for all three types of behavior;
- after 10 am (between 10 to 12 am) the values of the immobilization times increase in all cases, so the thymic status involutes towards depression during this time; this behavior is

valid for all psychoneuroendocrine types, becoming statistically significant ($p < 0.05$) in case of the opioid type;

- the peak of "depression" is recorded between 11 to 12 am in all cases and varies as follows: type O (maximum depression - Timob = 134.61 ± 46.70 sec) > TYPE A (Timob = 126.36 ± 36.60 sec) > type N (100.16 ± 21.89 sec);

- after 12 am (between 12 to 13 am) the values of the immobilization times decrease very much, quickly returning to the values recorded at 9 o'clock am (spectacular recursion of the thymic tonus); this issue was highlighted for all psychoneuroendocrine types, indicating that the balanced type distinguished itself significantly from the statistical point of view by the lowest values of the immobilization time (so the most important recursion of the thymic tonus): $p < 0.02$;

- in addition, the values of the immobilization times for the type N (at 12 am) were significantly lower (significantly greater thymic tonus) compared to type A ($p < 0.02$) and to type O ($p < 0.03$) from the statistic point of view.

Viewed through the chronovariability, during the study period, the thymic tonus is dynamic and dependent on the psychoneuroendocrine typology: it decreases gradually for all three psychoneuroendocrine types, between 9-11a.m and signals a "little depression" around the time 11.00 am. Subsequently, the thymic tonus recurs, quite fast, at the values of 9.00 am for all psychoneuroendocrine types under study.

Influence of the behavioural typology on the pharmacological response of some antipsychotic drugs

The experimental study aims the research of the thymic tonus for the three psychoneuroendocrine types after the chronic administration of the following antidepressants:

- imipramine - antidepressant that acts by inhibiting the noradrenaline and serotonin recapture;

- fluoxetine - selective inhibitor of serotonin recapture;

- lithium - normothymic antidepressant (probably) acting by altering the intracellular concentration of inozitoltriphosphate (IP_3).

In order to assess the variability of the antidepressant effect of the imipramine, fluoxetine and lithium carbonate for the three psychoneuroendocrine types, the initial groups of animals corresponding to types A, N and O have been redistributed, as follows:

1. Group 1A: the adrenergic type of animals, which were administrated a dose of 0.1ml/10g body ip normal saline solution in, for 10 days;

2. Group 2A: the adrenergic type of animals, which were administrated a dose of 10mg/kgbw ip imipramine, for 10 days;

3. Group 3A: the adrenergic type of animals, which were administrated a dose of 10mg/kgbw ip fluoxetine, for 10 days;

4. Group 4A: the adrenergic type of animals, which were administrated a dose of 10mg/kgbw ip lithium carbonate, for 10 days;
5. Group 1N: the intermediate type of animals, balanced which were administrated a dose of 0.1ml/10g body ip normal saline solution, for 10 days;
6. Group 2N: the intermediate type of animals, normal, which were administrated a dose of 10mg/kgbw ip imipramine, for 10 days;
7. Group 3N: the intermediate type of animals, which were administrated a dose of 10mg/kgbw ip fluoxetine, for 10 days;
8. Group 4N: the normal type of animals, which were administrated a dose of 10mg/kgbw ip lithium carbonate, for 10 days;
9. Group 1O: the opioid type of animals, which were administrated a dose of 0.1ml/10g body of ip normal saline solution, for 10 days;
10. Group 2O: the opioid type of animals, which were administrated a dose of 10mg/kgbw ip imipramine, for 10 days;
11. Group 3O: the opioid type of animals, which were administrated a dose of 10mg/kgbw ip fluoxetine, for 10 days;
12. Group 4O: the opioid type of animals, which were administrated a dose of 10mg/kgbw ip lithium carbonate, for 10 days.

The research on variability of the antidepressant effect of the three substances studied for the three psychoneuroendocrine types A, N and O was performed using the forced swimming test.

Thus, each animal in each group described above, was subjected to forced swimming in two stages:

- before starting the treatment (Timob1)
- after the administration of the three substances for 10 days (Timob2).

As it can be seen in figure 8, in the case of the adrenergic behavioural type, for all the three antidepressant drugs, after 10 days of treatment, the initial immobilization time decreased, resulting in an obvious antidepressant effect. The most important antidepressant activiy was registered for fluoxetine.

In the case of the normal behavioural type, for all the three antidepressant drugs, after 10 days of treatment, the initial immobilization time decreased, denoting an antidepressant effect. For the balanced psychoneuroendocrine type, the most important antidepressant activiy was registered for imipramine (figure 9).

	Group1		*Group2*		*Group3*		*Group4*	
Murine type	normal saline solution 0.1ml/10 g bw, ip		Imipramin 10mg/kgbw, ip		Fluoxetin 10mg/kgbw, ip		Lithium Carbonate 70mg/kgbw, ip	
	Timob1 (sec)	Timob2 (sec)	Timob1 (sec)	Timob2 (sec)	Timob1 (sec)	Timob2 (sec)	Timob1 (sec)	Timob2 (sec)
A type	M=53.36 ±20.28	M=53.72 ±20.64	M=51.5 ±12.17	M=32.9 ±10.54	(sec)	(sec)	(sec)	(sec)
N type	M=122.45 ±37.25	M=122.95 ±34.55	M=121.5 ±29.34	M=65.45 ±19.48	M=121.82 ±29.19	M=81.13 ±21.69	M=123.78 ±25.20	M=93 ±20.82
O type	M=135.27 ±26.37	M=137.54 ±30.02	M=138.18 ±28.79	M=83.45 ±19.90	M=136.45 ±34.25	M=59.18 ±14.66	M=137.25 ±31.47	M=107.7 ±21.5

Table 4. The average values of the immobility time during FST for the studied behaviour types, before starting the treatment (Timob1) and after the administration of the three substances for 10 days (Timob2).

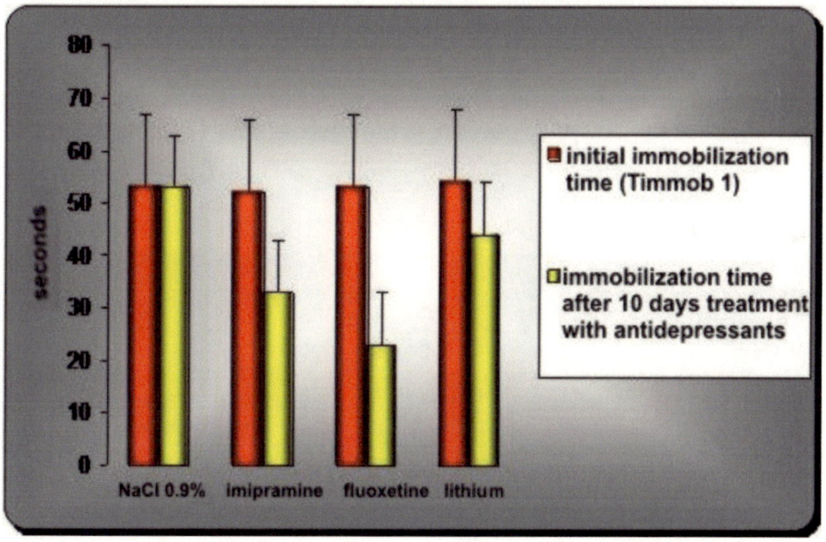

Figure 8. Adrenergic psychoneuroendocrine type. Graphic interpretation of the antidepressant effect of imipramine (10mg/kgbw, ip, for 10 days), of fluoxetine (10mg/kgbw, ip, for 10 days) and of lithium (70mg/kgbw, ip, for 10 ays)

Considering the opioid psychoneuroendocrine type, fluoxetine administered group of animals showed the most important results, decreasing efficiently the initial immobilization time (figure 10).

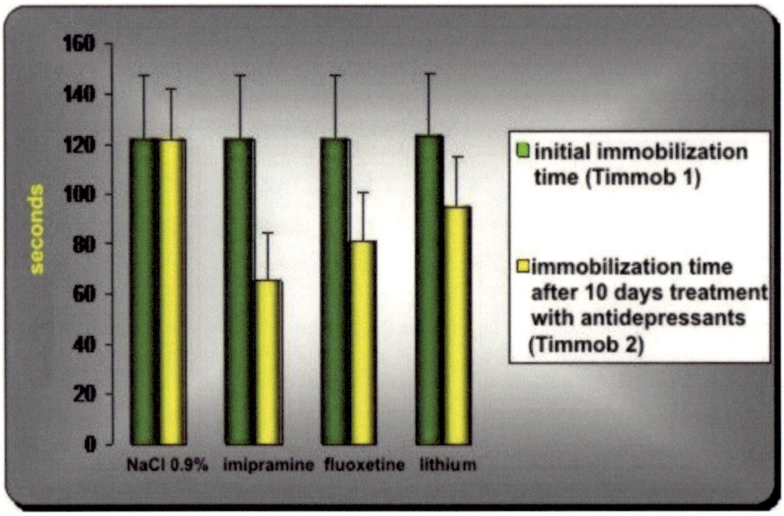

Figure 9. Balanced psychoneuroendocrine type. Graphic interpretation of the antidepressant effect of imipramine (10mg/kgbw, ip, for 10 days), of fluoxetine (10mg/kgbw, ip, for 10 days) and of lithium (70mg/kgbw, ip, for 10 days)

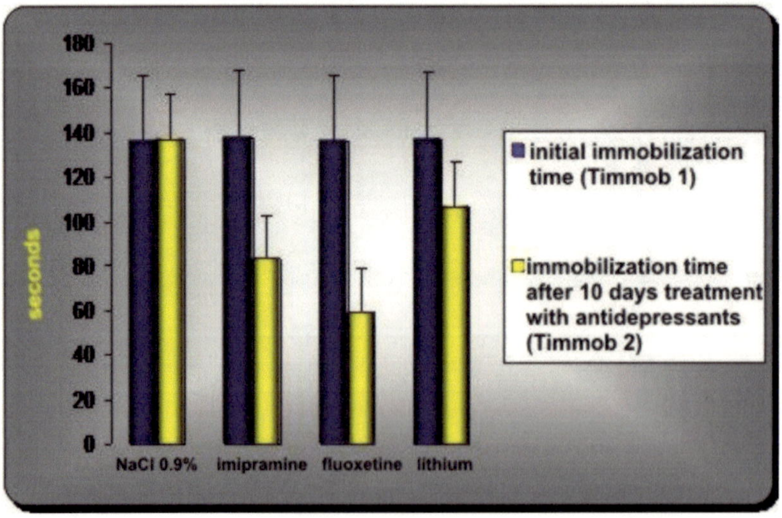

Figure 10. Opioid psychoneuroendocrine type. Graphic interpretation of the antidepressant effect of imipramine (10mg/kgbw, ip for 10 days), of fluoxetine (10mg/kgbw, ip for 10 days) and of lithium (70mg/kgbw, ip for 10 days)

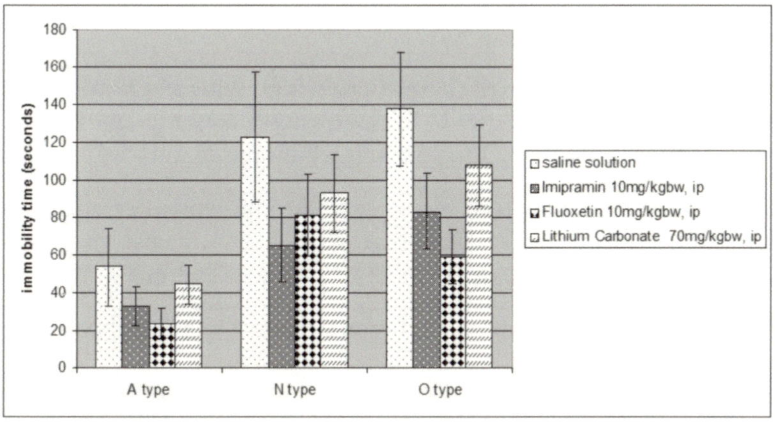

Figure 11. Graphic interpretation of the antidepressant effect of imipramine (10mg/kgbw, ip for 10 days), of fluoxetine (10mg/kgbw, ip for 10 days) and of lithium (70mg/kgbw, ip for 10 days) for the three psychoneuroendocrine types

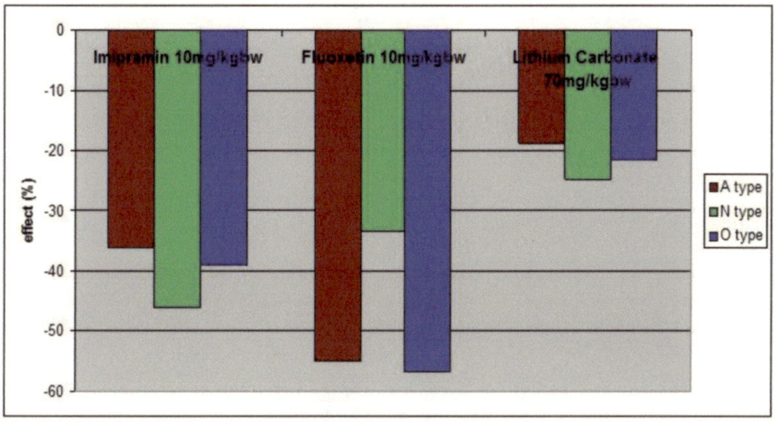

Figure 12. The percentual effect of imipramine, fluoxetine and lithium on murine behaviour in the FST

(Timob after 10 days of antidepressants treatment vs. Timob at the beginning of the experiment)

The effects of imipramine, fluoxetine and lithium on murine behaviour in the FST are shown in figure 12 and 13.

Analyzing the experimental results, we can highlight the following observations:

- in the case of the adrenergic psychoneuroendocrine type, the intensity of the antidepressant effect of the medications administrated (the effect varies inversely with the values of the immobilization times recorded through the "desperation" test) varies in the following order: fluoxetine (Timob = 23.8 ± 7.98sec) > imipramine (Timob = 32.9 ± 10.54sec) > lithium (Timob = 44.5 ± 10.4sec) (Fig. 12);

- in case of the normal, balanced psychoneuroendocrine type, the antidepressant effect of the medications administrated varies in the following order imipramine (Timob = 65.45 ± 19.48sec) > fluoxetine (Timob = 81.13 ± 21.69sec) > lithium (Timob = 93 ± 20.82sec);
- in case of the opioid psychoneuroendocrine type the antidepressant effect of the medications administrated varies in the same order as in type A, namely fluoxetine (Timob = 59.18 ± 14.66sec) > imipramine (Timob = 83.45 ± 19.90sec) > lithium (107.7 ± 21.5sec).

Fluoxetine developed the most important antidepressant effect, mostly in the extreme typologies:

- A type:
- 54.92% (Timob2 vs. Timob1, namely immobility time after 10 days of fluoxetine vs. immobility time at the beginning of the experiment);
- 55.69% (Timob2 vs. saline solution);
- O type:
- 56.62% (Timob2 vs. Timob1)
- 56.97% (Timob2 vs. saline solution).

On the other the intermediated, equilibrated N type was highly reactive to imipramine:

- 46.13% (Timob2 vs. Timob1)
- 46.76% (Timob2 vs. saline solution).

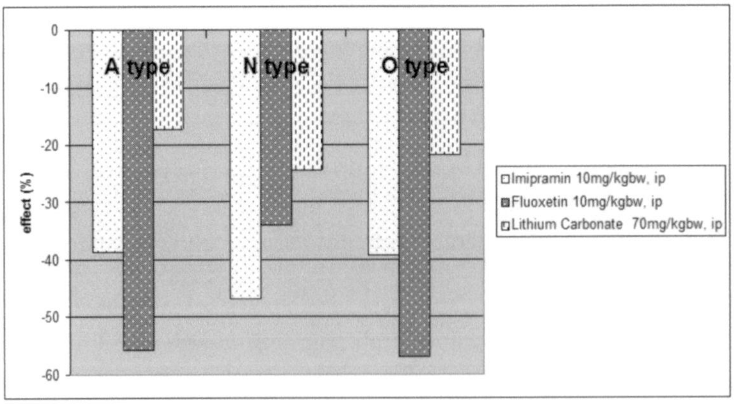

Figure 13. The percentual effect of imipramine, fluoxetine and lithium on the three psychoneuroendocrine types in the FST (Timob after 10 days of antidepressants treatment vs. saline solution)

Some interesting findings were revealed by the statistical analysis of the experimental data. Thus, the statistical comparison between the groups treated with the same antidepressant but coming from different typologies (e.g. Group A and Group O treated with fluoxetine) provided biological significance in all cases.

The statistical analysis of the results from the same psychoneuroendocrine typology but between groups of animals treated with various agents (e.g. Group O treated with imipramine and Group O treated with lithium) gave the biological significance in all cases except for the adrenergic type. In this case, the antidepressant effect of the different medications was statistically different only for Group A imipramine / and Group A lithium ($p < 0.05$).

6. Conclusions

All experimental observations presented support the theory of the pharmacological variability, as a manifestation of the biological variability imprinted by the psychoneuroendocrine typology. From this point of view, for an optimal pharmacological effect of antidepressant medications, one should take into consideration the following aspects:

- the adrenergic psychoneuroendocrine type has a very good general, basal thymic tonus;
- the opioid psychoneuroendocrine type has a low basal thymic tonus;
- the dynamics of thymic state is optimal, regardless of the psychoneuroendocrine typology, between 9-10 a.m. and 12-13 a.m.;
- there is a peak of "depression" daily, between 11-12 a.m., for all types of behavior;

From the antidepressant medication investigated, the extreme behavioural typologies (adrenergic and opioid types) have proven to be extremely responsive to the selective inhibitors of the serotonin recapture (as fluoxetine), while the balanced type reacted optimally to the group of nonselective inhibitors of the noradrenaline and serotonin recapture (as imipramine). These findings may be interestingly correlated with our previous reports regarding the monoaminergic status of the behavioural murine types. In this regard, we showed that the A and O types develop low amounts of serotonin and, therefore, become sensitive against antidepressants that selectively inhibit serotonin reuptake (like fluoxetine) [2].

Lithium, a controversial and incompletely elucidated antidepressant in terms of the action mechanisms, but with indication of choice in maniac-depressive syndrome, has proven the lowest effect in the case of the adrenergic psychoneuroendocrine type, but significant results in the intermediate type. Furthermore the study showed that extreme behavioural typologies are not suitable for lithium treatment.

A proper individualized neuropsychopharmacotherapy is submitted to many variables, like genetic and molecular status, and the behavioural typology seems to be important to be considered.

Author details

Andreea Letitia Arsene*, Niculina Mitrea, Dumitru Lupuliasa, Cristina Manuela Dragoi, Alina Crenguta Nicolae, Ion-Bogdan Dumitrescu, Dragos Florian Ciolan and Doina Draganescu

*Address all correspondence to: andreeanitulescu@hotmail.com

University of Medicine and Pharmacy "Carol Davila", Faculty of Pharmacy, Bucharest, Romania

References

[1] Appleton, K. M., et al. (2007). Type A behaviour and consumption of atherogenic diet: No association in the PRIME study. *Appetite*, 46.

[2] Arsene, A. L. (2011). Bipolar Disorder- A Portrait of a Complex Mood Disorder. *Rijeka: InTech.*

[3] Benfey, B. G., et al. (2001). Evaluation of sympathetic beta-receptor blockade by recording the rate of ventricular pressure rise in cats. *Br. J. Pharmacol*, 30, 23-29.

[4] Bergquist, J., et al. (2002). Catecholamines and methods for their identification and quantitation in biological tissue and fluids. *Journal of Neuroscience Methods*, 113, 1-13.

[5] Brian, Koehler. (2005). Bipolar Disorder, Stress, and the HPA Axis. Available from. http://www.isps-us.org/koehler/bipolar_stress.htm.

[6] Carolina-Rubalcava, López. (2012). Effects of Antidepressants. *Rijeka: InTech.*

[7] Cristea, A., et al. (1997). The nervous behaviour of the adrenergic and opioid types during several pharmacologic tests. *Farmacia*, 45(2), 71-79.

[8] Cristea, A., et al. (1994). The evolution of the painful sensitivity in acute and chronic stress. Rom. J. Phisyol. , 31(1-4), 75-79.

[9] De Nayer, A., et al. (2002). Venlafaxine compared with fluoxetine in outpatients with depression and concomitant anxiety. *The International Journal of Neuropsychopharmacology*, 5(2), 115-120, 1461-1457.

[10] Duffield, G. E., et al. (2002). Programs of transcriptional activation, signaling and protein turnover revealed by microarray analysis of mammalian cells. *Curr. Biol*, 12, 551-557.

[11] Eduardo, Vignoto. Fernandes. (2012). Effects of Antidepressants. *Rijeka: InTech.*

[12] Hache, G., et al. (2012). Antinociceptive effects of fluoxetine in a mouse model of anxiety/depression. *Neuroreport*, 23(9), 525-529.

[13] Haynes, S. G., et al. (1978). The relationship of psychosocial factors to coronary heart disease in the Framingham Study: Methods and risk factors. *Am.J.Epidemiol.*, 107.

[14] Herman, S., et al. (1981). Self ratings of type A (coronary prone) adults. *Psychosom. Med.*, 43(5), 405-413.

[15] Ipek, Komsuoglu. Celikyurt. (2012). Effects of Antidepressants. *Rijeka: InTech.*

[16] Jones, K. V. (1985). The thriel of victory: blood pressure, variability and type A behavior pattern. *J.Behav.Med.*, 8(3), 277-285.

[17] Le Melledo, J. M., et al. (2001). The influence of Type A behavior pattern on the response to the panicogenic agent CCK-4. *J. Psychosom. Res.*, 51.

[18] Masse, F., et al. (2005). M.α2-adrenergic agonistas antagonise the anxiolytic-effect of antidepressants in the four-plate test in mice. *Behav. Brain Research*, 52, 174-176.

[19] Meesters, C. M. G., & Smulders, J. (1994). Hostility and myocardial infarction in men. *Journal of Psychosomatic Research*, 38(7), 727-734.

[20] Nascimento, et.al. . (2005). Pilocarpine induced status epilepticus:Monoamine level, muscarinic and dopaminergic receptors alterations in striatum of young rats. *Neuroscience Letters*, 383, 165-170.

[21] Oedegaard, K. J., et al. (2006). Type A behaviour differentiates bipolar II from unipolar depressed patients. *J.Behav.Pharmacol.*, 90.

[22] Ortiz, J. G., et al. (2000). Plasticity of excitatory amino acid transporters in experimental epilepsy. *Epilepsia*, 41, 104-110.

[23] Owens, M., et al. (2008). Estimates of serotonin and norepinephrine transporter inhibition in depressed patients treated with paroxetine or venlafaxine. Neuropsychopharmacology 0089-3133X, 33(13), 3201-3212.

[24] Pacher, P., et al. (2001). Furst S.Serotonin Reuptake Inhibitors Fluoxetine And Citalopram Relax Intestinal Smooth Muscle. *Can.J.Physiol.Pharmacol*, 79, 580-584.

[25] Papakostas, G., et al. (2008). A meta-analysis of clinical trials comparing mirtazapine with selective serotonin reuptake inhibitors for the treatment of major depressive disorder. *Journal of Psychopharmacology*, 22(8), 843-848, 0269-8811.

[26] Petit-Demouliere, B., Chenu, F., & Bourin, M. (2005). Forced swimming test in mice: a review of antidepressant activity. *Psychopharmacology Berl*, 177(3), 245-255.

[27] Powell, L. H., et al. (1984). Can type A behavior be altered after myocardial infarction? A second year report from the Recurreent Coronary Prevention Project. *Psychosom. Med.*, 46.

[28] Rainer, Q., & Et, al. (2012). Functional status of somatodendritic serotonin 1A autoreceptor after long-term treatment with fluoxetine in a mouse model of anxiety/depression based on repeated corticosterone administration. *Molecular pharmacology*, 81(2), 106-112.

[29] Rhodewalt, F. (1984). Self involvment, self attribution and type A coronary-prone behavior pattern. *J.Pers.Soc.Psychol*, 47(3), 662-670.

[30] Rosenman, R. H. (1978). The Interwiew method of assessment of the coronary prone behavior pattern. *Dembronski, T.M., et al. eds., Coronary prone behavior, New York*, 55-70.

[31] Serretti, A., & Mandelli, L. (2008). The genetics of bipolar disorder: genome 'hot regions,' genes, new potential candidates and future directions. *Molecular Psychiatry*, 13(8), 742-771.

[32] Silvana, da Silva. (2012). Effects of Antidepressants. *Rijeka: InTech.*

Chapter 2

Depression and Glucose Metabolism (Diabetes Mellitus)

Dagmar Breznoščáková and Iveta Nagyová

Additional information is available at the end of the chapter

http://dx.doi.org/10.5772/53467

1. Introduction

The occurrence of depression with diabetes mellitus has been intensively researched for a number of decades now. It was Thomas Willis (1621 – 1675) who introduced the phrase diabetes mellitus (before then called Willis's disease) and associated it with what had already been known for decades – that patients with diabetes have glycosuria (sweet urine). He also noted that "sadness or excessive melancholy, similar to fits or other depressions and breakdowns of the animal spirit, give rise to or instigate this diseased condition (diabetes)". His follower J. C. Brunner (1653 – 1727) is known because of several studies with the pancreas. The large number of epidemiological studies documents the increasing interest in this problem.

Evidence of a bidirectional relationship between depression and diabetes has also been recently documented in large prospective studies. Comorbid depression is associated with an increased risk of poor glycaemic control, diabetes complications have also been found to be risk factors for subsequent development of depressive episodes

The importance of the research on depression and diabetes has been emphasized in recent years because of the modern-day epidemic of obesity and diabetes that is emerging in both high and low income countries. The direct medical and indirect personal and familial costs of this epidemic are starting to get international attention.

2. The epidemiology, risk factors and clinical features of depression and diabetes

2.1. The epidemiology of depression and diabetes

From the meta-analysis Petrak (2009) it follows that 9% of patients with DM have at the same time some form of affective spectrum disorder. If we also take the subclinical form of depression into consideration, then the number of patients with depression increases to 26%. diabetes mellitus (DM) doubles the risk of the occurrence of depression independently of the study design, the sample of patients and the methods of evaluating depression. Contemporary knowledge related to type 2 diabetes points out the worsening of depressive displays in individuals treated (but not those untreated) for type 2 diabetes. These findings could reflect stress or an association with management of diabetes and a large number of diabetic complications and co-morbidities in adults undergoing diabetic treatment in comparison with the untreated. Depressive displays occur in approximately 43 million people with diabetes, keeping in mind the overall prevalence of diabetes in the year 2000 (Wild et al., 2004). From the results of the study Sequenced Treatment Alternatives to relieve Depression (STAR-D), the largest study relating to depression carried out in the USA, the most common occurrence of the co-morbidity of depression and diabetes occurs in the elderly and in minorities (Hispanics and black African-Americans).

Clinically significant depressive symptoms occur in approximately 31% of patients with diabetes, more often in women (in a ratio of 1:1.8); the picture of severe depression (according to strict diagnostic criteria) occurs in 11% of patients with diabetes. With diabetes the risk of a depressive disorder arising is approximately 2 times higher than in the common population (OR = 2.0, 95% CI 1.7 – 2.2), independently of the type of diabetes or on the method of evaluating depressive symptoms (Katon et al., 2004). Approximately 30% of those ill with diabetes have a depressive disorder (28% of women with diabetes and 18% of men with diabetes – the preponderance of women with depression is similar as in the non-diabetic population). The risk of depression arising in patients with diabetes, whether insulin dependent or not, is higher by 15 – 20%. Depressive displays in the common population occur approximately in the age range from 27 to 35 years, but in patients with diabetes this already begins around the 22nd year. The relationship between demographic parameters, lifestyle and behaviour, anti-depressive treatment, BMI, diagnosis of diabetes, its duration and treatment and depressive symptoms were tested in 70,000 patients. Diabetes was identified in 21.7% and had a link with depressive symptoms (AOR, 1.24; 95% CI, 1.14-1.34). Demographic parameters, lifestyle and behaviour, BMI and anti-depressive treatment were more strongly linked with serious depression than a diagnosis of diabetes (Osborn et al., 2011). In a report, Gendelman et al. (2009) showed that prevalence rates were even higher if reports of elevated symptoms were combined with the use of antidepressant medication. This suggests that the available evidence should be considered with particular methodological differences in case ascertainment kept in mind.

In people diagnosed with type 1 or type 2 diabetes, depression increased the risk of lingering hyperglycemia, microvascular and macrovascular complications and overall mortality (Barnard et al., 2006; Ismail et al., 2007). It is interesting that complications and mortality in connection with diabetes are also observed even with less serious depressive displays. Older patients appear as a high-risk group, which is also reported by the result of a 7-year longitudinal study, which shows a five-fold growth in mortality without any significant differences of the impact of the seriousness between moderate and heavy displays of depression (Black et al., 2003).

http://dx.doi.org/10.5772/53467

2.2. Clinical symptoms

Depression is usually defined by the number of symptoms present, usually within the past two weeks. In order to diagnose major depression using DSM-IV or ICD-10 criteria, a clinical interview is conducted and a number of symptoms have to be present (table 1). Most epidemiological research on the prevalence of depression uses self-report instruments (for example Patient Health Questionnaire-9- PHQ-9) for detecting depression or depressive symptomatology, and most instruments that are used measure symptoms that approximate clinical levels of disorder (table 1). The specific symptoms for depression and diabetes are little difference as only for depression alone (table 2), (Lloyd et al., 2010).

DSM-IV criteria(at least five symptoms present nearly every day for 2 wk and causing significant distress or functional impairment
Depressed mood
Markedly diminished interest or pleasure in all or almost all activities
Significant weight loss/gain or decreased/increased appetite
Insomnia or hypersomnia
Psychomotor agitation or retardation
Fatigue or loss energy
Feelings of worthlessness/guilt
Diminished ability to concentrate/make decisions
Recurrent thoughts of death or suicide
Symptoms of depression measured using self-report instruments
Feeling sad/depressed mood
Inability to sleep
Early waking
Lack of interest/enjoyment
Tiredness/lack of energy
Loss of apetite
Feelings of guilt/worthlessness
Recurrent thoughts about death/suicide
DSM-IV criteria extracted from the Diagnostic and Statistical Manual of Mental Disorders, Fourth Edition, Text Revision, Copyright 2000. American Psychiatric Association

Table 1. Symptoms listed in the DSM-IV criteria for major depressive disorder and symptoms of depression measured using self-report instruments

Fatigue
Loss of weight, poor apetite
Psychomotor retardation
Insomnia
Pain
Gastrointestinal problems

Table 2. Common symptoms for depression and diabetes (free by Montano, 2004)

Salomé et al. (2011) evaluated the seriousness of depressive symptoms in patients with a diabetic ulcer of the shin area and determined that in 41 patients out of 50 depressive symptoms were present and in 32 of them found displays of moderate-severe depression with reduced self-evaluation, anorexia, disfigured body-image and a worse libido.

2.3. Risk factors associated with depression and with diabetes

Quality of life is worsened in regard to psychological, physical and social functioning (e.g. ability to work). Complications caused by diabetes are considered as the most serious, and treatment of diabetes is significantly more complicated and worse if depression is present at the same time. In a recent study patients with depression and diabetes were physically less active, smoked more, had fewer healthy dietary habits and were less inclined to diabetic treatment (Gonzales et al., 2008). Depression during diabetes, despite everything, often goes undiagnosed and untreated. In an American study, in which more than 9000 patients with diabetes took part – 51% of which had identified depression – only 43%of them used one or more antidepressants and only 7% took part in four or more psychotherapeutic meetings during a 12-month period (Katon et al., 2004).

2.3.1. Risk factors for depression in patients with diabetes

Through a number of epidemiological studies, aside from the prevalence of depression in patients with diabetes, it was also possible to identify a number of risk factors which are more or less associated with depression. These are the risk factors – demographic (female sex, younger age, lower education, poverty), clinical (seriousness of diabetes, duration of illness, complication of diabetes, high values of glycosylated HbA1c) and behavioral (smoking, obesity) (table 3). Their importance in relation to depression, however, is continuously being verified (Egede & Zheng, 2003). In connection with the presented results it was shown that the most significant association exists between depression, obesity and smoking. Obesity positively correlates with the growing prevalence of type 2 diabetes. It has been shown that smoking associates with increased insulin resistance and represents a risk factor for macrovascular complications in patients with diabetes mellitus. But we know that depression also increases the risk of smoking, which has been documented in several longitudinal studies in which it was confirmed that there are notably more smokers in the group of patients with depression than in the control group (Katon et al., 2004). In the study of Fisher et

http://dx.doi.org/10.5772/53467

al., 2011, in a group of more than 480 patients it was compared whether patients educated about regular observation of glucose monitoring, treatment and regimen also have better results in association with HbA1c and with glucose, which also confirmed at the same time the fact that improved depressive symptoms were not dependent on improved metabolic parameters or glucose. In a pilot randomized controlled study integrated treatment of type 2 diabetes and depression was more successful versus common treatment in improved HbA1c results and depression in older, perhaps 60 Afro-Americans. It follows from this that integrated treatment could be available and effective in real conditions taking into consideration certain limitations.

Although depression is not a part of normal ageing, prevalence rates of severe depressive episodes/major depressive disorder are higher amongst certain groups of older people, in particular, individuals with a co-morbid medical illness (Kovacs et al., 1997). However, to date, little epidemiological data has been available with which to examine rates of depression in older people with diabetes (Collins et al., 2009). To further complicate the picture, several studies have reported that depressive symptoms are more common in younger individuals, in both type 1 and type 2 diabetes (Fisher et al., 2008). Collins et al. (2009) also reported lower rates of depression in older individuals with type 1 diabetes, suggesting that age might have a protective effect. In a cohort of patients aged 70 -79 years followed for about six years, those with diabetes had an increased level of depression with attenuated after adjustment for diabetes-related co-morbidities, although this still represented a significantly increased risk compared to controls. In this study, HbA1c was a predictor of recurrent depression (Maraldi et al., 2007). The specific factors associated with recurrence of depression remain unclear. Gender has not been found to be associated with the number of episodes or the severity of recurrence or chronicity of depression, and the association between stress and depressive episodes appears to be less pronounced over time (Stroud et al., 2008). There is some evidence of a link between depression and the occurrence of diabetic complications and poorer glycaemic control. Painful neuropathy may be another trigger for depression. Diabetes can cause small vessel pathology in the brain that leads to subcortical encephalopathy, not unlike that seen in vascular depression. This may lead to both cognitive impairment and depressed mood (Baldwin, 2010).

Non-diabetic specific risk factors	Diabetes specific risk factors
Female gender	Manifestation of diabetes
Lack of social support	Occurrence of late complications
Low socioeconomic status	Persistent poor glycaemic control
Younger age; older age and physical health problems	Need for insulin therapy in type 2 diabetes
Occurrence of critical life events	Hypoglycaemia problems

Table 3. Risk factors for depression in diabetes

2.3.2. Depression - a risk factor for diabetes?

The link between depression and diabetes was made as early as the seventeenth century, when the famous English physician T. Willis (1621 -1675) noted that diabetes often appeared among patients who had experienced significant life stresses, sadness or long sorrow (Rubin & Peyrot, 2002). Whether depression increases the risk of type 1 diabetes is currently unknown. However, recent studies have suggested that people with depression are more vulnerable to the development of type 2 diabetes (Mezuk et al., 2008), thereby confirming Willis′ hypothesis. It is important to recognize that depression is not only associated with an increased risk for the development of type 2 diabetes, but is also an established risk factor for cardiovascular disease and several features of the metabolic syndrome, particularly hypertension, abdominal obesity and low HDL cholesterol (Vogelzangs et al., 2008). Several hypotheses have been put forward regarding the pathophysiological mechanisms that could explain the increased risk of type 2 diabetes in depressed subjects. For example, increased activity of the hypothalamic-pituitary-adrenal (HPA) axis and sympathetic nervous system might play a role; there are examined elsewhere in this volume (Lloyd et al., 2010).

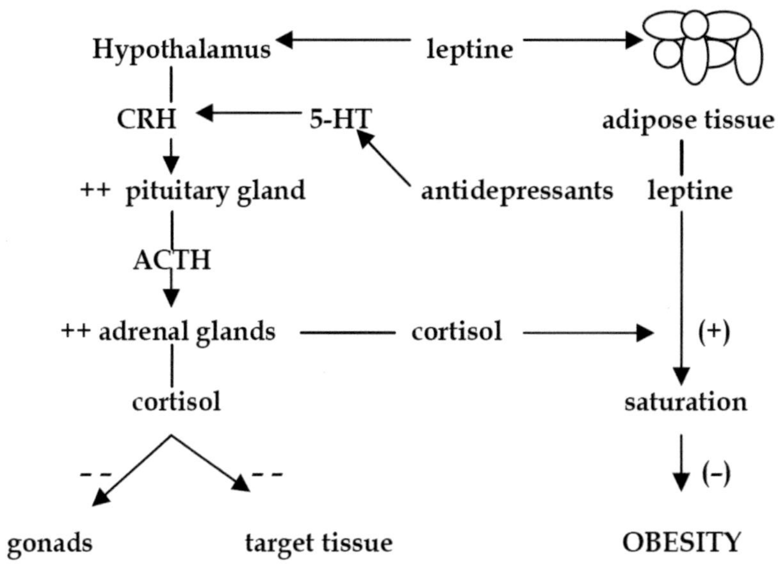

Figure 1. Pathophysiological abnormalities in HPA axis hyperactivity, which in response to elevated levels of CRH, ACTH production and secretion is increased, it stimulates the adrenal cortex to secrete cortisol, and cortisol concentrations inhibit secretion only other hormons, but it is also a signal for the (no) supersaturation

Depression may also increase the risk for type 2 diabetes via behavioural mechanisms. It is well known that the most important risk factor for type 2 diabetes is obesity, and that physical inactivity further increases this risk (Manson et al., 1991). Finally, the evidence to date suggests that depression may indeed increase the risk of developing type 2 diabetes. However, the mechanisms via which this may occur still require investigation. The link between depression and the development of type 1 diabetes remains unclear.

http://dx.doi.org/10.5772/53467

Anxiety is common in diabetes populations and is frequently associated with depression (Katon et al., 2007). A recent systematic review found that around 14% of people with diabetes have generalized anxiety disorder, but subclinical anxiety and symptoms were more common and affected 27% and 40% respectively (Grigsby et al., 2002). The presence of comorbid depression or anxiety has been associated with increased somatic symptoms of disease, which has important implications for treatment (Katon et al., 2007). Diabetic-specific psychological problems, such as fear of self-injecting insulin or self-testing blood glucose (which may or may not be full-blown needle phobia) and fear of complications, are all associated with anxiety and depression (Mollema et al., 2001). Fears regarding hypoglycaemia and psychological insulin resistance are also common, but their relationship with depression is less clear (Petrak et al., 2007).

3. The common pathophysiological mechanisms of depression and diabetes

Many etiological factors play a role in the pathophysiology of depression. Among them are the depletion of serotonin and other monoamines in areas of the brain which are connected with the managing of emotions, sleep and the taste for food. Another factor is the chronic activation of the hypothalamic-pituitary-adrenal axis with subsequent increased production of a corticotropic hormone (CRF). Depression can also originate as a consequence of insufficient plasticity of neurons as a response to different burdens, e. g. chronic stress (Wayne et al., 2004). Genetic influences also apply with depression and metabolic syndrome as well as unfavorable factors from the external environment. Among these, for example, are disorders of equilibrium in the autonomic nervous system with an inclination toward more rapid heart activity, reduced variability of heart frequency and increased level of catecholamines in peripheral blood. According to one of the theories of development of metabolic syndrome, an improper daily regimen (especially low physical activity during the day and intake of food in the late night hours) leads to disorders of equilibrium in the autonomic nervous system, with a preponderance of the sympathetic system in the area of the thorax and in the skeletal muscles, with a subsequent increase in blood pressure, insulin resistance in the muscles and, in contrast, to increased activity of the parasympathetic system in the stomach area, which leads to hyper secretion of insulin and the accumulation of visceral fatty tissues, which can lead further to increased risk of origin of metabolic syndrome, type 2 diabetes, dyslipidemia, hypertension and visceral obesity (Zeman & Jirák, 2008). In patients with a metabolic syndrome, as well as in patients with depression, oxidation stress is shown to be increased with subsequent destruction of neurons in the hippocampus, whose smaller volume we find also in patients with depression (Sapolsky, 2000). An association between symptoms of depression and metabolic syndrome was shown in a study tracking pairs of male twins (McCaffery et al., 2003). In the population tracked in NHANES III (Third National Health and Nutrition Examination Survey) the prevalence of metabolic syndrome among women with depression was double that of women without depression (Kinder et al. 2004).

In the study of Poulsen et al. (2001) 303 older twins were tracked, and significantly higher glucose intolerance was found along with obesity and low HDL-cholesterol among monozygotic versus dizygotic twins, which shows the genetic impact on the development of these phenotypes. They observed a higher genetic influence on glucose intolerance and systolic pressure and a lower genetic influence on low HDL-cholesterol and diastolic pressure in male twins versus female twins. Pouwer & Snoek (2001) observed in more than 1500 patients for the first time significant associations between depression and HbA1c in women with type 2 diabetes. The values of estrogen and the daily regimen could play a significant role in these associations.

With type 1 diabetes the development of an endocrine disorder precedes the first episode of depression. Anderson et al. (2001) in a meta-analysis of 27 clinical studies (a total of 5370 patients) found a statistically significant relationship between depression and diabetic complications (diabetic retinopathia, nephropathia, neuropathia, macrovascular complications and sexual dysfunction) ($p<0,0001$, $z=5,94$). Pro-inflammatory cytokines also show a clear association of both disorders (Tůma, 2005). Cytokines, interleukins and TNF alpha are increased with both disorders and can associate with some depressive displays (Tůma & Hubeňák, 2007).

From a biological point of view depression and diabetes overlap on a number of levels. Among endocrine and neurotransmitter changes are a lower concentration of catecholamines, primary serotonin (Kuzmiaková et al., 1998), stimulation of the production of glucocorticoides, growth hormone and glucagon, which work counter-regulationally against the hypoglycaemic effect of insulin. Increased levels of cortisol are observed equally in patients with diabetes and depression, similarly glucose intolerance disorder and the origin of insulin resistance (Lustman et al., 2000). In many patients with depression, glucose intolerance linked with hyperinsulinemia and insulin resistance develops (Okamura et al., 2000). According to Zimmet et al. (1991) metabolic changes with depression evoke the destabilization of a preexisting metabolic imbalance in individuals with a risk of developing type 2 diabetes. An abnormality of serotonergic neurotransmission localized in pre-synaptic and post-synaptic areas plays an important (thought not the only one) role in the pathogenesis of depression (the so-called serotonin hypothesis of depression). Substances which have a serotonergic effect (serotonin precursors, fenfluramine, SSRIs) conditioned a clinically significant improvement in depressive symptoms. In this association the results of human studies are known: 6 weeks of issuing certain SSRIs (paroxetine, fluoxetine and sertraline) to patients with both depression and diabetes led to a drop in weight, a fall in triglycerides and cholesterol in the blood, a drop in HbA1c and improved compliance (Talbot & Nouwen, 2000; Rubin & Peyrot, 2002).The positive effect of serotonergic substances on depressive mood as well as on a number of disease parameters of diabetes points to a possible etiological relationship.

The conjoined occurrence of depression and diabetes is not a chance phenomenon which evokes consideration about their possible relationship. Scientific authorities present several hypothetical interpretations: 1. Depression arises as a primary consequence of neurochemical – biochemical changes which associate with diabetes; 2. Depression is a consequence of psychosocial factors which associate with the disease or its treatment; 3. Depression is an independent risk factor for the origin of diabetes.

3.1. Depression with diabetes: result of biochemical factors

Current knowledge supports the presence of a relationship between depression, depressive symptoms and possible growth of the risk for the development of type 2 diabetes. In contrast, type 1 diabetes leads to the later development of depression. Kovacs et al. (1997) determined that the first year from the origin of type 1 diabetes was the most risky for the origin of depression. Lustman et al. (1988) observed that the values of glycaemia in individuals with DM improve simultaneously with improvements in remission of depression. In double-blind randomized studies the hypoglycemic effect of antidepressant treatment was confirmed. The origin of depression is a later result of type 2 diabetes, but depression can increase the risk of its development. Results are similar for type 1 diabetes. Control of DM improves simultaneously with the remission of depression, but also without a clear explanation of the mechanism for this assumption.

Depressive phases are more common in individuals with diabetes (Fava & McGratth, 2003, Berken et al., 1984) and have longer duration (Bogner et al., 2007). In a 5-year monitoring Lustman et al. (1988) found that in 22 of 28 patients with diabetes the occurrence of some kind of depressive disorder was found, while depression was not manifested in only 2 of 20 individuals with diabetes. No differences between type 1 diabetes and type 2 diabetes in this regard were observed. According to all, a longer duration of the depressive phase is more associated with type 1 diabetes, although the differences between type 1 diabetes and type 2 diabetes were not observed in relation to inducing remission after the first depressive episode. Peyrot & Rubbin (1989) also observed a longer duration of depressive symptoms in 245 individuals with type 1 diabetes and type 2 diabetes during a 6-month study, and 73% were identified as having depressive symptoms. On the other hand Lustman et al. (1988) did not find any differences in relation to the course and length of duration of depression between both types of diabetes. They found a higher risk for longer duration of depression only in patients with type 2 diabetes who were not treated with insulin. Wellset al. (1993) did not find any significant differences between the course and the duration of the depressive phase in patients with or without a case history of type 1 diabetes or hypertension. It's possible to say that depression and depressive symptoms have a higher recurrence and duration in patients with diabetes.

3.2. Depression with diabetes: the result of psychosocial factors in relation to DM

With an increasing number of complications in diabetes, the probability of depressive symptoms is also higher (Peyrot & Rubbin, 1997). In a study carried out by Davis et al. (1988) it was shown that the social consequence of existence with DM (e.g. on traveling, active leisure time, relationships) is connected with an increased risk of mortality, although no causal association was demonstrated. A significant relationship was shown between overall and specific social support and depressive symptoms with diabetes (Littelfield et al., 1990).

The presence of positive family history of depression occurs more often in patients with depression in comparison with individuals with diabetes without depression *(27 vs. 3%)*. Depression in mothers was found as a specific risk factor for the origin of depression in their children type 1 diabetes at a low age with (Downey & Coyne, 1990). Kovacs et al. (1997) did not find any significant differences in relation to sex and the origin of depression, but young women with diabetes had a 9-times higher risk for the recurrence of depression compared with young men with diabetes.

3.3. Depression with diabetes: a risk factor for the origin and worsening course of the result of DM

Brande & Egede (2008) followed the long-term impact of depression on the control of glycaemia in more than 11,000 people with type 2 diabetes with an average age of 66 years with relatively well controlled diabetes (HbA1c = 7.3%), while depression was identified in 6% of the them. A significant relationship was consequently found between depression and control of glycaemia by measuring the HbA1c values, which were persistently higher (on average by 0.13, 95%CI, 0.03-0.22, p=0.008) with each measurement at 3 months during a 4-year study of patients with diabetes and concurrent depression.

Akbaralya et al. (in Barclay, 2008) monitored more than 5000 patients age 41-61 years with depressive symptoms from 1991 to 1993 and then again 6 years later by using the 30-item subscale General Health Questionnaire; metabolic syndrome was determined on the basis of criteria from the National Cholesterol Education Program. They found that the presence of metabolic syndrome was linked with the increased risk of possible depressive symptoms (OR, 1.38, 95%CI, 1.02-1.96). Central obesity, increased triglycerides and HDL (but not other components of metabolic syndrome) were predictors of manifestation of depressive symptoms. These findings are thus consistent with the hypothesis that depressive symptoms could be a consequence as well as the reason for metabolic syndrome.

In a study by Backes et al. (2007) of more than 11,000 women with gestation diabetes, depression was retrospectively found in up to 15.2% of women in the period of the last 6 months of gravidity up to a year after giving birth, versus only 8.5% of women without diabetes. These findings support the existence of a relationship between the two diseases – diabetes and depression – namely, that both are frequent during gravidity and after birth, and it is relevant, that post-partum depression is treatable but often goes unrecognized. It is known that women with diabetes (keeping in mind the (non)use of insulin) have during gravidity approximately two-times the risk of depression arising versus women without diabetes (OR 1.85 (95%CI)).This is similar with the occurrence of depression in women with diabetes in the post-partum period (OR 1.69 (95%CI)).

We can say that particularly late rising of depression could be the result of micro or macrovascular changes, and the origin of depression often precedes predominately type 2 diabetes by a number of years. The newest findings support the consideration regarding the reciprocal interaction among depression and diabetes, because depressive symptoms could increase the risk of origin of type 2 diabetes and the diabetic complications associated with it.

4. The treatment of comorbidity depression and diabetes

Referring to some evidence that depression has an adverse psychological impact than the "well being" as a diabetes, we can say that the treatment of depression in diabetes can directly improve the psychological as well as medical parameters. Improving depressive symptoms and induce remission, the main objectives related to psychological parameters. The treatment of diabetes involves improving glycaemic control and reducing the risk for the occurrence of either short or long-term complications of diabetes and premature mortality.

Based on mainly anecdotal evidence and a handful of randomized controlled trials, monoamine oxidase inhibitors (MAOIs) and tricyclic antidepressants (TCAs) are considered to have a hyperglycaemic effect, which is in keeping with their noradrenergic and(or appetitogenic effects, while selective serotonin reuptake inhibitors (SSRIs), such as fluoxetine and sertraline, are more likely to be anorectic, improve insulin sensitivity and reduce glucose levels, probably because the central serotoninergic pathways are important in the regulation of food intake and food preferences (Ismail, 2010).

The common mechanisms etiopathogenetic diabetes and depression to some extent highlights the fact that intensive treatment of depression leads to improved disease manifestations diabetes (eg. decrease glucose) and vice versa, effective treatment for diabetes determines retreat depressive symptoms. Selective serotonin reuptake inhibitors (SSRIs - sertraline, paroxetine, fluoxetine, fluvoxamine, citalopram) due to a beneficial effect on a number of pathological parameters diabetes - decrease glucose levels, weight loss, decreased serum cholesterol and triglycerides - and given the antidepressant effect comparable with TCAs and MAOIs are in the treatment of depression in diabetes first-line drugs.

The use of TCAs in patients with diabetes is mainly limited to their cardiotoxicity. TCAs may increase serum concentrations of glucose and increased craving for sweets. Considerably better is to use antidepressants - SSRIs or SNRIs later, while in patients with diabetes on this treatment was demonstrated the hypoglycaemic effect. From the observation of about 2% of 40 000 patients (Derijks, Heerdink et al., 2008) that the use of antidepressants is associated with an increased risk of hypoglycaemia, but if they are used in patients with diabetes for more than 3 years, the risk of hypoglycaemia is almost three times, it is important to monitor the symptoms of hypoglycaemia and blood glucose. The use of antidepressants was associated with hyperglycaemia (ROR 1.52 (95% CI: 1.20 to 1.93) and hypoglycaemia (ROR 1.884 (95% CI: 1.4 to 2.42). Connection with hyperglycaemia was risky for antidepressants with affinity for serotonergic reuptake transporter (Derijks, Meyboom et al., 2008), the published data show that in terms of impact on the metabolic parameters between SSRIs differences. Paroxetine abdominal obesity leads to more frequent administration than other SSRI antidepressants (Reader, Bjelland et al., 2006).

The other antidepressants should mention bupropion, venlafaxine and nefazodone, which are favorable for their pharmacological properties in terms of comorbid conditions also convenient - to have a neutral effect on body weight and glucose metabolism. Among the nine antidepressants especially in pursuit of their effects on the gastrointestinal, central nervous system and sexual life come out with the best profile of bupropion and soon fluvoxamine (Dewan, Ananad, 1999). Weight gain is a common adverse side effect of acute and long-term treatment with antidepressants. TCAs and MAOIs are probably more common cause of weight gain than SSRIs and newer antidepressants, except mirtazapine, which is in this respect between SSRIs and TCAs. Also, paroxetine causes higher weight gain compared to other SSRIs preparation for longer-term therapy and bupropion or nefazodone cause less weight gain over the longer-term treatment (Fava, 2000).

According to several studies being less effective in patients with depression and diabetes mirtazapine, in view of a higher risk of gaining weight. The case study series of patients receiving doses of mirtazapine and 15 mg were observed gain weight during 5 months 16 kg, with obesity and by all important risk factor for glucose dysregulation (Fisfalen, Hsiung et al., 2003).

TCAs (Carney, 1998) and MAOIs should be administered only as a last option (Nickelson, Box, 1999) for the treatment of depression in patients with diabetes. TCAs are associated with weight gain (Nakra, Rutland et al., 1977, Berken, Weinsthein et al., 1984) and taste the sweet and carbohydrate (Paykel, Mueller et al., 1973, Harris, Young et al., 1984), which can be problematic for patients with increased consumption of calories (Goodnick, Henry et al., 1995, Carney 1998). TCAs can worsen hyperglycaemia and glycaemic control during longer treatment (Nickelson, Box 1999, Carney, 1998) and their anticholinergic, cardiovascular and musculoskeletal adverse side effects may worsen symptoms in relation to diabetes (constipation associated with diabetic gastroparesis) (Carney, 1998, Lane, 1993). MAOIs can aggravate hypoglycaemia and delay the restoration of normal glucose concentrations when taken with insulin or sulfonylurea (Cooper & Ashrocft., 1966). In addition, treatment with MAOIs is associated with weight gain and the need for strict dietary restrictions, which certainly complicates the diet such as in patients with diabetes (Carney, 1998).

In 80 patients with depression Kopf, Westpal et al. (2004) observed values of lipoproteins, insulin sensitivity and cortisol in saliva before and after 35 days of treatment with amitriptyline or paroxetine. The main findings were that patients with depression and weight in the standard have insulin resistance corresponding to the HPA axis, overweight patients had total and LDL cholesterol out of standard antidepressant treatment led to an improvement in lipoprotein and cholesterol levels, changes in triglyceride metabolism affected by the treatment and weight three important factors control lipid parameters depending on the presence of the metabolic state: weight, hypercorticolism and insulin resistance. This study first examined the detailed lipid profile in patients with diabetes and depression.

Bupropion contrast in patients with diabetes suited to the fact that side does not sexual reactions and decreases body weight in obese patients had more than placebo (Jain, Kaplan et al. 2002). Lustman, Williams et al. (2007) in a group of 90 patients with type 2 diabetes and depression and taking over 16 months bupropion found decrease BMI, total fat, and HbA1c (p

≤ 0.01 for all parameters). Reduction of BMI and severity of depression independently predicted lower HbA1c after treatment of the acute phase of depression, while only reducing the severity of depression (p≤0.001) affected on HbA1c with the passage of time. Sawhney et al. (2007) observed the good effect of TCAs administered in low doses in depressed patients suffering from chronic vomiting, did not respond to prokinetic therapy. Antidepressant duloxetine is recommended for the treatment of diabetic neuropathy (Švestka, 2005).

Data from a large study of over 4800 patients with diabetes enrolled in a health maintenance organization (HMO) found that approximately 70% of those with comorbid depression (based on scoring ≥ 10 on the PHQ-9) had experienced affective symptoms for two years or longer(Katon et al., 2004). Patients with diabetes tend to be older, and recent primary care data have shown that the average length of an episode of depression in older primary care patients is approximately 18 months, whereas in mixed-aged populations the mean length of an episode is approximately 4 - 6 months (Vuorilehto et al, 2009).

The tendency for depressive symptoms to be chronic in patients with diabetes is also shown by recent data from a five-year follow-up study of approximately 2700 patients with diabetes. Approximately 82% of patients who met DSM-IV criteria for major depression at five-year follow-up had minor or major depression at baseline (Katon et al., 2009). Finally, the recurrent course of depression was shown in a longitudinal study, which found that 79% of patients with diabetes who had major depression relapsed over a five-year follow-up period, with a mean of four episodes per patients (Katon, von Korff et al. 2004).

Several systematic reviews have been completed exploring effect sizes of psychotherapeutic as well as pharmacological treatments of patients with comorbid depression and diabetes (Petrak 2009; van der Feltz-Cornelis et al. 2010). Efficacy trials generally evaluate intensive treatment of a carefully selected patient group by highly trained staff. Patients with clinically significant psychiatric comorbidities, such as panic disorder of medical comorbidities, are often excluded from these trials. An important question for researchers and clinicians is whether evidence-based pharmacotherapies and psychotherapies that have proven effective in populations of patients with depression with minimal medical illness would be as efficacious in patients with diabetes.

A systematic review of efficacy trials performed in 2009 yielded 11 randomized clinical trials, five on psychotherapeutic interventions and six on pharmacological treatments. Most trials were small, with only one recruiting more than 100 patients and the others including 60 or fewer patients. Most trials were completed on patients with type 2 diabetes with serious depressive symptoms or major depressive disorder, and effect sizes were specified for depressive symptom severity as well as for glycaemic control.

4.1. Pharmacological studies

As shown Table 4, the pharmacotherapeutic interventions had moderate effects on depressive symptoms, and small effects on glycaemic control. The effect on depressive outcomes was very similar, but the effect on glycaemic control was smaller than that of the psychotherapeutic studies, many of which had explicit interventions aimed at improving glycaemic control. The pharmacologic trials were also small, mostly under 100 patients enrolled. The small numbers of patients enrolled in both psychotherapy and pharmacologic efficacy trials limits the generalizability of the findings.

Study	N (completers), diabetes type, mean age	Intervention conditions, follow-up (FU)	Outcome assessment (depression, diabetes	Effect size
Lustman et al., 1997b	N=28, type 2-50% 49-49,2ys	nortriptyline vs placebo,FU- 9 ws	Depression: BDI (p=0.03), DM: HbA1c, n.s., no outcome reported	Depression: Δ -0.868, DM: Δ 0
Lustman et al., 2000	N=54,type 2- 56% 45-47ys	fluoxetine vs placebo, FU- 8 ws	Depression: HAMD (p<0.04), DM: HbA1c (p=0.13, n.s.)	Depression: Δ -0.573, DM: Δ 0.419
Paile-Hyvärinen et al., 2003	N=13, type 2-100%, 61-62ys	paroxetine vs placebo, FU- 4ws	Depression: MADRS (p=0.25,ns.), DM:GHbA1c (p=0,08, n.s.)	Depression: Δ -0.68, DM: Δ 1.07
Xue et al., 2004	N=48, type 2-85%, 21-65ys	paroxetine vs placebo	Depression: HAMD-17 (p<0.01), DM: HbA1c (p=0.25, ns.)	Depression: Δ -0.78, DM: Δ 0.34
Gülseren et al., 2005	N=23, type 2-100%, 58ys	fluoxetine vs paroxetine	Both groups improved –HDRS (p=0.003, s.f.), HbA1c – n.s. both	No significant difference between the two conditions
Lustman et al., 2006	N=152, type 2-65%, N/A	sertraline (flexible doses) vs placebo	n. s. between groups	
Paile-Hyvärinen et al., 2007	N=49, type 2-100%, 59ys	paroxetine vs placebo	Depression: HADS (p=0.45, n.s.), DM: HbA1c (p=0.7, n.s.)	Depression: Δ -0.26, DM: Δ 0.14

Table 4. Overview of the most important trials with antidepressant treatment under: BDI-Beck Depression Inventory, HAMD-Hamilton Asberg Montgomery Depression Scale, ns- no significant

Due to the lack of data in our conditions in relation to the comorbidity of depression and disorders related to glucose and lipid metabolism and at the same time of the presented high prevalence independently existing of these disorders, we decided to work-up a pilot study on the impact of antidepressants primarily on glucose and lipid metabolism in patients with depression. We found changes in lipid – HDL, LDL, triglycerides, glucose, HbA1c and BMI parameters in patients with depression during antidepressive treatment without diabetes. The assess changes of treatment with two groups of antidepressants – SSRI´s and SNRI´s in flexible doses. It was prospective study of outpatients and in-patient's file hospitalized at the 1st Dept. of Psychiatry University Hospital and University of P. J. Šafárik, Košice (2010 – 2011). Hypothesis was that SSRI´s and SNRI´s do not deteriorate theese metabolic parameters, HbA1c will be decrease, HDL will be increase and compare the differences between groups. After six months 74 patients completed follow-up (65% women with MDD, DSM-IV). We used scales: MADRS, Beck Anxiety Inventory, Zung Depression Scale, statistical program IBM SPSS (version 20. 0). The consent to research granted Ethics committee of School of Medicine of University of P. J. Šafárik in Košice.

http://dx.doi.org/10.5772/53467

Scale	Groups SSRI´s/SNRI´s	N	Mean
Beck Anxiety Inventory - baseline	SSRI/SNRI	38/36	23,29/ 24,14
Beck Anxiety Inventory - final	SSRI/SNRI	38/36	15,18*/16,50*
Zung Depression Inventory- SDS-baseline	SSRI/ SNRI	38/36	67,26/ 66,83
Zung Depression inventory – final	SSRI/SNRI I	38/36	49,39*/ 52,44*
MADRS baseline	SSRI/SNRI	38/36	37,21/ 36,89
MADRS final 1	SSRI/SNRI	38/ 36	16,95*/ 17,89*
BMI baseline	SSRI/SNRI	38/ 36	25,54/ 26,76
BMI final	SSRI/SNRI	38/ 36	26,22/ 27,1

* the mean difference is significant at the,05 level

Table 5. Score in some scales

In both groups dominated by women (three times) – 27/9 (SSRI's group); 28/10 (SNRI's group) and on the other hand, less presumptive SNRI medication type were deployed globally in patients with a higher mean age (SNRI's = 52,7/28-73/; SSRI's = 41,7 /20-64/). There was an improvement in the scales in both groups: MADRS, Beck Anxiety Inventory, Zung Depression Scale (s. f., table 5). Similar, the results in study Songar et al. (1993) indicate that some relations exist between anxiety and the worsening of metabolic control (mainly in HbA1c). The HDL cholesterol values have improved after six months antidepressive treatment in both groups (1.31 vs 1.4 /SNRI's/ 1.38 vs 1.5 /SSRI's/), which corresponds to the data Svačina et al. (2006) and Hardy et al. (2007). These findings are particularly important because from this one that is most closely connected with cardiovascular risks play mainly LDL and HDL components. The triglycerides values have improved statistical significant after six months SSRI treatment vs SNRI treatment (Mann-Whitney U=496,000 Asymp. Sig. (2-tailed)=0.042 = $p \leq 0.05$), which correlates with the monitoring Flechtner-Mors (2008) also in SSRI preparations, which is important from the point of view that higher levels of triglycerides are considered primary in the aetiology of disorders that are related to oxidative stress and increased levels of LDL. As we expected, HbA1c improved in the SNRI's (5.55 vs 5.24, n. s.) and SSRI's group (5.23 vs 5.18, n. s.) which corresponds with the results of several pharmacological studies (Lustman et al., 1997b, 2006; Gülseren et al., 2005). On the other hand can not draw definite causal conclusions regarding the limitations on file size and especially the length of the monitoring itself. We confirmed the hypothesis that SSRI's and SNRI's do not deteriorate metabolic parameters – HDL, LDL, triglycerides, HbA1c, BMI, even HbA1c will be decrease (n. s.), HDL will be increase (n. s.), triglycerides were improved in SSRI's group (s. f.), but in addition the differences between groups we didn't find similar as Gülseren et al. (2005).

4.2. Psychotherapeutic interventions

The effect size of the psychotherapeutic interventions were moderate to large for improvement of depressive symptoms, and moderate to large for improvement of glycaemic control. Three of the five psychotherapy trials compared an evidence-based depression psychotherapy and diabetes education to diabetes education alone. Therefore, it is unclear whether improvements in glycaemic control were due to the beneficial effect of the depression-focused psychotherapy or the combination of both depression therapy and diabetes education.

Study	N (completers), diabetes type, mean age	Intervention conditions, follow-up (FU)	Outcome assessment (depression, diabetes	Effect size
Lustman et al., 1998	N=41, type 2-100%, 53-56,4ys	CBT+ diabetes education vs diabetes education alone, FU- 11ws	Depression: BDI (p<0.001)in CBT group, DM: HbA1c in CBT group (p<0.03)	Depression: Δ -1.112, DM: Δ -0.704
Huang et al., 2002	N=59,type 2-100%, N/A	Antidiabetics + diabetic education + psychological +relaxation vs antidiabetics only, FU- 3mo	Depression: SDS (p<0.05), DM: HbA1c (p<0.05)	Depression: Δ -0.521, DM: Δ -0.521
Li et al., 2003	N=120, N/A, 50,5-52,3ys	Antidiabetics + diabetic education + psychological treatment vs antidiabetics only, FU- 4ws	Depression: SDS (p<0.01), DM: FBG(p<0.05)	Depression: Δ -0.478, DM: Δ -0.362
Lu et al., 2005	N=60, type 2-100%, 65ys	Diabetes and CVA education + electromyographic treatment + psychological treatment vs usual care, FU- 4ws	Depression: HAMD-17 (p<0.01), DM: FBG (p<0.05)	Depression: Δ -0.688, DM: Δ -0.517
Simson et al., 2008	N=30, type 2-80%, 60,5ys	Individual supportive psychotherapy vs usual care, FU- discharge (3-20ws)	Depression: HADS (p=0.018), DM: PAID mean (p=0.008)	Depression: Δ -0.918, DM: Δ -1.043

Table 6. Overview of the most important trials with psychotherapeutic interventions under table: CBT - Cognitive-behavioral therapy, BDI- Beck Depression Inventory

5. Discussion

The probability of the occurrence of depression in patients with diabetes is higher, because depression in patients with diabetes is often unrecognized and therefore also untreatable and the association between depression and glycaemic control is small in cross-sectional

http://dx.doi.org/10.5772/53467

studies and almost disappears in most of the handful of prospective studies (Lustman et al., 2000a). It is interesting that complications associated with diabetes and mortality are already observed with less serious depressive displays (Black et al., 2003). The comorbidity of depression and obesity worsens the course of diabetes, and furthermore, depression worsens the adherence to a diabetic diet and treatment and predicts low compliance in diabetological programs (McKellar et al., 2004). From the results of several studies (Katon et al., 2004) it follows that the relationship between depression and obesity runs in both directions. From several studies it follows that the course of depression in individuals with diabetes is not causally dependent on diabetes. Depression in individuals with diabetes represents a more complex phenomena following from interactions between genetic, biological and psychosocial factors, which could significantly influence the recurrence and longer duration of depression. In the case of type 2 diabetes it is unlikely that the first episode of depression would be as a consequence of diabetes. The development of depression often precedes the manifestation of type 2 diabetes by many years. Depressive symptoms could increase the risk of development of type 2 diabetes and its complications. It is shown that depression ranks among the most important risk factors for the development of type 2 diabetes and is not merely a secondary emotional response to a chronic and complicated bodily illness, but that an independent risk factor for the origin of type 2 diabetes is involved (Lustman et al., 2006). Despite all, we today still do not have sufficient proof about confirmation of the hypothesis relating to the occurrence of depression as a consequence of biochemical changes following directly from diabetes or its treatment or from psychological factors. But these factors can influence the increasing of insulin resistance and the reduction of glucose as a result of changes during depression.

6. Conclusion

The occurrence of depression with bodily diseases represents an unfavorable prognostic indicator. It worsens the therapeutic response and the course of the bodily disease, makes regaining health and rehabilitation more difficult, prolongs hospitalization, weakens the ability of the ill individual to care for his or her own needs, represents a risk of suicidal behaviour and as a final consequence increases the costs for treatment and demands on the health care system. Its timely recognition and adequate treatment are exceptionally important. Depression in patients with diabetes mellitus represents a complex phenomenon which is the result of complicated interactions between biological, genetic and psycho-social factors. There has been the hypothetical assumption that depression originates as a direct consequence of neurochemical changes with diabetes mellitus. More proof, however, supports the so-called inverse hypothesis, according to which depression represents a risk for the origin of type 2 diabetes mellitus as well as its complications.

The fact that intensive treatment of depression leads to improved disease displays of diabetes (e.g. a drop in glucose levels) and the reverse, that effective treatment of diabetes conditions the regression of depressive symptoms, points to common etiopathogenic mechanisms to a certain measure point. There is high prevalence of depressive and anxiety disorders in patients with diabetes, and these disorders adversely affect diabetes self-care, disease control and clinical outcomes. Complications of diabetes resulting in functional impairment can also precipitate a depressive episode. Efficacy data have demonstrated that both evidence-based psychotherapies and pharmacotherapies are effective treatment modalities for depression in patients not only with diabetes. The choice of antidepressant medication for the patient with diabetes and depression remains one in which the clinician needs to individualize therapy to the specific needs of the patient. There are strong data showing that the specific initial choice of antidepressant, with the aforementioned exceptions, may be less crucial than the duration of appropriate therapy, the coordination of psychiatric and medical care, and the input of the clinician in modification of dose or choice of medication dependent upon the response to therapy. The patient´s tolerance to a specific antidepressant is not predictable, in part due to genetic variations in the metabolism of specific medications, as well as other less well studied aspects of biologic variability.

To what measure treatment of comorbid depression reduces morbidity and mortality of diabetes mellitus and to what measure treatment influences the unfavorable consequences of depression still remain an open question.

Author details

Dagmar Breznoščáková[1] and Iveta Nagyová[1,2]

1 1st Department of Psychiatry, Faculty of Medicine, Šafárik University, Košice, Slovak Republic

2 Institute of Public Health – Department of Social Medicine, Faculty of Medicine, Šafárik University, Košice, Slovak Republic

Graduate School Košice Institute for Society and Health, Faculty of Medicine, Šafárik University, Košice, Slovak Republic

References

[1] Backes K et al. (2007). Diabetes Linked to Pregnancy-Related depression in Low-Income Women, JAMA, 301: 842- 847

[2] Baldwin R (2010). Depression in Later Life. Oxford University Press, 978-0-19-959126-8, Oxford, UK

[3] Barclay L et al. (2008). Metabolic Syndrome May Predict Depressive Symptoms. Diabetes Care, Published online December 23, www.medscape.com/viewarticle/586355

[4] Barnard KD, Skinner TC, Peveler R (2006). The prevalence of comorbid depression in adults with type 1 diabetes: systematic literature review. Diabet. Med., 23: 445-448

[5] Berken GH, Weinstein D, Stern WC (1984). Weight gain: a side effect of tricyclic antidepressants (letter), J. Affect Disord, 7: 13

[6] Black SA, Markides KS et al. (2003). Depression predicts increased incidence of adverse health outcomes in older Mexican Americans with type 2 diabetes. Diabetes Care, 26: 2822-2828

[7] Bogner HR, Morales KH et al. (2007). Diabetes, depression and death: a randomized controlled trial of a depression treatment program for older adults based in primary care (PROSPECT). Diabetes Care, 30: 3005-3010

[8] Brande NM, Egede L (2008). Depression in individuals with type 2 diabetes is associated with higher blood glucose levels with time, new research suggests, Gen Hosp Psychiatry, 30: 509-514

[9] Carney C (1998). Diabetes mellitus and major depressive disorder: an overview of prevalence, complications and treatment, Depres Anxiety, 7 (4): 149-57

[10] Collins MM, Corcoran P, Perry J (2009). Anxiety and depression symptoms in patients with diabetes, Diabet. Med., 26: 153-161

[11] Cooper AJ, Ashrocft G (1966). Potentiation of insulin hypoglycaemia by M.A.O.I. antidepressant drugs. Lancet I: 407-9

[12] Davis WK, Hess GE, Hiss RG (1988). Psychosocial correlates of survival in diabetes, Diabetes Care, 11: 538-545

[13] Derijks HJ, Heerdink ER, Koning FH et al. (2008). The association between antidepressant use and hypoglycaemia in diabetic patients: a nested case-control study. Pharmacoepidemiology and Drug Safety, 17:336-344

[14] Derijks HJ, Meyboom RHB, Heerdink ER et al. (2008). The association between antidepressant use and disturbances in glucose homeostasis: evidence from spontaneous reports, Eur J Pharmacol, 64:531-538

[15] Dewan MJ, Ananad VS (1999). Evaluating the tolerability of the newer antidepressants, J Nerv Ment Dis, 187(2): 96-101

[16] Downey G, Coyne JC (1990). Children of depressed parents: an integrative review, Psychol Bull, 108: 50-76

[17] Egede L, Zheng D (2003). Independent Factors Associated With Major Depressive Disorder in a National Sample of Individuals with Diabetes. Diabetes Care, 26(1): 104-111

[18] Fava M (2000). Weight Gain and Antidepressants, J Clin Psychiatry, 61(suppl 11): 37-41

[19] Fava M., McGratth PJ (2003). Reboxetine Study Group. Switching to reboxetine: anefficacy and safety study in patients with major depressive disorder unresponsive to fluoxetine. J Clin. Psychopharmacol., 23: 365-369

[20] Fisfalen ME, Hsiung MD (2003). Glucose Dysregulation and Mirtazapine Induced Weight Gain Am J Psychiatry, 160: 797-799

[21] Fisher L, Skaff MM, Mullan JT et al. (2008). A logitudinal study of affective and anxiety disorders, depressive affect and diabetes distress in adults with type 2 diabetes, Diabet. Med., 25: 1096-1101

[22] Flechtner-Mors M et al. (2008). Metabolism in adipose tissue in response to citalopram and imipramin treatment – An in situ microdialysis study. Journal of Psychiatric Research, 42: 578-586

[23] Gendelman N, Snell-Bergeon JK, McFann K et al. (2009). Prevalence and correlates of depression in individuals with and without type 1 diabetes. Diabetes Care, 32, 575-579

[24] Gonzalez. J., Delahanty L. et al. (2008). Differentiating symptoms of depression from diabetes-specific distress: relationships with self-care in type 2 diabetes. Diabetologia, 51: 1822-1825

[25] Goodnick PJ, Henry JH, Buki VMV (1995). Treatment of depression in patients with diabetes mellitus, J. Clin. Psychiatry, 56 (4): 128-36

[26] Grigsby AB, Anderson RJ, Freedland KE et al. (2002). Prevalence of anxiety in adults with diabetes: a systematic review. J. Psychosom. Res., 53: 1053-1060

[27] Gulseren L, Gulseren S, Hekimsoy Z, Mete L (2007). Comparison of fluoxetine and paroxetine intype 2 diabetes mellitus patients. Arch. Med. Res., 36: 156-165

[28] Hardy T et al. (2007). Does treatment with duloxetine for neuropathic pain impact glycemic control ? Diabetes Care, 30(1): 21-26

[29] Harris B, Young J, Hughes B (1984). Changes occurring in appetite and weight during short-term antidepressant treatment, Br J Psychiatry, 145: 645-8

[30] Huang X, Song L, Li T et al. (2002). Effect of health education and psychosocial intervention on depression in patients with type 2 diabetes. Chin. Ment. Health J., 16: 149-151

[31] Ismail K (2010). Unraveling the Pathogenesis of the Depression-Diabetes Link. In Katon W, Maj M, Sartorius N. Depression and Diabetes, John Wiley & Sons Ltd., 978-1-4443-5026-5, Chichester, UK

[32] Ismail K., Winkley K. et al. (2007). A cohort study of people with diabetes and their first foot ulcer: the role of depression on mortality. Diabetes Care, 30: 1473-1479

[33] Jain AK, Kaplan RA, Gadde KM, Wadden TA (2002). Bupropion SR vs. placebo for weight loss in obese patients with depressive symptoms. Obes Res, 10: 1049-1056

[34] Katon W, Lin EH, Kroenke K (2007). The association of depression and anxiety with with medical symptom burden in patients with chronic medical illness. Gen. Hosp. Psychiatry, 29: 147-155

[35] Katon W, Maj M, Sartorius N (2010). Depression and Diabetes, John Wiley & Sons Ltd., 978-1-4443-5026-5, Chichester, UK

[36] Katon W, Russo J, Von Korff M et al. (2009). Depression and diabetes: factors associated with major depression at 5-year follow-up. Psychosomatics, 50: 570-579

[37] Katon W., Simon G. et al. (2004). Quality of depression care in population-based sample of patients with diabetes and major depression. Med Care, 42: 1222-1229

[38] Katon WJ, Von Korff M, Lin EH et al. (2004). The Pathways Study: a randomized trial of collaborative care in patients with diabetes and depression. Arch. Gen. Psychiatry, 61: 1042-1049

[39] Kinder LS, Carnehon MR, Palaniappan LP et al. (2004). Depression and the metabolic syndrome in young adults: findings from the Third National Health and Nutrition Examination Survey. Psychosom. Med., 66: 316-322

[40] Kopf D, Westphal S, Luley CW, Ritter S et al. Lipid Metabolism and Insulin Resistance in Depressed Patients, J Clin Psychopharmacol, 2004, 24:527-531

[41] Kovacs M, Obrovsky DS, Goldston D, Drash A (1997). Major depressive symptoms and occurrence and outcome, Diabetes Care, 20: 45-51

[42] Kroenke K, Spitzer RL, Williams JB (2001). The PHQ-9: validity of a brief depression severity measure. J. Gen. Intern. Med., 16: 606-613

[43] Kuzmiaková M., Horáček J., Anděl M (1998). Tryptofan, jeho metabolizmus a funkce v lidském těle (s ohledem na metabolické choroby a depresívny syndrom). Vnitřní lékařství, 44(5): 288-293

[44] Li S, Li M, Song S et al. (2003). The effect of psychological intervention in treating the diabetic patients with negative emotion. Shandong J. Psychol. Med., 16: 148

[45] Littelfield CH, Roin GM, Murray MA, Craven JL (1990). Influence of functional imapairment and social support on depressive sympoms in persons with diabetes, Health Psychol, 9: 737-749

[46] Lloyd CE, Hermanns N, Nouwen A et al. (2010). The epidemiology of depression and diabetes: in Katon W, Maj M, Sartorius N (2010). Depression and Diabetes, John Wiley & Sons Ltd., 978-1-4443-5026-5, Chichester, UK

[47] Lu S, Lu B, Gu X (2005). Cognitive therapy in combination with electromyographic feedback in treatment of diabetes patients with depression after cerebral infarction. Chin. J. Clin. Pharm., 13: 215-216

[48] Lustman PJ, Anderson RJ, Freedland KE et al. (2000a). Depression and poor glycaemic control. A meta-analytic review of the literature. Diabetes Care, 23: 934-942

[49] Lustman PJ, Clouse RE, et al. (2006). Sertraline for prevention of depression recurrence in diabetes mellitus: a randomized, double-blind, placebo controlled trial. Arch Gen Psychiatry, 63: 521-529

[50] Lustman PJ, Griffth LS, Clouse RE (1988). Depression in adults with diabetes: results of a 5 – year follow-up study, Diabetes Care, 11: 605-612

[51] Lustman PJ, Griffth LS, Clouse RE et al. (1997a). Effects of nortriptyline on depression and glycemic control in diabetes: results of a double-blind, placebo-controlled trial. Psychosom. Med., 59: 241-250

[52] Lustman PJ, Griffth LS, Clouse RE, Freedland KE, et al. (2000b). Fluoxetine for Depression in Diabetes, Diabetes Care, 23(5): 618-623

[53] Lustman PJ, Griffith LS, Freedland KE, Clouse RE (1997b). The course of major depression in diabetes. Gen. Hosp. Psychiatry, 19: 138-143

[54] Lustman PJ, Griffith LS, Freedland KE et al. (1998). Cognitive behavior therapy for depression in type 2 diabetes mellitus. A randomized, controlled trial. Ann. Intern. Med., 129: 613-621

[55] Lustman PJ, Williams MM, Sayuk GS et al. (2007). Factors influencing Glycaemic Control in Type 2 Diabetes During Acute-and Maintenance-Phase Treatment of Major Depressive Disorder With Bupropion. Diabetes Care, 30: 459-466

[56] Manson J, Rimm E, Stampfer M et al. (1991). Physical activity and incidence of non-insulin-dependent diabetes mellitus in women. Lancet, 338: 774-778

[57] Maraldi C, Volpato S et al. (2007). Diabetes mellitus, glycaemic control, and incident depressive symptoms among 70- to 79-year-old-persons: the health, aging, and body composition study. Archives of Internal Medicine, 167: 1137-44

[58] McCaffery JM, Niaura R, Todaro JF et al. (2003). Depressive symptoms and metabolic risk in adult male twins enrolled in the National Heart, Lung, and Blood Institute Twin Study. Psychosom. Med., 65: 490-497

[59] McKellar JD et al. (2004). Depression increases diabetes symptoms on adherence, function and costs. Arch. Internal Medicine, 160(2): 3278-3285

[60] Mezuk B, Eaton WW, Albrecht S, Golden SH (2008). Depression and type 2 diabetes over the lifespan: a meta-analysis. Diabetes Care, 31: 2383-2390

[61] Mollema ED, Snoek FJ, Adér HJ et al. (2001). Insulin-treated diabetespatients with fear of self-injecting or fear of self-testing: psychological comorbidity and general well-being. J. Psychosom. Res., 51: 665-672

[62] Montano CB (2004). Recognition and treatment of depression in a primary care. J Clin Psychiatry, 55 (12): 18-34

[63] Nakra BRS, Rutland P, Verna S, et al. (1977). Amitriptyline and weight gain: a biochemical and endocrinological study, Curr Med Res Opin, 4: 602-6

[64] Nickelson L, Box R (1999). Treating depression in diabetic patients, J Pharm Practise, 12 (2): 128-35

[65] Okamura F, Tashiro A et al. (2000). Insulin resistance in patients with depression and its changes during the clinical course of depression: minimal model analysis. Metabolism, 49: 1255-1260

[66] Osborn CY, Patel KA, Liu J, Trott HW, Buchowski MS et al. Diabetes and Co-morbid Depression among Racially Diverse, Low-income Adults. Ann Behav Med. 2011 Jun; 41(3):300-9.doi: 10.1007/s12160-010-9241-1

[67] Paile-Hyvarinen M,Wahlbeck K, Eriksson JG (2003). Quality of life and metabolic status in mildly depressed women with type 2 diabetes treated with paroxetine: a single-blind randomised placebo controlled trial. BMC Fam. Pract., 4: 7

[68] Paile-Hyvarinen M,Wahlbeck K, Eriksson JG (2007). Quality of life and metabolic status in mildly depressed patients with type 2 diabetes treated with paroxetine: a double-blind randomised placebo controlled 6-month trial. BMC Fam. Pract., 8: 34

[69] Paykel ES, Mueller PS, De La Vergne PM (1973). Amitriptyline weight gain and carbohydrate cravings: a side effect, Br J Psychiatry, 123: 501-7

[70] Petrak F (2009). Treatment of Depression in Diabetes: an Update. Curr Opin Psychiatry, 22(2): 211-217

[71] Petrak F, Stridde E, Leverkus F et al. (2007). Development and validation of a new measure to evaluate psychological resistance to insulin treatment. Diabetes Care, 28: 2543-2545

[72] Peyrot M, Rubbin RR (1989). Determinants of depression among diabetic adults (Abstract), Diabetes, 38 (Suppl. 1): 9A

[73] Poulsen P., Vaag A., Kyvik K (2001). Genetic versus environmental aetiology of the metabolic syndrome among male and female twins, Diabetologia, 44: 537-543

[74] Pouwer F., Snoek F. J (2001). Association between symptoms of depression and glycaemic control may be unstable across gender. Diabet. Med., 18: 595-598

[75] Reader MB, Bjelland I, Vollset SE, Steen VM (2006). Obesity, dyslipidemia and diabetes with selective serotonin reuptake inhibitors: The Hordaland Health Study. J. Clin Psychiatry, 67: 1974-1982

[76] Rubin RR., Peyrot M (2002). Was Willis right? Thoughts on the interaction of depression and diabetes. Diabetes/Metabolism Res. Rev, 18(3): 173-175

[77] Salomé GM, Blanes L, Ferreira LM (2011). Assessment of depressive symptoms in people with diabetes mellitus and foot ulcers. Rev Col Bras Cir. Oct; 38(5): 327-33

[78] Sapolsky RM (2000), The possibility of neurotoxicity in the hippocampus in major depression: a primer on neuron death. Biol Psyhiatry, 48: 755-765

[79] Sawhney MS, Prakash C, Lustman PJ, Clouse RE (2007). Tricyclic antidepressants for chronic vomiting in diabetic patients. Dig Dis Sci, 52: 418-424

[80] Simson U, Nawarotzky U, Friese G et al. (2008). Psychotherapy intervention to reduce depressive symptoms in patients with diabetic foot syndrome. Diabet. Med., 25: 206-212

[81] Songar A, Kocabaşoğlu N, Balcioğlu İ et al. (1993). The relationship between diabetics' metabolic control levels and psychiatric symptomatology. Integrative Psychiatry, Vol 9(1): 34-40

[82] Stroud C, Davila J, Moyer A (2008). The relationship between stress and depression in first onsets versus recurrences: a meta-analytic review. J Abnorm. Psychol, 117: 206-213

[83] Svačina Š (2003). Lipidy a psychofarmaka. In: Ateroskleróza, 7(3): 118-121

[84] Švestka J (2005). Duloxetin – duální specifický inhibitor reuptake serotoninu a noradrenalinu v léčbě akutní depresivní poruchy. Psychiatrie, 9(1): 23-30

[85] Talbot F., Nouwen A (2000). A Review of the Relationships Between Depression and Diabetes in Adults. Diabetes Care October,volume 23, number 10: 156-1562

[86] Tůma I (2005). Deprese a diabetes. Vnitř Lék, 51(S2): S94-S98

[87] Tůma I., Hubeňák J. (2007), Diabetes Mellitus and Mental Disorders, Psychiatrie, 11 (4): 235-239

[88] Vogelzangs N, Kritchevsky SB, Beekman ATF et al. (2008). Depressive symptoms and change in abdominal obesity in older persons. Arch. Gen. Psychiatry, 65: 1386-1393

[89] Vuorilehto MS, Melartin TK, Isometsa ET (2009). Course and outcome of depressive disorders in primary care: a prospective 18-month study. Psychol. Med., 39: 1697-1707

[90] Wayne KJ, Korff M, Lin EH (2004). A Randomized Trial of Collaborative Care in Patients with Diabetes and Depression. Arch Gen Psychiatry, 61: 1042-1049

[91] Wells KB, Rogers W, Burnam MA, Camp P (1993). Course of depression in patients with hypertension, myocardial infarction, or insulin-dependent diabetes, Am J Psychiatry, 150:632-638

[92] Wild S., Roglic G. et al. (2004). Global prevalence of diabetes: estimates for the year 2000 and projections for the year 2030. Diabetes Care, 27: 1047-1053

[93] Xue H (2004). Paroxetine for depression in diabetes: a randomizedcontrolled trial. Chin. Ment. Health J, 18:735-737

[94] Zeman M., Jirák R (2008). Metabolic Syndrome and selected mental illnesses, Psychiatr prax, 9 (4): 176-180)

[95] Zimmet P, Dowse G, Bennedett P (1991). Hyperinsulinemia is a predictor of non-insulin-depended diabetes mellitus. Diabetes Metab, 17: 101-108

Chapter 3

Depression: Classification, Culture and the Westernisation of Mental Illness

Kenneth Walsh and Wendy Cross

Additional information is available at the end of the chapter

http://dx.doi.org/10.5772/54176

1. Introduction

In this era of functional MRIs, neurobiology and the sequencing of the human genome, it is easy to forget that the complex phenomenon of mental illness is to some degree socially constructed. The trend towards globalisation has seen a Western social bias (one could even say an American bias) towards the classification and treatment of mental illness.

In this chapter we argue that the homogenisation of the experience, classification and treatment of mental illness, whilst having some benefits, has also done harm and that this is especially true of the complex phenomenon of depression.

The chapter examines:

- the effects of the Diagnostic and Statistical Manual on the homogenisation and simplification of mental illness and in particular depression,
- the phenomenology of depression across cultures in light of the Westernisation of mental illness, and,
- the role of "Big Pharma" in pathologising the cultural expression of sadness.

In addition, the chapter will suggest some ways forward to a more nuanced approach to the diagnosis and treatment of depression.

1.1. Introduction: Surface symptoms and aetiology

Sarah's depression

Sarah had been diagnosed with depression following the death of her much loved father some eighteen months previously. Her symptoms were severe enough for her to be diagnosed with the DSM-IV category of Major Depression. The prescribed medication had helped somewhat but some two and a half years after her father's death her depression and its accompanying anxiety saw this once confident woman lose her business and her marriage.

Sarah was eventually referred to a group and individual psychotherapy program. In this program Sarah told the story of her father's death. Her father had been scheduled for a hip replacement. The surgery was delayed and his eventual admission coincided with Sarah's scheduled move to a distant city to set up a new business. The surgery went ahead but Sarah's father developed postoperative pneumonia. Not wishing to alarm Sarah and necessitate her unnecessary return, her sister Jane, expecting their father to recovery quickly, kept the information from Sarah. However their father's condition deteriorated and by the time Sarah was notified it was too late and her father died whilst she was on a flight home.

All of this was explored in therapy but Sarah's symptoms remained. Then some months into therapy Sarah was notified that her mother had suddenly become ill and had been admitted to the same hospital. Sarah arrived at the hospital in good time and was able to be with her mother up until her death. Shortly before her death her mother began talking to her dead husband as if he were in the room with them.

On returning back to therapy following her mother's funeral Sarah seemed to have changed. Sarah related that when her mother was talking to her dead father Sarah remembered her last conversation with him: something she had hitherto forgotten. She had gone to see him prior to his operation and her travel interstate. Her father, who had never been in hospital before, appeared anxious and said to Sarah, "You are leaving me here to die". She assured him that he would be fine and back on his feet in no time.

Reflecting on this in therapy Sarah was surprised that she had forgotten the comment and reflected on the fact that she had indeed left him to die, albeit unknowingly. In the following weeks Sarah went over this comment time and again; she had not meant to leave him to die, it was not deliberate. Sarah then went through a period of grieving for both her parents and the grief turned to a period of mourning at their passing. Gradually over the following months Sarah's depression and anxiety lifted. At six and twelve months follow-up her depression and anxiety had not returned.

Carolyn's agoraphobia

Carolyn's Agoraphobia had begun without any identifiable cause. Following a panic attack in a supermarket checkout queue she found it increasingly difficult to go out in public. Cognitive Behaviour Therapy (CBT) and anxiolytics had helped a little but her anxiety and accompanying depressive symptoms persisted.

Carolyn was eventually referred to individual and group psychotherapy. Progress was slow and Carolyn's anxiety made it difficult to travel to therapy. Some weeks after commencing group therapy, a group member brought up the topic of loss. This client spoke of the loss of a child as being the greatest loss one could suffer. Carolyn broke down and began crying uncontrollably. Over the next few sessions she recounted how twenty-five years previously she had been admitted to hospital following complications of her

http://dx.doi.org/10.5772/54176

first pregnancy and subsequently suffered a late miscarriage. She recounted how today it would have been considered a still birth, how she had not been allowed to see the baby and how she was told to forget about it and try to get pregnant again. Her husband and her family never mentioned it again.

Over subsequent group therapy sessions Carolyn recounted the days and months following the "miscarriage". She recounted how she had tried to put on a brave face and not cry and how secretly she went back to the hospital and asked where the child's grave was, only to be told there wasn't one. She had not spoken to anyone about it from that day to this. Over the following weeks she cried, "Twenty five years worth of tears". Gradually, Carolyn's symptoms of anxiety and depression subsided and she found herself once more able to go out in public without fear of a panic attack.

What do these two stories have to say about depression? In both cases the clients had been diagnosed and treated with medication which had some affect on the symptoms but did not bring about a resolution of the problem. In the case of Carolyn, Cognitive Behaviour Therapy was used and once again had some affect but did not resolve the problem. Both the medication and the CBT were used to treat the surface symptoms. As Darian Leader puts it, the consequence of treating the surface symptoms is that, "The interior life of the suffer is left un-examined, and priority given to medicalizing solutions…The problem has to be got rid of rather than understood (Leader, 2008:2)". Medication in this case aimed to restore presumed chemical imbalances in the brain. CBT was aimed at restoring presumed faulty cognition. In both cases the underlying loss was left untouched and in fact remained hidden. In Sarah's case the guilt associated with her father's death and the loss of her identity as a dutiful daughter remained hidden even from her. In Carolyn's case the surface symptoms which were predominately of anxiety, meant that grief and loss were not even associated with her case and were masked as much by the diagnosis as anything else. This concentration on the appearance, diagnosis and surface symptoms effectively blocked a deeper and more wide ranging explanation of the symptoms.

The other interesting element of both cases is that the surfacing of the underlying loss and its subsequent resolution took time. Time is one thing we often do not have for clients in today's world: time for them to explore their reality and, as the experts of their own experience, to teach us. Indeed in some countries psychiatrists spend on average two hours per year in face-to-face dialogue with clients (Leader, 2011). Sarah and Carolyn's recovery also took place within an alliance with others. Both women underwent a period of public (albeit within the group) mourning in which both appeared to integrate their experiences into their life story.

In this chapter we shall explore the consequences of classifying and treating depression based upon the surface symptoms. We shall also explore how culture and context influence surface symptomatology. We suggest a way forward which acknowledges our shared humanity and the need to look beyond surface symptomatology in the treatment of depression.

2. The effects of the diagnostic and statistical manual on the homogenisation and simplification of mental illness and in particular depression

Naming something does not explain it.

In the 1960s many school biology classes taught that the Platypus was a "freak of nature": as it suckled its young and laid eggs it was neither a mammal nor a reptile. Of course because something does not fit neatly into a human classification system does not make it a "freak of nature". To believe so is to believe that by naming something we have explained it. Yet to some extent this is what we are doing when, using a diagnostic system based on surface symptoms or descriptions, we classify human behaviour as this or that disorder: the diagnosis becomes the explanation for the symptoms. Whilst there are undoubted advantages to standard classification systems (communication between clinicians; ability to examine the natural history of a disorder and develop targeted treatment regimens) the major disadvantage is that the individual, their experience, their inner life, their uniqueness, their humanity culture and context, can be overlooked or ignored and the surface symptoms alone treated.

The debate about psychiatric classification and its consequences is not new. The debate has generally revolved around description versus aetiology. Kraepelin believed that pure description would eventually lead to and be replaced by a system based on aetiology (Zigler & Phillips, 1961). Unfortunately this has not happened.

The danger with an emphasis on description is that it may leave little room for the interpretation of psychopathology (Zigler & Phillips, 1961). In addition if the descriptions are drawn from one dominant cultural perspective then from the beginning their cross-cultural universality should be questioned. In such a system, the manifestations of mental illness may be forced to fit preconceived frameworks and paradoxically the zeal for classification may see more and more human behaviour pathologised.

The dominant classification system in the world is the American Psychiatric Association's (APA) Diagnostic and Statistical Manual (DSM) of Mental Disorders: now about to be released in its fifth version. Whilst the DSM has assisted clear communication between physicians when discussing mental illness and its treatment, it has also been accused of medicalising (and therefore pathologising) an ever-increasing range of behaviours (Flaskerud, 2010). The original DSM I, which was first published in 1952, contained 103 diagnoses; by the publication of DSM-IV-TR in 2000 this had grown to 365. This growth in diagnostic categories has not been without its critics. The APA has been accused of manufacturing madness by pathologising a wider and wider spread of human behaviour. This has been achieved, say the critics through devising new diagnostic categories and broadening the criteria for the old ones. The most recent controversy surrounds the suggestion by the APA that the new edition of the DSM remove the bereavement exclusion in the diagnosis of major depression and add complicated grief as a new diagnosis (Frances et al, 2010).

That the DSM is a descriptive classification system is clear. The DSM-IV-TR (APA, 2000) in addition to listing surface symptoms, also discusses prevalence, course, familial pattern

http://dx.doi.org/10.5772/54176

and differential diagnosis but not aetiology. As a consequence of its purely descriptive stance there have been those who argue that the DSM lacks validity as it is a classification system without a theoretical/explanatory basis or an agreed upon scientific model other than a general assumption of a biological causation of mental illness (Thakker & Ward, 1998; Flaskerud, 2010).

According to Gary Greenberg (2010, p. 15) "the DSM is an unparalleled literary achievement. It renders the varieties of our psychospiritual suffering without any comment on where it comes from, what it means, or what ought to be done about it".

Criticisms of the DSM are abundant and we do not propose to outline them all here. However there are some points of critique which are of relevance to this chapter. The first is the imposition of a North American/Western European perspective on mental illness and the relegation of other cultural perspectives to curiosity status. The second is the mistake of thinking we are describing stable entities when what are really being described are also socio-political constructs.

That the DSM has a North American/Western European bias is evident. The DSM-IV-TR (2000) relegates non-western syndromes to an appendix called "culture-bound syndromes (APA, 2000: 897-903)". This ignores the fact that the DSM itself is culture bound and a product of North American Western European culture (Flaskerud, 2010). It further assumes the universality of its primary syndromes, some minor culture bound influences aside (Thakker and Ward, 1998). The socio-political construction of the DSM, even within its own cultural paradigm, is well illustrated by the fact that the mental disorder of homosexuality was cured with a stroke of a pen when it was eliminated from the DSM II in 1974 (Flaskerud, 2010). Prior to this societal change, homosexuality was deemed a mental illness and treated by various means including aversion therapy.

A mental disorder is defined as the "existence of a clinically recognisable set of symptoms or behaviour associated in most cases with distress and with interference with personal functions" (ICD-10, World Health Organisation (WHO), 1992, p. 5). A person is considered to have a mental illness when the clinical presentation meets the criteria defined either in the DSM-IV (APA, 2000) or the ICD-10 (WHO, 1992). Conversely, a mentally healthy person will not exhibit clinically recognisable symptoms, behaviours or functional distress.

Importantly, the diagnostic process for any person is concerned with the accurate assessment by the clinician. This assessment occurs through the interaction between the clinician and the client and is based on an interrogatory process. Any examination of the rates of mental illness within a given community rests on the assumption that the diagnosis is accurate. Forming an accurate diagnosis is based on a number of factors including cultural variances in the expression of mental illness and cross-cultural communication patterns. Self-disclosure by the client in the assessment procedure is a communication variable that influences the nature and amount of information the clinician is able to secure during the interview. Clinicians therefore, need to be culturally sensitive to the differences in communication practices within cultures that affect self-disclosure as well as the cultural differences in illness expression and help-seeking behaviour.

According to Marsella (1981) any ideas relating to mental health must be viewed in the context of what constitutes "the self". Given that cultures ascribe and define notions of self, reality and illness, it is fundamental to study mental health and illness in a holistic framework with regard to social, contextual and cultural history (Marsella & White, 1982). "Cultural conventions about the self, reality, social rules, and patterns of emotional expression, for example, simply make universal criteria of psychiatric illness difficult to attain and the idea itself problematical" (Fabrega, 1987, p. 386).

Burr and Chapman (1998) argue that psychiatry has pathologised culture by perpetuating cultural stereotypes as definable categories and failing to acknowledge the institutionalised racism that exists. Moreover, these authors argue that,

---

"Health carers seem to be characterised as either cultural translators or functionaries, whose practice is largely circumscribed by a social system characterised by social and economic inequality" (Burr & Chapman, 1998, p. 435).

Historically, there have been challenges to the assumptions that cross-cultural similarities in abnormality exist. Earlier, cultural anthropologists suggested that abnormality was relative and should be addressed in conjunction with the cultural norms and deviations tolerated relative to that society (Kleinman, 1996). Since these early warnings questioning the validity of applying non-specific diagnostic criteria to non-Western social groups, a number of studies have empirically demonstrated the need to define concepts of normality and abnormality according to normative standards relevant to reference populations (Kleinman, 1996).

The concept of mental health has traditionally been embedded in psychological and behavioural characteristics. According to MedlinePlus (2012) "Mental health is how we think, feel and act as we cope with life. It also helps determine how we handle stress, relate to others and make choices. Like physical health, mental health is important at every stage of life, from childhood and adolescence through adulthood". Somatic expressions have until recently largely been ignored mostly due to the scientific models that have defined illness. Models of causality are now including epistemological and ontological paradigms, which interact to identify mental illness across many cultures (Marsella, 1981). Although some (APA, 1994; Gaw, 2001, Weller & Baer, 2008) would argue that there are identifiable and unique "culture-bound syndromes", these syndromes are also found across quite disparate cultures.

In parallel with the rise of a descriptive nosology has been the rise of the biomedical model of causation of mental illness. This model assumes that mental illness including depression arises from chemical imbalances in the brain, which in turn may have a genetic cause. The consequence of this pairing of a descriptive nosology with a biological causation has been that contextual factors or the life world of the patient as well as their inner life world are seen as much less important to both understanding and treating depression. It has also seen the rise and rise of pharmacological treatments especially since the advent of the SSRIs starting with Prozac in 1988. Of this more later.

http://dx.doi.org/10.5772/54176

Regier (2004, p. 25) describes the problem: Various critics of the current diagnostic system have characterised the expansion of diagnostic categories as a "guild" attempt to justify payment for any condition a psychiatrist might see in practice, or as fabrications of the pharmaceutical industry to justify the sale of their products".

3. An "Epidemic" of depression?

According to the World Health Organisation (2012), depression is the leading cause of disability as measured by years lived with disability (YLD) and the 4th leading contributor to the global burden of disease in 2000 (WHO 2012). By 2020 depression is projected to be the second highest ranked cause of years of productive life lost due to disability (DALYs). Various reasons for this apparent epidemic have been posited varying from the rise of individualism (Ehrenreich, 2007) and dissolution of a sense of community (Levine, 2008) to, paradoxically, the use of anti-depressants as front-line treatment for depression (Whitaker, 2011).

However, behind the alarming statistics and the posited causes, the influence of a descriptive classification system, depression awareness campaigns and the marketing of antidepressants by drug companies, makes the picture even less clear.

As previously stated, the classification of depression is based upon surface symptoms from a predominately North American/Western European perspective. The term depression has come to replace earlier terms such as "melancholia" and "mourning" which subsumed depressive symptoms within them and at least hinted at contextual factors. The DSM has elevated depression from a symptom to a disorder. Whilst the DSM has a definition and set criteria for depression, the term has a variety of meanings to the general public; both figurative and literal (Summerfield, 2006). Coupled with this is the global campaign to raise awareness of the disease so that treatment can be effected and the "epidemic" fought.

In Australia, the spearhead of this campaign is the not for profit organisation "Beyond Blue" (www.beyondblue.org.au). The Beyond Blue website contains symptom checklists some of which are so broad that many people may be concerned that they are in fact depressed. For example, the website contains the SPHERE symptom checklist which is a "... scale developed as part of a national mental health educational project aimed at increasing GP's rate of identification, effective treatment and management of common psychological disorders like depression" (Beyond Blue website). The scale contains 27 items grouped under behaviours, thoughts, feelings and physical symptoms. On entering four symptoms at random into the checklist ("not getting things done", "it's my fault", "indecisive" and "tired all the time") the site advised that: "If you scored 3 or more of the [27] symptoms, you *probably have a depressive illness* [emphasis added]", and should see a doctor. Contextual factors are not taken into consideration.

The doctor that most people undertaking such a symptoms test will see will likely be a General Practitioner (GP). Dumit (2005) states that in the USA 75% of all prescriptions for antidepressants are written by non-psychiatrists. GPs are increasingly facing clients armed with symptom checklists, often supplied by drug companies, which may influence prescribing behaviour (Dumit, 2005). The situation in the UK is similar. Summerfield (2006) states that whilst there is little empirical evidence for an epidemic of depression, with prescriptions for antidepressants rising in the UK in the 1990s from 9 million to 21 million, there is evidence of an epidemic of prescribing. We are now seeing the diagnosis of depression and the prescription of SSRIs rising in non western countries.

4. The phenomenology of depression across cultures and the westernisation of mental illness: The case of Japan

Depression is a complex phenomenon. It is experienced by different individuals in different ways. The phenomenology of depression is also influenced by the cultural context. For example, in the West people diagnosed with depression are likely to present with predominately psychological symptoms. That in other parts for the world somatic symptoms tend to dominate has long been known (Ryder, 2008; Tanaka-Matsumi & Marsella, 1976). That different cultures view depression and the expression of sadness in different ways is also well known. Indeed, until recently this was also the case in Japan. Sadness and depression were often positively viewed as "... yielding enhanced awareness of the transient nature of the world (Kirmayer, 2002)". Up until the 1990s "Utsubyô" (the Japanese term for depression) was considered a severe but rare disorder (Watters, 2010). Other lesser forms of depression were seen as a personal affliction which did not require treatment (Kirmayer, 2002).

However, the Japanese attitude to depression changed dramatically in the late 1990s when Japan saw a 46% increase in cases of depression diagnosed between 1999 and 2003. In 2005 it was estimated that 2 million Japanese suffered from depression as defined by the DSM (Schulz, 2004). Although the rate of suicide in Japan is much higher than other countries (twice that of USA and four times that of UK), the prevalence of depression is still lower than the USA and only 53% of suicides are attributed to depression (Sado et al 2011). Nevertheless the Japanese experience mirrors reports in the professional and popular press of an "Epidemic of Depression" (Levine, 2008). This epidemic of depression has set alarm bells ringing in Japan not least because on the economic front alone it has been estimated that the total cost of depression in Japan in 2005 was ¥2 Trillion (Sado, et al 2011).

Interestingly this rise of depression in Japan coincided with the rise in the use of the DSM and the marketing of SSRI antidepressants.

The DSM 111 was introduced to Japan in 1980 but its uptake was slow. The conventional classification of mental illness had been influenced by German neuropsychiatry of the early 20th century (Someya, 2001, Kirmayer, 2002). However, by 2000 there was a general acceptance and use of the DSM by the younger generation of psychiatrists (Someya, et al 2001).

Whilst there is some evidence that the cardinal symptoms of depression as described in the DSM appear as clusters or syndromes in many cultures, there are many other symptoms that reflect cultural idioms of distress and "ethnophysiologies" (Kirmayer, 2002). As globalisation takes hold and a degree of cultural homogenisation takes place there may well be a shift in these culture bound manifestations which reflect a shifting globalised perspective on distress and the individual's place in society. Such homogenisation may see the descriptive nosology of the DSM adopted as the standard across cultures. As Kirmayer puts it,

---

"The notion that a comprehensive or complete nosology can be created without regard to culture and context can be sustained only by adopting a reductionistic perspective that ignores the fact that human beings are fundamentally cultural beings (Kirmayer, 2005:193)".

---

5. Westernisation of depression the role of "big pharma"

Given Japanese cultural views of depression, it is not surprising that Japan was not seen as a large market for antidepressants. However, that changed in the late 1990s when drug company GlaxoSmithKline began marketing its new SSRI, Paxil (Watters, 2010).

The campaign began with the GlaxoSmithKline convening a group of experts in cross cultural psychiatry in order to promote the concept of depression in Japan and reconceptualise somatic symptoms and social anxieties as indicators of an illness amenable to pharmacological treatment (Kirmayer, 2006). One more cynical aspect of this campaign was the marketing of depression as a "kokoro no kaze": cold of the soul (Watters, 2010) for which the remedy was a kind of psychic Aspirin; an SSRI.

Whilst the upshot of this campaign may well have been the treatment of Japanese people who had hitherto been undertreated or not treated at all for depression, the subsequent drug company community information media campaign aimed to broaden the market for SSRIs in Japan. This was achieved by presenting depression as "…intentionally ambiguous and ill-defined, applicable to the widest possible population and to the widest possible range of discomforts (Kitanaka, 2006 quoted in Watters, 2010: 226)". Whilst in no way a cynical or a deliberate attempt to mislead, the symptoms checklists seen on the Beyond Blue website may have a similar effect in that three or more vague discomforts of the common lot for humanity which coincide with a two week period of depressed mood are seen as "probably" indicating depression.

The GlaxoSmithKline community information campaign in Japan may have also been aimed to overcome another barrier to the diagnosis and treatment of depression: stigma. Again, this may have been of benefit for some Japanese suffers of depression as stigma is a barrier to many individuals who would otherwise seek treatment (Cross and Walsh; 2012). Dumit, however, takes a more cynical view: "Marketers see stigma as inhibiting self recognition of patient status and therefore reducing prescription demand (Dumit, 2005)". Indeed Dumit believes that differences in diagnosis between races or genders are seen by drug marketers as an opportunity to achieve "parity". In this way the lesser market [Japan for example] is seen as 'undertreated'. Efforts to open up the market and achieve parity are characterised by "...the funding of epidemiological studies, the introduction and invention of new languages and the creation of websites explaininis seen by drugg the symptomatology of the conditions (Dumit, 2005:11)". This has seen an interesting shift from previous expressions of illness and suffering in which the patient's experience of suffering and identification as a sufferer took primacy over one where it is possible for the patient to be a sufferer without knowing it. Indeed the patient may need to be assisted to develop insight into their state by public service campaigns, drug company information, experts in the field, symptoms checklists and diagnostic manuals. Objective opinion takes precedence over subjective experience.

Overall there appears to be a lowering of the threshold for symptomatic treatment of depression. For some commentators this amounts to "disease mongering" which interferes with the individual's coping mechanisms and culturally appropriate ways of dealing with distress (Das, 2011).

The increasing pathologising and medicalising of human behaviour has been well documented (Greenberg, 2010). Some see this as evidence of the rise of the medical-industrial complex (Das, 2011) and the manufacturing of illness (and attendant cures). However, it also brings into question notions of happiness and expectations of the human condition in contemporary society.

6. A way forward

In North American/Western European societies the story of depression is illustrative of a deeper malaise which in turn is being exported to other cultures. This malaise includes: an uncritical adoption of a descriptive nosology of mental illness; the gradual broadening of what constitutes mental distress; simplistic genetic and biological models of causation with attendant simplistic pharmacological treatments.

This has had a number of consequences. The gradual broadening of the definition of mental disorders and the lowering of thresholds for diagnostic categories has seen hitherto unpathologised human experience pathologised (Atrens, 2011). This has brought about a fundamental change in expectations of what life should bring and in fundamental notions of happiness, suffering and what it means to be human. This situation is nicely satirised by a slogan on the T shirt seen recently: "I used to care but I take a pill for that now.' Not only is there change in the expectations of what constitutes suffering and the human experience, there is another more insidious effect. If the cause of our problems resides in our biology, our neurones and our genetics, then it is, at its core, a problem of the individual. This splitting of the individual from their society and context is analogous to the focus on surface symptoms discussed earlier. The surface symptoms of the deeper malise in our societies is the disorder of the individual. The cure then is to treat the individual rather than explore the part that society, culture and context plays and therefore need for social reform.

There is little doubt that the suffering and disability (and indeed mortality) caused by severe depression needs to be alleviated wherever possible and in all cultures. It is however less

http://dx.doi.org/10.5772/54176

clear that lesser forms of unhappiness, dissatisfaction or distress require a medical diagnosis and pharmacological treatments. This is even more the case where cultural and other differences are poorly understood. Collectivist societies (such as those commonly found in Asia and Africa) will differ markedly in their expression of sadness and depression and will often require a different approach to individualist societies. Nevertheless, it could be argued that underlying issues of separation and loss are common across cultures (Leader, 2008) but the culture then shapes the expression of the surface symptoms.

Descriptive nosologies, simplistic biological models of causation and the attendant emphasis on pharmalogical treatments may not be helping to alleviate mental distress but may be making it worse (Atrens, 2011).

As Kirmayer states:

Health and illness reside not just in the individual but also in networks of relationships that are culturally defined. The creation of discrete disorders involves bracketing off social context. A comprehensive psychiatric nosology must reserve a place for human predicaments. Rather than focusing exclusively on problems presumed to be intrinsic to the person, or even to the central nervous system, we need to continue to develop and refine a typology of the range of human predicaments (Kirmayer, 2005:195).

Author details

Kenneth Walsh[1,2] and Wendy Cross[3]

1 University of Wollongong, Australia

2 Illawarra Shoalhaven Local Health District, NSW and Canterbury Christchurch University, UK

3 School of Nursing and Midwifery, Monash University, Melbourne, Australia

References

[1] Atrens, D. 2011. Big Pharma and the manufacture of madness. *Quadrant*, Jan–Feb: 50-55.

[2] American Psychiatric Association. 2000. *Diagnostic and Statistical Manual of Mental Disorders (4th ed., text rev.)*. APA. Washington, DC.

[3] Burr, J. A. & Chapman, T. 1998. Some reflections on cultural and social considerations in mental health nursing. *Journal of Psychiatric and Mental Health Nursing*, 5, 431 - 437.

[4] Cross, W & Walsh, K. 2012. Star Shots: Stigma, self-disclosure and celebrity in Bipolar Disorder (Chapter 10). In Barnhill, J. (Ed) *Bipolar Disorder*. Intech Publishing, Rijeka.

[5] Das, A. 2009. Pharmaceutical industry and the market: The case of Prozac and other antidepressants. *Asian Journal of Psychiatry*. 4: 14-18.

[6] Dumit, J. 2005. The Depsychiatrisation of Mental Illness. *Journal of Public Mental Health*. 4(3): 8-13.

[7] Ehrenreich, B. 2007. How we learned to stop having fun. The Guardian, April 2nd.

[8] Fabrega, H. 1987. Psychiatric diagnosis: A cultural perspective. *The Journal of Nervous and Mental Diseases*, 175(7): 383 - 394.

[9] Flaskerud, J. 2010. DSM Proposed Changes, Part I: Criticisms and Influences on Changes. *Issues in Mental Health Nursing*, 31: 686-688.

[10] Frances, A., Pies, R., & Zisook, S. 2010. DSM5 and the Medicalization of Grief: Two Perspectives. *Psychiatric Times*. 27(5): 334-340.

[11] Gaw, A. C. 2001. *Concise guide to cross-cultural psychiatry*. Washington, DC: American Psychiatric Publishing Inc.

[12] Greenberg, G. 2010. *Manufacturing Depression: The secret history of a modern disease*. Bloomsbury, London.

[13] Kirmayer, L. 2002. Psychopharmacology in a Globalizing World: The Use of Antidepressants in Japan, *Transcultural Psychiatry*, 39: 295-332.

[14] Kleinman, A. (1996). How is culture important for the DSM-IV? In J. E. Mezzich, A. Kleinman, H. Fabrega & D. L. Parron (Eds.), *Culture and Psychiatric Diagnosis: A DSM-IV perspective* (pp. 15 - 25). Washington, DC: American Psychiatric Press.

[15] Leader, D. 2008. *The New Black: Mourning, melancholia and depression*. Penguin, London.

[16] Leader, D. 2011. *What is Madness?* Penguin, London.

[17] Levine, 2008. Depression is becoming epidemic in consumer societies. *CCPA Monitor*, 15(1): 36.

[18] Marsella, A. 1981. Cross-cultural research on severe mental disorders: issues and findings. In A. Marsella & P. B. Pedersen (Eds), *Cross-cultural Counseling and Psychotherapy* (pp. 7 -22). Pergamon, New York.

[19] Marsella, A. & White, G. (Eds.)(1982). *Cultural Conceptions of Mental Health and Therapy* (pp. 361-389). Reidel, Boston.

[20] MedlinePlus (2012) http://www.nlm.nih.gov/medlineplus/mentalhealth.html Accessed September 2012

[21] Regier, D.A. 2004. State-of-the-art psychiatric diagnosis. *World Psychiatry* 3 (1): 25-26.

[22] Ryder, A. Zhu, X., Yao, S., Yi, J., Yang, J., Heine, S. & Bagby, M. 2008. The cultural shaping of Depression: Somatic symptoms in China, psychological symptoms in North America. *Journal of Abnormal Psychology*, 117(2): 300-313.

[23] Schulz, K. 2004. Did antidepressants depress Japan? *New York Times,* August. 22nd.

[24] Someya, T., Takahasi, M. & Takahasi, S. 2001. Is DSM widely accepted by Japanese clinicians? *Psychiatry and Clinical Neurosciences*. 55: 437-450.

[25] Tanaka-Matsumi, J. & Marsella, A. 1976. Cross-Cultural Variations in the Phenomenological Experience of Depression : I. Word Association Studies. *Journal of Cross Cultural Psychology*, 7: 379- 396.

[26] Thakker, J. & Ward, T. 1998. Culture and Classification: The cross cultural application of the DSM. *Clinical Psychology Review*. 18(5); 501-529.

[27] Watters, E. 2010. *Crazy Like Us: The globalisation of the American psyche.* Scribe, Melbourne.

[28] Weller, S.C., & Baer R.D. (2008). Susto and Nervios: Expressions for Stress and Depression. *Culture, Medicine & Psychiatry* 32, (3): 406-420.

[29] Whitaker, R. 2011. The Anatomy of an Epidemic: Magic Bullets, Psychiatric Drugs, and the Astonishing Rise of Mental Illness in America. Crown Publishing, New York.

[30] World Health Organization, 1992. The ICD-10 classification of mental and behavioural disorders: Clinical descriptions and diagnostic guidelines. WHO, Geneva.

[31] http://www.who.int/mental_health/management/depression/definition/en/

[32] www.Beyondblue.org.au.

[33] Zigler, E & Phillips, L. 1961. Psychiatric Diagnosis: A critique. *Journal of Abnormal and Social Psychology*. 63(3): 607-618.

Chapter 4

Cognitive Behavioral Therapy (CBT) of Depressive Disorders

Irene Lehner-Adam and Bertalan Dudas

Additional information is available at the end of the chapter

http://dx.doi.org/10.5772/54200

1. Introduction

Depressive disorders belong to the most frequent psychiatric disorders in Western Europe and the U.S.A. and are associated with high recurrence rates, high resistance to therapy, morbidity and mortality [1-4]. Currently, depressions have a share of 6.1% in total DALYs (DALY = Disability-Adjusted Life Year = as measure for disease burden), and thus are ranked at the 4th place in worldwide causes of disease [4]. It is expected that unipolar depression will become the main health-related cause of death in developed countries by 2020 [5,6]. In the E.U. alone, 18.5 million people have been diagnosed with major depression [7].

Depression involves numerous personal, family-related, social and economic consequences. Due to a high psychological burden, this disorder no longer allows the usual conduct of life; furthermore, not only does it represent a burden on the quality of life of the affected persons and close relatives but it is also connected to a significant economic impact. In the U.S.A. the costs incurred by treatment, morbidity and mortality amount to 83 billion USD per year [8]; in the United Kingdom the annual depression treatment costs for adults amount to 636 million euros [9]. In Europe, 28 billion euros are spent on treatment of affective disorders [10]. The socio-economic costs of depression for society as a whole amount to approx. 1% of the gross domestic product. However, the largest part of economic expenses is generated outside of the health system [11] and is related to the loss of work productivity, leisure-time opportunities and early mortality due to suicide [12,13].

During the past twenty years, there has not only been an enormous growth in the number of depressed patients, but the selection of antidepressant medication has been dramatically increased. Despite major advances in depression research and development of new antidepressant substances, the high rate of therapy-resistant and/or recurrent patients was not improved [14,15].

Although there is a general consensus that, based on evidence-based psychotherapy research in past decades, both antidepressants and psycho-therapeutic procedures are effective for treatment of depressive disorders [16-20], psycho-pharmacological treatment still represents first-choice therapy. However, clinical studies show that only approximately 30% of the patients show remission after first treatment with antidepressants [21]. In case of a severe and acute depression, stabilizing the patient through medication clearly takes precedence; however, in case of slight to moderate depression (without symptoms of delusions) the focus of treatment should initially be placed on psycho-therapeutic methods due to the limited success of psycho-pharmacological therapy [22,23]. There is an increasing number of patients who do not desire pharmacological treatment (pregnant women, children), or do not tolerate such treatment due to undesired side effects and/or interactions (cancer, pain, geriatric patients). In these cases, psychotherapy should be preferred [24-30]. Whilst psychotropic drugs act biologically, psychotherapy is effective via patient self-efficacy by changing cognitions and behavior. To numerous depressed patients, the cause of their disorder is explained as being a chemical imbalance that can only be treated with medication. It can be assumed that the probability of mobilizing self-coping mechanisms in terms of fighting disorders is particularly low in this patient group. The high recurrence rate (50% within one year after treatment) of depressed patients who received pharmacological treatment in the past seems to support this notion [31].

Rush et al. [32] compared the effectiveness of cognitive behavioral therapy (CBT) to pharmacotherapy in a group of depressed patients treated as out-patients and ascertained that CBT is superior to pharmacotherapy. Bellack and colleagues [33] came to similar conclusion in their study and pointed out that combination therapy - which is preferred by some researchers - even shows negative results because pharmacotherapy has an inhibiting effect on behavioral therapy in connection with depression. Kovacs et al. [34] showed that the recurrence rate with behavioral therapy is significantly lower as compared to pharmacotherapy; CBT also shows the termination of therapy less frequently, and, after a one year follow-up, CBT-treated patients show significantly greater favorable progress as compared to patients with antidepressant treatment [19,35-36]. However, in-patient depression treatment in Western Europe indicates a growing trend towards the combination of both approaches.

CBT is a scientifically founded, active, problem- and target-oriented, structured, temporally limited psychological treatment method that shows high effectiveness against both psychiatric disorders (anxiety, phobias, compulsions, addictive disorders) and physical disorders including eating disorders, pain disorders and tinnitus [29,37-38]. During the past four decades there has been a number of scientific studies supporting the significance and effectiveness of CBT in connection with affective disorders, particularly depression [17,19,39-41].

The primary goal of the following section is to provide an overview of the history of CBT as well as its clinical features and the behavior-therapeutic diagnostics of depressive disorder. In the subsequent sections the psychological disorder models of depression and corresponding therapeutic approaches will be explained by using clinical cases. The presented methods represent treatment fundamentals of depressive disorders requiring a competent therapist.

The specific order of the presented elements of treatment does not represent a rigid sequence of treatment steps, but rather a recommendation of therapy. Certain therapeutic elements can only be determined if the patient provides certain basic information, e.g., with severe depression the patient is expected to activate behavioral strategies before the introduction of cognitive techniques [31]. The intensity of depression, current symptoms, cognitive levels, motivation as well as current patient problems determine the speed and the systematic progress of therapy.

The correct duration and sequence of CBT is pivotal for successful treatment. CBT for unipolar depression requires 15 - 30 sessions [42]. In case of moderate and severe depression it is recommended to have two sessions per week for 4 - 5 weeks, followed by weekly sessions during the next 8 - 12 weeks and then sessions every other or every third week. Relatively infrequent contacts are sufficient for the maintenance of therapy success. The described strategies are performed in single-person settings but can be adapted to group and pair therapies. The same applies to age groups: CBT proved to be successful in the treatment of depression in children [43] as well as in aged patients [44,45,46].

2. Symptoms of depression

Depressive disorders are included in the group of affective disorders in the major classification schemes (WHO – ICD-10, APA – DSM-IV). Affective disorders are psychiatric disorders where major symptoms include changes of mood or affectivity. The mood change is accompanied by change of activity levels in most cases (ICD-10). Although the terms "affect", "mood" and "emotion" are defined differently in most cases, many of these concepts exhibit similarities [47-48]. Here, affect is defined as an umbrella term that includes mood and emotion [49].

Feeling depressed does not particularly represent an onset of a disorder. However, depression is more than only a temporal change of mood or short-term sluggishness. The characteristic condition of a depressed patient is most commonly represented by the following symptoms:

Physical symptoms: Most patients with a depression suffer from sleep disturbances ranging from problems with sleeping through the night up to constant tiredness. Decreased or increased appetite, constipation and loss of libido are also characteristic of depression. The patient often complains of feeling of tension, coldness or diffuse pain in the head, back or gastrointestinal tract.

Cognitive symptoms: Depressed patients feel weak and powerless, and they lose most of their interests in people or activities they used to enjoy. These patients feel overwhelmed and they hesitate to make decisions. Their power of concentration decreases; many patients exhibit a decrease in cognitive performance as well. Recurrent negative thoughts are common and may be extremely disturbing, often leading to suicide attempts.

Emotional symptoms: Persistent gloom, feelings of despair, hopelessness, loneliness, forlornness, emotional void, anxiety, feelings of guilt and the feeling of inferiority are often present.

Behavior-specific symptoms: Speaking in a low-key voice, monotonous language, the lack of eye contact, powerless or bent posture, and slow movements are characteristic of depression. In contrast some patients can exhibit psychomotor unrest and agitation often manifesting in tremor or ergomania. Most patients retreat to isolation resulting in decreased communicative and social abilities as well as conflicts in close relationships. Daily activities such as personal hygiene and chores are often neglected. Some patients with depression correspondingly consume large amounts of alcohol, medication or drugs to make their mood more tolerable.

3. Epidemiology and co-morbidity of depressive disorders

Point prevalence of 2.3-4.9% [50-52] and lifetime prevalence between 13.3% and 17.1% have been identified for major depression in the general population [53]. Recent studies estimate that as many as 40% of women and 30% of men suffer from at least one episode of major depression during their life [54-56]. Although prevalence of bipolar disorders is identical in both genders in the western world [57], dysthymia, a relatively mild form of chronic depression, occurs almost twice as much in women as compared to men [53,57]. Significant gender-specific differences do not only apply to the frequency of occurrence of depressive disorders, but rather to their symptoms and accompanying diseases in adults [58-59]. Depressive disorders have also become more frequent in children of less than 11 years of age [56,60,61]; meta-analysis shows a prevalence rate of depression amounting to 2.8% in individuals younger than 13 years, and a rate of 5.7% in persons 13-18 years of age [62]. The symptoms are described similarly in both genders (depressed mood, concentration disorder, sleep problems); only after puberty can gender-specific differences be observed [58,63]. The prevalence rate of depression significantly increases with age and it is closely connected to family status and socio-economic circumstances [64]. However, the highest rate is present in 25-45 years old married women who have at least one child [65,66].

Disturbances of affective experience, such as anxiety, panic disorders, certain personality disorders and mourning sorrow, often show co-morbidity with depression. Depressive disorders are most frequently accompanied with panic disorders (40-80%), generalized anxiety disorder (50%), obsessive-compulsive disorder (3-30%), alcohol and drug abuse (30%), attention deficit disorder and suicide [67-70]. According to previously published data, 56% of the patients affected by serious depression have at least one suicide attempt, and 15% of the affected commit suicide [71]. Previous studies suggested that as much as 30-88% of suicides can be linked to depressive disorders in Europe [72].

http://dx.doi.org/10.5772/54200

4. Classification and diagnostics of depressive disorder

Currently, there are two major classifications commonly used in describing the severity of depressive disorders. One is established by the Diagnostic and Statistical Manual of Mental Disorders (DSM) of the American Psychological Association (APA) and the other one by the International Classification of Diseases (ICD-10) of WHO (Table 1). The differences between these classification systems are primarily in the number of the listed core symptoms which should be present for at least two weeks in both classifications, and in the classification of additional accompanying symptoms. If five of the described symptoms are present for more than two weeks, DSM-IV refers to the condition as "major depression". If only two to three symptoms have been simultaneously present for at least two years, DSM-IV diagnoses "dysthymia". In addition to diagnosing depressive disorders, both classification systems also determine its **polarity** (unipolar or bipolar), **course** (recurrent, partially remittent or remittent) and, depending on the number of core/additional symptoms, the **degrees of severity** of the disorder (slight, moderate, severe) as well as **additional symptoms** (with or without psychotic/somatic/catatonic/melancholic characteristics).

According to ICD-10, at least 2 core symptoms and 2 other symptoms should be present for the diagnosis of a slight episode; a moderate depressive episode requires at least 2 core symptoms and 3-4 additional symptoms, and a severe episode can be diagnosed by the presence of at least 2 core symptoms and at least 4 other symptoms with less severity.

DSM-IV (296.xx)	**ICD-10 (F32.xx; F33.xx)**
At last 5 of the following symptoms that are present almost every day for two weeks	at least 2 core symptoms simultaneously that are present for two weeks
1. depressive mood 2. significantly decreased interest/joy 3. tiredness, loss of energy 4. sleeplessness/increased sleep 5. psychomotor unrest, slowing 6. significant weight gain/loss 7. worthlessness, improper feelings of guilt 8. decreased cogitation, concentration problems, decreased decision-making ability 9. recurrent thoughts of death imagination of suicide without plan, or detailed planning of suicide	1. depressive mood 2. loss of interest, loss of joy 3. increased fatigability plus at least two to four of the following symptoms: 1. sleep disorders 2. worthlessness, feelings of guilt 3. decreased concentration and attentiveness 4. decreased appetite 5. suicidal thoughts or acts 6. pessimistic view of future

Table 1. Diagnosis criteria for major depression as per DSM IV [73] and a moderate depressive episode as per ICD-10 [74].

These symptoms cause clinically significant impairments in the social, occupational or other fields of life in the most frequent cases, and cannot be explained by the direct effect of pharmacological treatment, substance abuse, another disease or simple sorrow.

5. Brief history of CBT

In the 1950s, psychology as a scientific theory and practice underwent a major development. During this period, the first steps of behavioral therapy (BT) were developed independently in the USA and in England based on the knowledge gained in experimental psychology and subsequently developed learning theories. Right from the beginning, BT was a collective term for a variety of different therapeutic procedures. The common feature of these procedures is that, unlike personality, behavior - including cognitive, emotional and physical responses - can be built, reduced and modified during the lifetime of the individual [75].

The roots of cognitive BT and behavioral learning theories go back to ancient times. Epictetus, a Greek stoic philosopher, who is considered one of the major influences in the development of psychotherapy, wrote: "Men are disturbed, not by things, but by the principles and notions which they form concerning things". Freud (1900/1953) was the first modern-day scientist addressing the perception that symptoms and feelings are based on unconscious thoughts. Alfred Adler [76], who was an important proponent of individual psychology, noted that humans actually do not suffer from an experienced trauma, but rather from the perception of personal interpretation of the event. In the beginning of the 19th century, the phenomenological direction of philosophy had a great impact on the development of psychology and the maturation of CBT, as authors including Kant, Heidegger and Husserl established their theory on the control of conscious experiences [77].

The principal element of CBT, classical conditioning, is a behavioral learning theory founded by Russian physiologist I. P. Pavlov (1849-1936), stating that new and conditioned reflexes can be added to natural, mostly inherited, unconditioned reflexes by means of learning. Based on the knowledge of classical conditioning it is also possible to generalize or erase behavioral patterns [78]. John B. Watson, who is considered to be the founder of classical behaviorism, described mental processes, e.g. thoughts, as responses to the autonomic nervous system on external stimuli, and he attempted to explain behavior on the basis of conditioned reflexes described by Pavlov. He wrote: "*Give me a dozen healthy infants and I will train them to become any type of specialist I might select*" [79].

Contrary to classical conditioning, operant conditioning theory stated that spontaneous behavior is promoted or inhibited by the consequence that follows. In the 1950s, Burrhus Frederic Skinner further developed the concept of operant or instrumental conditioning. Skinner's approach was to positively or negatively impact behavior by means of subsequent consequences. Based on this theory, behavior is supported by positive consequences, while negative consequences result in reduction or deletion of certain behavioral elements. This concept corresponds to an S-R-C model, with a stimulus (S) followed by the response (R), and the consequences (C). The S-R-C model is considered to be one of the crucial elements of CBT even today [80]. The 1950s were also significantly influenced by the work of Mowrer (learning theory, 1947) and Dollar & Miller [81; 82], who created the first therapeutic models.

Initially, BT gave a very mechanistic idea of the human mind. Consciousness psychology limited itself to the externally observable human behavior and was based on the idea that such behavior could be shaped by environmental influences without taking genetic circumstances into consideration. Thus, the fundamental statement of BT was that behavior is learned by learning processes, and thus, incorrect behavior can be unlearned while desired behavior can be acquired by learning.

In the 1960s, as part of the so-called cognitive change, thoughts, emotions and attitudes progressively moved to the focus of CBT as principal approaches for explanation and treatment. One of the major sources of this paradigm shift was the integration of cognitive techniques in CBT; consequently, CBT became a valuable tool focusing primarily on strengthening the patient's independent ability to solve problems. The cognitive method described first by Beck addresses negative modes of thoughts and the resulting schemes as the source of psychiatric disorders [77]. The emotion theory of Schachter and Singer [83] was followed by the A-B-C concept by Albert Ellis, the father of the rational-emotive therapy, determining that emotions are triggered by interpretation the current situations. Consequently, by changing the attitude and perception of the event, the emotion/mood can also be altered [84]. In addition to Beck and Ellis, the second wave of BT was also influenced by authors including Jacobson, Eysenck, Wolpe, Bandura, Lazarus, Meichenbaum and Ullrich, whose concepts of model learning, relaxation exercises, stress management, self-instruction and self-assurance training complemented the various methods of CBT.

From the 70s until today,, behavioral therapy has been subject to substantial development based on emotion-focused approaches, methods of self-regulation and training of specific skills, including Dialectical Behavior Therapy (DBT; [85]), Acceptance and Commitment Therapy (ACT; [86]), Cognitive Behavioral Analysis System of Psychotherapy (CBASP; [87], Mindfulness-Based Cognitive Therapy (MBCT; [88]), Positive Psychology, [89] and Scheme Therapy [90].

In contrast to the psychoanalytical approach, CBT does not perceive psychiatric disorders as consequences of suppression or expression of mental conflicts, but rather as consequences of maladjusted attitudes and errors in reasoning expressed through disturbed behavior. Thus, the disturbed behavior itself represents the problem that requires changing as a response to certain conditions.

Behavioral therapy offers an approach to enhance the patient's own capacities. Its primary objectives include, amongst others, making the patients aware of counterproductive attitudes and disturbing thought patterns. These goals are identified via learning processes performed in the therapeutic situation and then modified step by step until the adequate behavior is generated. In the therapeutic process, the relation of therapist and client represents a pivotal factor. At the onset of therapy, the therapist offers a particularly high amount of support by helping clients with identification and solving their problems, and then increasingly delegating responsibilities and correspondingly promoting the patient's ability to solve problems as well recognizing processes that eventually lead to self-determination and social competence. As Hautzinger stated: *"The current level of CBT is based on the scientific results of years of therapy studies in the USA as well as Great Britain, Germany and Australia, and finally is the result of a productive development of the originally highly behavioristic stimulus-response approach into an explanatory approach of psychiatric disorders, which also includes internal processes such as cognitions and emotions."* [41].

6. Diagnostics of depressive disorders in behavioral therapy

Behavioral therapy intends to change problematic behavior by applying therapeutic methods. Disturbed behavior should be described precisely in order to enable differentiated use of these methods.

Despite the fact that clinical-psychological diagnostics is focused primarily on the collection of personality characteristics preferably across time and situation by means of clinical-psychological testing procedures, precise descriptions and quantification of behavior started only towards the end of the 1960s [91]. The diagnostics of depressive disorders in behavioral therapy is based on:

1. Criteria diagnostics (ICD-10, and DSM-IV; DSM-V as of May 2013)
2. Test-psychological diagnostics by using self-assessment and external assessment scales (e.g. **BDI** - Beck Depression Inventory [92]; **HAMD** – Hamilton Rating Scale for Depression [93]; **MADRS** – Montgomery Asberg Depression Rating Scale [94]; and structured clinical interviews, (e.g. **CIDI** - Composite International Diagnostic Interview [95]; **SCID** – Structured Clinical Interview for DSM-IV Axis 1 Disorders [96]; **ADIS** – Anxiety Disorders Interview Schedule for DSM-IV [97]; **IMPS**- Inpatient Multidimensional Psychiatric Scale [98]. Special procedures may gather additional psychopathologic symptoms on cognitive and motivational levels such as helplessness and hopelessness as well as on somatic, motor and interaction levels.
3. SORCK model of behavioral analysis

As a detailed description of behavioral-therapeutic diagnostics would exceed the scope of this chapter, we limit ourselves to a brief presentation of the SORCK model. Problem analysis is based on Skinner's learning theory and represents a diagnostic process crucial in behavioral therapy. Problem analysis connotes that the human behavior is controlled by preceding (triggering) and succeeding conditions. This represents the first components of the behavioral-diagnostic SORCK model: S-O-R-C = Stimulus – Organism - Response – Consequence. These conditions should be modified during therapy by using various methods [99]. Thus, behavioral diagnostics gather the patient's responses during various situations of life as well as from the maintaining conditions and the cognitive schemes conditional to problems. Then the patient's own coping efforts are determined, followed by the identification of the method that can be used to alter the disturbed behavior.

http://dx.doi.org/10.5772/54200

6.1. SORCK model of behavioral analysis

The first step of behavioral analysis is to describe in detail the problematic behavior or response (R) with regard to its topography, intensity and duration [100]. **Topography/intensity** refers to the cognitive, emotional, physiological and motor components of the symptoms [101]. **Frequency** is to determine whether an actually proper behavior occurs too rarely (e.g. communication with autistic persons) or too frequently (e.g. obsessive washing), if the behavior is dysfunctional (anxiety in a department store), or if there is a complete lack of the particular behavior.

In the next step, the conditions preceding the disturbed behavior - the so-called triggering situations (S) - and the subsequent conditions - the so-called consequences (C) - are determined. Kanfer and Saslow [102] expanded the SRCK models proposed by Lindsley [103] by adding the variable "O" ("Organism" meaning biologic conditions of behavior). This includes relatively permanent (e.g. brain damage) and short-term functional disorders (e.g. consequences of increased alcohol consumption) [99]. According to Lindsley, every stimulus or situation (S) is followed by a response (R), correspondingly resulting in behavior-supporting or behavior-penalizing consequence (C) and a contingency (K) as long as the consequences follow the behavior. The above described SORCK model has been a subject of further development within the scope of the diagnostic process and has been complemented by the determination of dysfunctional thoughts controlling the behavior.

This model differentiates four types of consequences [104]:

C+ (positive reinforcement)

C- (direct punishment)

Ȼ+ (indirect punishment by omitting positive reinforcement)

Ȼ- (negative reinforcement by omitting direct punishment)

During problem analysis the therapist may collect sufficient information to formulate the intended objective together with the patient.

7. Psychological generation models of depressive disorders

Depressive disorders are characterized by a multifactorial pathogenesis. Thus, above all psycho-social factors (such as stresses and strains, role conflicts, lack of social support), biological factors (genetic predisposition, neuroendocrine regulation), personality factors (introversion, inclination towards melancholy, "typus melancholicus", etc.), outside factors (deprivation of light, etc.) as well as traumatic events all may play an important role. Detailed discussion of these factors would certainly exceed the scope of the present chapter; therefore, in this section we focus primarily on the three psychological generation models as these are mainly relevant for behavior-therapeutic treatment.

The hypothetic causes of generation and maintenance of a depressive syndrome that can be effectively treated with behavioral therapy are linked either to the behavior or the cognition of the patient.

7.1. Cognitive models

7.1.1. Cognition-theoretical explanation model according to Beck

According to the cognition-theoretical explanation, the basis of each depressive development is represented primarily by cognitive dysfunction; the thinking pattern of the depressed patient is characterized by logical errors such as selective perception, random drawing of conclusions, exaggerations, etc. Negative, burdensome life experiences, which manifest themselves as cognitive schemes, are triggering conditions leading to dysfunction by developing a set of negative perceptions (also called "cognitive triads"; [77]) regarding the

- identity ("I am of no worth")
- environment ("nobody loves me; everybody is against me")
- future ("there is no point, nothing will improve").

The cognitive triad forces the depressed individual to deal with irrational negative thoughts that are plausible to him/her over and over again. The patient experiences these thoughts as being automatic, intractable, persistent and unintended. Such thoughts are always about topics such as hopelessness, low self-esteem or suicide. Beck holds this cognitive disorder responsible for all psychiatric features of depression. Depressed individuals usually aim very high and believe that the world always imposes insurmountable obstacles for them. They tend to make their own deficits or low level of ability responsible for unpleasant experiences. Thus, one of the primary goals of therapy is to teach the patients that in addition to their first-person observation (usually actually based on self-contempt), there are other principles of self-control such as self-reinforcement. Depressed individuals show the tendency to consider their thoughts as being a given fact without cross-checking them with reality. When following this theoretical model, the searching, questioning and modifying of automatic, unperceived thoughts - i.e. the basic attitude of the patient characterizing his/her behavior, emotions and thinking - will become the primary objective of therapy as detailed in section 8.3.

For the sake of completeness, it should be mentioned that some authors regard cognitive dysfunctions as being consequences and not the causes [105]. Tringer describes this theory as the theory of "uniform structure" (depressive-cognitive structure – DCS; [106]).

7.1.2. Irrational beliefs according to Ellis

The concept of Ellis regarding the generation and maintenance of depressive symptoms [107] is very similar to Beck's concept. Ellis assumes that irrational thinking will result in psychiatric disorders and that both rational and logical thinking can be learned, correspondingly resulting in reduction of psychological stress. The main purpose of cognitive therapy according to Ellis is also the change of cognition and irrational beliefs (section 8.3), correspondingly changing emotions and disturbed behaviors. According to Ellis' theory, emotions develop as a result of highly distorted attitudes and assessments accompanied by severe physical reactions and often trigger negative actions by the affected person due to past experiences.. These emotions are often maintained by means of talking to oneself (soliloquies; [107]).

7.1.3. Learned helplessness as per Seligman

If events are deemed to be uncontrollable (i.e. if self-behavior and its consequences are perceived independently from each other within the environment) and this perception is generalized, the individual gets into the stage of "learned helplessness", a term invented by Martin E. P. Seligman in 1967. According to Seligman, depression is co-induced by feelings of helplessness that follow apparently uncontrollable, unpleasant events. The causes a person attributes to the event are decisive for the experienced controllability of the events. In 1978, Abramson, Seligman and Teasdale modified the helplessness model and included into their system an attribution style determining how the non-controllability of situations is processed. In this system, attribution styles are categorized as internal vs. external, global vs. specific, and stable vs. instable. Internal attribution is based on the assumption that the cause of personal helplessness is within the individual itself. Thus, this dimension is also responsible for decreased self-esteem. Global attribution represents a rather general description of the causes of non-controllability; specific attribution is limited to well-describable elements. The stable attribution style includes persistent and/or recurrent uncontrolled conditions and may result in chronic helplessness. According to Seligman, depressed patients interpret failures internally, soundly and globally (e.g. "I am stupid"). In contrast, success is attributed to external, unstable and specific causes ("the good grade was by accident" or "this task was difficult at all"), resulting in feelings of helplessness, and eventually leading to depression [108].

Based on this theoretical model, the first step of therapy is to identify the attribution style of the depressed patient. Then, cognitions should be carefully examined in order to reveal the degree of reality, followed by an attempt to re-attribute them in order to alter the basic attitudes (section 8.3).

7.2. Learning and behavior-theoretical models

While the cognitive models state that the conscious change of cognition will alter behavior and the experience, behavior-theoretical models assume that the change of behavior will modify cognition and mood.

7.2.1. Reinforcement model according to Lewinsohn

According to Lewinsohn, depressive disorders are generated as a consequence of the loss of positively reinforcing feedback from close environment. This model is connected to operant learning theory and based on the following assumptions:

A low rate of behavior-contingent positive reinforcement has a triggering effect on depressed behavior and maintains depression.

The total amount of positive reinforcers depends on three factors: (1) the scope of potentially reinforcing events and activities; (2) the quantity of reinforcers available at a certain point in time; and (3) the repertoire of the individual behavior to receive reinforcers.

Reduction of the usual positive reinforcers results in reduction of activity, correspondingly resulting in depressed mood, which in turn leads to increased avolition (lack of motivation to pursue meaningful goals) that further decreases normal activity and reduces the effect of positive reinforcers. In the course of time, the ability of positively interpret the reinforcers may significantly decrease due to the lack of "training". This will correspondingly trigger a vicious cycle, a downward spiral [109].

The depressed behavior will also be maintained and positively reinforced, at least in the short term, by social attention. Attention is usually paid to those complaining. However, the social reinforcement of the depressive symptoms may also turn against the depressed person; individuals that complain a lot will eventually be avoided, leading to more frequent complaining and correspondingly being avoided even more.

This theory can be utilized in crucial therapeutic approaches, i.e. promotion of activity level, increase of positive behavior-contingent reinforcers, reduction of depression-promoting activities (section 8.1) and the augmentation of certain social abilities (section 8.2).

7.3. Integrative models

Integrative models, as the term indicates, integrate both approaches mentioned above (cognitive and behavior-theoretical) and assume that depressive symptoms are conditioned both by dysfunctional cognitions as well as by reduction of the activity rate [41]. According to this model, behavior and cognition are in complex interaction with each other. Depressed patients sees themselves as being a good-for-nothing due to their own passivity and listlessness. This negative self-perception (cognition) contributes to a further reduction in activity rate (behavior), thus, further promoting negative self-opinion. When increasing their activity rate (behavior), patients will see that their mood will improve and their thoughts will change.

More recent multi-factor models [110, 111] extract six significant factors contributing to the generation and maintenance of depressive disorders (triggering events, vulnerability, increase of self-attentiveness, aversive conditions, disturbed automated behavioral patterns, and dysphoric prevailing mood). Moreover, the interpretation of this explanatory model can yield the three major pillars for depression therapy – support of pleasant activities (section 8.1), change of dysfunctional cognitions (section 8.3) and social competence training (section 8.2).

8. CBT in depressive disorders

Since depression is a multi-factorial disorder, its treatment requires a multi-factorial approach. In addition to the stabilization of the patient during a severe acute episode or in case of slight to moderate depression addressed by chemotherapy, psychological approaches are increasingly utilized. Cognitive and behavior-therapeutic techniques are applied depending on the basic theoretical model described above, on the severity of depression and on present problems. Therapy is based on the identification and elimination of disorder-triggering and disorder-maintaining factors in the patient's behavior or cognition. Treatment also has an indirect influence on emotional, somatic and motivational effects of the disorder [41].

CBT integrates behavior-modifying and cognitive techniques. Therapy of depression with CBT is based on three principal pillars:

- building up daily activities (section 8.1);
- training of social competencies (section 8.2); and
- cognitive techniques (section 8.3).

The chapter at hand provides a collection of cognitive behavioral therapeutic strategies that can be utilized in the treatment of depressive disorders. There is a common consensus that the first therapeutic step is to increase the activity level of the unmotivated patient; after an increase in activity, the therapeutic effort can be focused on dysfunctional thoughts and low self-esteem of the patient by introducing cognitive techniques. However, the sequence of the presented methodical steps should be considered as suggestions for therapy only, and addressing the individual problems and requirements of the patient should remain a major focus during course of therapy.

8.1. Building-up daily activities

Most depressed patients reduce their activities dramatically; they seldom participate in enjoyable activities and they usually withdraw themselves into isolation. These patients lose valuable social relationships and also deprive themselves of the possibility of having positive experiences. Such pathological processes often result in a vicious circle; the loss of pleasant events (positive reinforcement) increases depressed moods, tiredness and listlessness, consequently leading to the loss of ability and motivation to engage in activities and in isolation from the rest of the society. Paradoxically, depressed patients justify their self-isolation by the fact that their activity is useless and they only represent a burden to other people.. As a result of this attitude they reduce activities they used to perform in the past without any problems, and even if they start an activity, they will not finish it due to the lack of belief in a successful outcome [31].Thus, building up of activities that have a positive reinforcing effect on the patient (pleasant activities) and creation of a daily structure remains the first basic step of behavioral therapeutic treatment.

When the connection between maintaining a balanced activity level and self-controlled management of depression symptoms depression is established, the patient becomes conscious of the relationship between activity/passivity and mood. On the other hand, based on the basic principles of learning, the consequences of behavior have a significant impact on the frequency of repetition of these particular activities in the future, and consequently, activities with pleasant consequences will be performed more frequently in the future as compared to activities with unpleasant consequences. The principle of reinforcement can be systematically used to modify the patient's behavior and to introduce new elements of behavior. Active build-up of daily activities improves one's mood; a positive mood will contribute to pleasant activities and thus the vicious circle is broken. Furthermore, patients will be aware of the feeling of being able to actively control their own life.

In the initial part of the therapy the theoretical background of the concept of reinforcement as well as the importance of therapeutic exercises at home between individual sessions is explained to the patient. For successful treatment it is extremely important that the affected person understand that activity/passivity and mood are interacting factors. Depressed patients usually spend a lot of time with unyielding, empty activities such as speculation or activities that are absolutely necessary (cleaning, laundry), but don't have any positive reinforcing effect and/or are not pleasant. A low activity level suppresses mood and forces the patient to retreat even more to a passive attitude, correspondingly reducing the probability of having positive experiences (i.e., lack of positive reinforcers). The reduction in frequency of pleasant experiences leading to increasingly suppressed mood eventually results in passivity and self-isolation. However, this downwards spiral can be reversed by systematically emphasizing that performing pleasant activities generates a positive mood and also increases the probability of planning further activities [41].

Depressed patients often report that they feel like they are in a continuous pointless and meaningless condition. According to Beck and colleagues [31], the most important purpose of the activity-increasing exercises is to give a structural content to the time spent in order to reduce the feeling of aimlessness. Recording the daily activities is crucial and often demonstrates the distorted cognition of the patients stating: *"I have not done anything the whole day."*

The building up of activities is usually done gradually, in small steps by interrupting the patients' passivity and achieving a proper activity level. In the first step, the patient is asked to systematically observe his/her usual daily activities during the week. By using "activity diaries", the activities are recorded along with the associated mood. First-person observation is an important BT technique as it enables both the therapist and the patient to consciously observe a change in the patient's condition, eventually resulting in the identification of depression-supporting behavior that can be corrected by therapy. By utilizing this method, patients learns to observe himself/herself and to associate activity level and the emotions; this provides momentum to the next step, i.e. the targeted increase of the positive activities.

Below there is an example for an activity diary filled in for three days, based on the research of Hautzinger [41]. For recording the mood and the attitude, the scale -5 to +5 is commonly used, with 0 being neutral mood, - 5 being severest negative mood and + 5 being highest positive mood.

Monday	Tuesday	Wednesday	Thursday	Friday	Saturday	Sunday
9 am - 11 am		Awake since 5 am, still in bed (-5)	Awake since 6 AM, breakfast in bed (-4)	Awake since 4 AM (-5)		
11 am - 1 pm		Bathroom, breakfast (-2)	Cleaning, ironing (-1)	Fallen asleep (-4)		
1 pm - 3 pm		Sofa, TV (-2)	Lunch with granddaughter (+2)	Eating (0)		
3 pm - 5 pm		Visit of a colleague (+1)	Shopping, snoozing in bed (0)	Sofa, TV (-2)		
5 pm - 7 pm		Dinner, TV (0)	Sofa, TV (-3)	TV in bed, no hunger (-4)		
7 pm - 9 pm		Bed, speculating (-4)	Bed, speculating (-4)	TV in bed (-5)		
9 pm - 11 pm		Bed, speculating (-4)	Fallen asleep	Speculating until 2 am (-5)		

Table 2.

In the following therapy session, the weekly plan is assessed by the therapist and the connection between the activity and corresponding mood is explained to the patient by using personal examples.

Example. Therapist: *"Let's have a look at Wednesday and Thursday. I see that your mood on Wednesday at 1 pm was much worse as compared to Thursday. Do you have any idea why there is such a difference?"*

In the second step, a list of activities generating positive mood is created together with the patient. Then the patient attempts to integrate as many activities as possible from this list into the next weekly plan. This individual list is also used as a collection of potential reinforcers as therapy progresses [41].

At the next stage, an activity plan for the whole next week, including activities that the patient wants to perform, is created together with the therapist. This time the schedule is more detailed and includes information regarding the place and the people associated with positive activities as well as the corresponding mood.

Some patients may voluntarily participate in some activities without enjoying them. This may be due to the fact that 1) they did not perceive these activities as being pleasant even before the depressive episode; 2) negative cognitions suppress any feelings of happiness; or 3) these feelings are disregarded selectively [31]. The exercise described above helps the patient to experience happiness again.

The activities should be defined by the patient (important for intrinsic motivation); the therapist may support the patient's objective by requesting activities enjoyed in the past and/or by using a pre-defined list of pleasant activities [41,112]. Many depressed patients feel that they are not able to perform a particular activity. This should be accepted by the therapist; however, the therapist should motivate patients to perform minor activities and explain to them that since passivity has been of no help in the past, another strategy should be tried. Cognitive testing (imaginative exercise) of certain activities is a good compromise with highly unmotivated patients.

After successfully performing the activities defined as in the daily or weekly plan, the patient then records the mood changes in the diary. It is particularly important to schedule activities that are not performed alone in order to maintain social contacts and improve social skills (described in the next section).

When in a negative mood, depressed patients tend to set unrealistically high expectations for themselves; therefore, often they won't even start the activity because of fear of failure. Consequently, if they do not achieve a particular goal, they attribute the lack of success to their own inability. Often patients start an activity but won't finish it. An activity started but not completed is regarded as a failure by the patient. Therefore, the therapist's task is to make patients understand that it is unlikely that they will be able to perform as originally planned and that even an attempt is much better than doing nothing; additionally, it is important to emphasize that completing an activity depends both on external factors (weather, other people's availability, etc.) as well as internal factors (concentration, fatigue).

Objectives of these activities are generally based on the SMART principle [113]:

Specific: concrete goals in writing

Measurable: achieving the objective should be verifiable

Action-oriented: concrete acts of realization

Realistic: achievable goals that are attractive, challenging, but not scary

Time-bound: setting a definite time frame

Examples for setting of objectives [41]:

Example 1. Objective: I want to look more attractive.

First, the patient should provide a definition of attractiveness. Activities for achieving this objective are integrated into the weekly plan, e.g. going to the hairdresser, participating in a make-up class, going to the gym, performing sports (which?), buying more trendy clothes, etc.

Example 2. Objective: I want to have more contact with friends.

Activities for achieving this objective: Inviting friends for dinner, planning an evening with friends at the movie theatre, inviting friends for a game night, doing sports together with friends etc.

Example 3. Objective: I want to learn a foreign language.

Activities for achieving the objective: Get language books, get a private teacher, take a language class, go abroad, etc.

Introduction of positive reinforcers

The patient needs to learn how to deal with unpleasant experiences. During the course of therapy, the patient needs to understand that certain not very pleasant activities may actually be fun and satisfactory. However, additional reinforcers need to be integrated into weekly activity plans in order to achieve this goal. The patient must learn that some activities have direct pleasant consequences but will have negative consequences in the long term. In contrast, some activities have immediate unpleasant consequences but positive effects in the long term. The problem is that patients suffering from depression tend to have a short-term view on things and therefore, as therapy advances, activities that are less pleasant in the short term but have positive effects in the long term need to be integrated into the weekly plan. Following each activity the patient will record the associated mood and, even more importantly, the reward after successful performance of each activity (from the individual list of pleasant activities). A positive reward for successfully performed but less pleasant activities will increase motivation to start an unpleasant activity with unpleasant short-term but pleasant long-term consequences. The reward or reinforcer becomes the source of positive emotions.

Example 1: A depressed, short-sighted female patient has a counseling interview with an ophthalmologist who can offer laser treatment to improve her short-sightedness. This intervention would give her the opportunity, in the long term, to get rid of her glasses that have highly affected her self-esteem since childhood. In the short term, scheduling an appointment and surgery are connected to aversive emotions. In case of this successfully performed activity (i.e., if the patient actually participates in the counseling interview), she should reward herself immediately (e.g. by buying a new book, a blouse, or a new perfume she has wanted for a long time).

Example 2: A depressed, 30-year old female patient wants to get her driving license in order to be more independent of her husband. The upcoming driver's course (which she already postponed three times) is connected to aversive emotions, costs money and also occupies free evenings. However, in the long term, the patient could move more freely and her self-esteem would increase as well. She could reward herself after each unit of the course.

Example 3: Identifying and correcting depression-supporting behavior.

The patient wakes up every morning at 10 a.m., has breakfast in bed, does not leave bed but instead watches TV or doesn't think about anything specific. During her therapy session it is agreed that she will get up at 8 a.m., has breakfast in the kitchen and then takes a short walk outside for at least half an hour. In this case, depression-supporting behavior has been replaced by positively perceived activities.

8.1.1. Euthymic therapy

Parallel to the modification of the problematic behavior, it is recommended to develop a cognitive, physiologic and motor behavioral repertoire that corresponds to positive experiences and utilizes the elements of so-called euthymic therapy. During this therapy the patient again learns to consciously enjoy positive experiences without negative emotions. The emphasis is on being happy without any remorse, since most depressed patients feel that they do not get and do not deserve anything positive out of life. Consequently, these patients will do anything, usually subconsciously, to block out positive experiences. Euthymic therapy was used with great success during the treatment of depressed patients in the Psychiatric Clinic in Mannheim, Germany, in the 1980s; since then the method has also been used to treat other psychiatric disorders.. During therapeutic sessions patients learn to focus their attention on sensory perception and consciously enjoy various visual, auditory, tactile, gustatory and olfactory stimuli according to the instructions of the therapist and in order to learn to focus on and enjoy the present moment [114]. This therapy eventually increases patient self-confidence and self-perception. The learned pleasant experiences can be utilized during daily activities by developing a list of pleasant experiences the patient mentioned during sessions.

8.1.2. Happiness diaries

The use of so-called 'happiness diaries' has proved to be extremely successful in depression therapy. At the end of the day patients should review their daily activities and record the ones they enjoyed and their corresponding positive thoughts and events. This method is based on 'positive psychology' according to Seligman [89]. With this approach happiness in life depends on conscious optimistic perception that can be learned through practice. Happiness diaries play two pivotal roles in the treatment of depression. The first role is consciously focusing on positive experiences in the present. The second role of happiness diaries is particularly useful when the patient's mood is low. In this case the patient can replay former positive experiences. Since the imagined situation triggers similar physiological processes to the ones that were induced by real events, this method can dramatically improve the patient's mood.

8.2. Social competence training

Introduction to this method

In psychology, social competency has become a very frequent term that is only rarely defined in a clear manner. This term subsumes abilities and skills such as self-confidence, enforcement of desires, denial of requests, emotional freedom, assertiveness, socializing

http://dx.doi.org/10.5772/54200

and cultivating contacts, communication skills etc. [115]. While Wolpe and Salter state that social problems are the result of inhibiting personality characteristics [116,117], Lazarus indicates that these problems may be rooted in incorrectly learned social behavior [118]. Ullrich de Muynck and Ullrich [119] complemented these theories with cognitive variables such as the attitude towards oneself and social perceptions. They define social competence as 'self-confidence' that includes recognizing and enforcing the needs and demands of the individual [120].

Therapeutic examination reveals that depressed people often organize their interpersonal interactions in an impeding manner. They complain constantly, hide their positive emotions, look for contacts with others less actively, are more sensitive to criticism and rejection, do not or only improperly support their own opinion, and lack confidence and assertiveness. These interaction characteristics, combined with unfavorable non-verbal communication forms such as a quiet voice, bent posture, infrequent eye contact, may result in social isolation. Often patients are faced with painful experiences in the beginning of behavioral therapy when experiencing drawbacks in interpersonal interactions during new daily activities.

Example 1: Mr. F. visits an old friend for an evening of games as part of his BT activity planning. Although he is very happy about having been invited he keeps complaining about his bad health so that the other guests soon stop talking to him. Mr. F. feels hurt and decides that he will never participate in such an activity again. The lack of positive reinforcers in this case result in the generation of continued problems with social interactions and make individuals socially isolate themselves as their depressed mood is sustained.

The objective of social competence training is to support the patient's self-confident behavior. During the course of therapy patients learns to properly communicate, to state their wishes, opinions and positive emotions, to use services offered by others, to develop problem-solving skills, and to understand the connection between mood and self-esteem.

8.2.1. Performance of social competence training

Practicing social competence includes several methods that are based on teaching socially expected behavior via modelling and role play. Social competence is composed of skills that include, among others, self-confident behavior, problem solving and communication competencies, the ability to express one's own wants and feelings, and proper reaction to criticism. It has been previously reported that practicing certain behavioral sequences (behavior rehearsal) as well as role plays help to create and maintain socially competent behavior [121]. After explaining the social problem to the patient, a realistic role play situation is designed and verbal (expression, volume), non-verbal (mimic), interactive (such as active listening) and motor components (posture, etc.) of the proper behavior are determined [122]. Following the initial analysis of the strengths and weaknesses of the patient's behavior, the desired outcome of the situation is identified together with the participation of the therapist, and the problematic situation is practiced with any required corrections within the therapeutic setting until the required behavior is achieved. Then the learned behavior is transferred to everyday situations and tested regularly.

Example 1. Mr. M. works as salesperson at a DIY store. Due to his depressive disorder he has problems approaching customers. Most of the time he is alone in the corner of the store and only helps customers who approach him. The objective of the training is to achieve self-confident active behavior [41].

In the first behavior-therapeutic role play, the therapist takes the role of the customer and Mr. M. plays his own role as the salesperson. The therapist observes the strengths and weaknesses of the patient. Mr. M. approaches the customer but maintains a distance, stops with his side facing towards the customer and talks to the customer in a quiet voice. At the end of role play the therapist gives feedback to Mr. M. First, the therapist describes the positive aspects of behavior.

Therapist: *"Being a customer, I felt welcome because you actively approached me and asked if I need any help."* Then the therapist focuses on the behavioral deficits of the patient observed during the role play. Therapist: *"During the second role play, could you try to speak louder and establish eye contact with me? If you stand closer, the customer would feel that you have the motivation and desire to help him."*

Prior to the role play the therapist explains the verbal and nonverbal aspects of a self-confident behavior (eye contact, relaxed posture, articulate speech, etc.) and emphasizes the importance of repeated positive self-instructions ("I will succeed", "I have a right to do this", "I will be convincing", etc.). After the play it is crucial to acknowledge the enthusiasm and the progress of the patient; it is also important to emphasize that the learning process takes time and effort.

Example 2. Ms. F. is a part-time worker at an office, where she shares a desk with a colleague (who works on alternate days). When Ms. F. does her work at the office, her 2-year old son stays with her mother-in-law. Ms. F. has problems in the following areas and describes them as follows: As Ms. F. uses the desk together with her colleague, it often happens that there is no paper in the printer, the stapler is empty, markers are open and dried out, and there are empty paperclip boxes and non-filed invoices on the desk when Ms. F. arrives. Often she has to start by organizing the desk and completing work that was begun by her colleague. These activities take time from her actual work. Ms. F. gets angry about her colleague's unfairness and wants to talk to her. The objective of the training is to define and enforce self-confidence and self-assured behavior regarding Ms. F.'s own wants.

Ms. F.: *"Since I am at the office twice a week only for three hours, there is a lot of paper work; I have to sort the mail of the entire company weekly. This task alone takes almost three hours. When my colleague does not refill the missing stationery and the desk is not tidy, I have to do this work first before I start with my responsibilities. I do not want to stay longer at the office for this reason, because I do not get paid for overtime and I want to be at home in time to pick up my son from my mother-in-law as soon as possible."*

An additional problem emerges during Ms. F.'s communication of with her mother-in-law. Ms. F. wants her son to take a nap after lunch and does not want him to eat sweets. During her time off, she can control this by herself; however, on workdays, when her son is with her mother-in-law, her son eats sweets and he can refuse the nap. Ms. F. wants to present her will properly to her mother-in-law.

In this case, two different problem situations are role-played and practiced. In the first role play, the behavior of Ms. F., when interacting with her colleague at the office, is identified by the therapist playing the role of the colleague. Ms. F. is instructed to ask the colleague nicely to refill the stationery by herself during her work time. During the role play, the therapist observes the strengths and weaknesses in Ms. F.'s behavior as she insecurely explains to him with a quiet voice that she does not want the mess on the desk. After the end of the role play, the therapist gives feedback on Ms. F.'s performance. First, the strengths of the patient are highlighted.

Therapist: "*It is courageous that you told me that the mess on the table is disturbing for you although we barely know each other due to our alternating work hours.*"

Then, the therapist focuses on the elements of Ms. F.'s behavior that need correction.

Therapist: "*Being a colleague, I could understand better if you give reasons why do the mess and the missing stationery disturb you. Please try to state the aspects given before, i.e. that you want to pick up your son in time. Please try to speak up a little as this sounds more self-confident, and explain that you also refill stationery if it becomes empty during your work time. Please describe your desires in detail, i.e. that you want both of you tidy up the desk and refill stationery at the end of work so that the other colleague can leave in time.*"

In the second role play, Ms. F.'s behavior and communication with her mother-in-law are practiced. The therapist asks Ms. F. to clearly state her desires.

Ms. F.: "*I do not want my son to eat sweets, and he should also have an after-lunch nap.*"

The therapist explains to Ms. F. the importance of positively formulating the desires and objectives (to not state the things that you do not want, but the things you want).

Ms. F. tries again: "*I want my son to have a healthy diet, stay physically fit, have healthy teeth and enough sleep. When I am at home with my son, this is not a problem. I also want my mother-in-law to have him go to bed after lunch, and I want to make sure that she does this also in case he cries or tries to throw a fit. I also want my mother-in-law to offer fruits to him, but not sweets, and that she would say no when he would request sweets.*"

Therapist: "*That was perfect, Ms. F. Now, let us play that I am your mother-in-law, and you try to argue the way stated before. Could you please try to have eye contact during the whole discussion?*"

Using this technique the problematic situation is practiced with the required corrections until the targeted behavior of the patient is fully achieved. The patient's "homework" is to test the learned behavior in everyday situations.

In this session we have discussed the one of the most crucial component of the social competence for the depressed patient, the training of the self-confident behavior. As we have previously described, social competence includes several other skills as well that are not detailed in this chapter. Obviously, the patient's individual shortages are in focus during the therapy of depression (learn how to say no to an unpleasant request, start a conversation with a stranger, reveal emotions, etc.). These elements are practiced using the similar methodology to the one mentioned above.

8.2.2. Problem-solving training

Problem-solving training belongs to the standard methods of behavioral therapy. It is highly structured didactically and it is usually combined with other therapeutic methods. The various concepts of this method do not differ significantly from each other. In the following, we will present the 5-level model described by D´Zurilla.

According to D´Zurilla and Goldfried [123], problem-solving is a behavioral process, including cognitive operations, that elaborates a number of efficient possible actions for problematic situations and that supports decision for one of these alternatives [120]. For this reason this method is classified as a cognitive strategy by some authors, while others mention it among the behavior-modifying elements. However, the current trend of CBT does not draw a strict boundary between these two fields.

With depressed patients the repertoire of their problem-solving abilities is often insufficient and their motivation to actively deal with problems is inadequate. Patients perceive these problems as being unsolvable per se and they do not attempt to address them because of the possibility of failure. Problem-solving training helps patients identify and name their problems, develop alternatives for problem solving, make decisions and to correspondingly decrease their feeling of hopelessness and at the same time increase self-efficacy.

D´Zurilla and Goldfried [123] describe a 5-level training model for gaining skills in solving problems:

1. The first level is used for general orientation by patients realizing their 'problems.' As this term is quite complex, Fliegel and colleagues [120] proposed the word "difficulties' in a therapeutic context and they state that burdensome situations connected to patient uncertainty, dissatisfaction or anxiety should be avoided.

2. After successful recognition of the problem, the next level includes detailed identification of the 'difficulty' and comprehensive analysis of the problematic situation. During this stage the therapist will ask patients about their own experiences concerning the troublesome situation and their thoughts and emotions. At this point patients should also formulate their own objectives, i.e. describe the desired status so that the situation is not burdensome any more, but instead rather pleasant or at least acceptable. Patients should also consider what they are willing to do to achieve this desired status as well as the impacts or side effects of the new situation.

3. In the next step, alternatives for actions required for achieving the objective are elaborated and recorded. The more practical and problem-solving strategies are developed by the patient, the higher the possibility is that at least one useful idea will be identified to solve the problem.

4. At the decision stage all alternative actions are recorded with their short-term and long-term consequences impacting the patient and the patient's environment. Considerations can be presented as a matrix that simplifies the presentation of the alternative actions and their corresponding consequences.

5. In the last step, the most favorable solution is selected and imposed. Imagination techniques are helpful for improving patient decision-making skills. As stated in section 8.1, patients are instructed to perform the activity in their mind first (compare it with 'covert modelling' Rational-Emotive-Therapy by Ellis [107]) since imagining the situation usually triggers the same physical reaction and emotions as the ones associated with the real situation.

Example. Problem-solving training

A 27-year old female patient wants to move in with her fiancé. Her fiancé's parents own a large rural house that would also offer enough space for the couple and it would only impose a slight financial burden for utility costs. However, the patient and her fiancé work in a city approximately 20 kilometers away and they need to use a car or a bus for commuting. Furthermore, the patient is worried about being forced to helping her parents-in-law with their farm work during her spare time in order to express the couple's gratitude for housing, or to nurse his parents in case of illness, as this is customary in rural regions. She considered a town apartment as the first alternative action. Although the apartment is expensive the couple would not have to commute and they would be independent from his parents. The second possibility would be the rural house of the parents-in-law, which is more favorable in terms of costs but would include the necessity of commuting and also pose a threat of conflicts with his parents and correspondingly with her partner. She also considered a third possibility where the couple would live in the parents' house and pay a reasonable rent in addition on top of utility costs. This solution would also include a contract in the agreement regarding any work she would be willing/not willing to do on the farm. After considering the pros and cons, the patient selected the first solution.

If realization of the most favorable action strategy does not generate the desired benefit for the patient the next best alternative can be tried and the matrix can be supplemented with new aspects.

8.2.3. Helping behavior

Providing help to others offers several benefits regarding the treatment of depression. First, this competence-oriented exercise increases the feeling of personal efficacy; second, self-centered ways of thinking which are typical for depression (speculating on the patient's own problems and sadness) is changed as the affected person focuses on the problems of others [124].

The following section focuses on therapy that is based on the principles of cognitive learning. Nevertheless it must be emphasized that the most accepted structure of CBT does not make a strict separation between classical behavioristic methods and cognitive techniques. Experience shows that these two components a closely correlated and complement each other.

8.3. Cognitive techniques

During life, each individual attains - by learning and undergoing experiences - certain cognitive patterns that are typical for situations – so-called schemes – and that may differ with each person, but that are relatively constant interpersonally. These cognitive patterns define our expectations, attitudes and beliefs that are mainly unconscious and contribute to the structure and assessment of the conscious self.

Psychopathologic conditions such as depression are characterized by dysfunctional schemes that manifest in dysfunctional basic attitudes and are expressed by means of uncontainable negative thoughts (this sequence also corresponds to the cognitive hierarchy according to Beck [31]. If such schemes are activated, they have a major effect on cognitive information processing, on the type and quality of the experience and eventually on the behavior.

Depressed patients tend to exhibit errant, one-sided, absolutist ways of thinking, so-called cognitive distortions, that are expressed through exaggerations, generalizations, black and white thinking, understatement as well as over-generalizations. Cognitive techniques can be utilized to detect and correct such improper cognitions (automatic thoughts) and their corresponding basic assumptions that result in the disturbed behavior and that are connected to oppressive emotions. Learning cognitive techniques helps the patient replace dysfunctional cognitions with ways of thinking appropriate for a particular situation and to identify and use the central role of cognition for adjusting emotions. Thus, the objectives of the cognitive therapy include manipulating negative expectations and abnormal self-perceptions by means of the identification of abnormal belief systems.

In the cognitive stage of therapy there is a comparatively high amount of verbal communication between the patient and the therapist that enables the therapist to collect sufficient information in order to be able to enter into the patient's world and understand his or her organization of reality. The therapist must clearly understand the patient's thought pattern associated with his or her symptoms as well as the way the patient assesses these symptoms. It is also crucial for the therapist to explain to the patient that they will jointly examine these thoughts that are by no means objective representations of reality, as experience shows that cognition is seriously distorted in depression. The therapist also needs to explain that a particular situation can be interpreted differently depending on the observer. Depressed individuals tend to evaluate situations negatively and thoughts, emotions and behavior generate a chain reaction. The patient must understand that a disorder is created by the way one assesses a situation.

In summary, the objectives of cognitive techniques can be identified as follows. The patient learns

- not to accept his/her thoughts as facts,
- how thoughts, emotions and behavior are connected to each other,
- and how to develop a more objective and distant view concerning his/her own problems.

Cognitive restructuring is a gradual approximation based on the principles of cognitive hierarchy. In the first step, the patient's negative automatic thoughts causing the unpleasant emotions are identified, as this can be determined most easily. After identifying distorted cognitions, the arduous situation is re-interpreted. Finally, the patient's dysfunctional basic attitudes which are based on deeper levels of consciousness and which are responsible for maintenance of depression can be identified and altered.

8.3.1. Identification of automatic thoughts

8.3.1.1. ABC technique

The ABC technique described by Ellis [107] is intended to differentiate thoughts, emotions and real facts, representing a very important step for identification of dysfunctional automatic thoughts. Using the ABC technique, the affected person learns that a situation or an event can be explained differently depending on the point of view and any consequent emotions depend on the interpretation of the event. In the ABC technique "A" refers to acting event, "B" to beliefs, thoughts and interpretation of the situation, and "C" to consequences, i.e. the emotions that are triggered by the thoughts and beliefs and that determine the subsequent behavior.

Example:A. Situation: The neighbor passes by without saying hello.

B. Thoughts: "She does not like me."

C. Emotions: Feeling depressed.

Using this example, patients realize that their own thoughts actually trigger the negative emotion. The patient may ask: *"Does this thought help me to feel the way I want to feel?"*

In the next step the patient may try to develop helpful alternative thoughts instead of dysfunctional cognitions:

Example:A. Situation: The neighbor passes by without saying hello.

B. Thoughts: "She did not see me."

C. Emotions: Neutral.

8.3.1.2. Socratic dialogue

The Socratic dialogue is a cognitive CBT intervention technique described by Beck. Instead of didactic explanations and persuasive attempts by the therapist, the objective of this technique is to encourage the patient to uncover his or her own unprofitable way of thinking. This kind of verbal communication scarcely causes resistance since targeted questions enable patients to see their own problems from a different point of view and helps them learn to dissociate from distorted cognitions while gaining an objective view of the situation. As depressed individuals have a deficient ability of adequately understand certain problems, the open-question technique enables patients to see the correlation between mental structures (thoughts, emotions and behavior) and their personal experiences via self-awareness. The therapist uses Socratic questions to collect information regarding a problem and gives feedback to the patient by means of a brief summary showing that the therapist actively listens and correctly understands the patient. The Socratic dialogue is based on so-called negative automatic thoughts (NAT) that imply dysfunctional attitudes and that can be changed during the course of the therapy. In a first step these dysfunctional attitudes and persuasions are recognized by identifying negative automatic thoughts with the therapist carefully pointing out the embedded conflicts. Eventually, the questioning results in a new and more realistic perception of the problem.

NATs are highly distorted defects (over-generalization, dichotomous thinking), and one of the primary goals of therapy is to verify their degree of reality by the patient explaining a number negatively interpreted past situations. In addition to the Socratic dialogue, recording the patient's troublesome thoughts in writing is a common method for identifying NATs. For depressed patients it is often difficult to describe their cognitions; in this case the therapist should point out that changes of emotions are good indicators for NATs. Experience shows that patients can identify negative emotions more easily than cognitions.

Example. Identifying negative emotions: *("How did you feel when... ?")*

Therapist.: *"Identify the emotion you felt when your neighbor was not saying hello…?"*

Patient: *"I was sad."*

The patient should also assess the intensity of his or her emotions on a scale from 1 to 100% and understand that certain emotional variations are not pathological. The patient should also focus on emotions with the intensity of more than 40% since NAT generally associated with intense affects [125].

Example. Questions for NATs identification:

"What did you think when you were sad?"

"What does this mean to you?"

"What is particularly disturbing about this situation?"

If the patient cannot name the depressive cognitions, it may be helpful to illustrate the troubling negative situation in a **three-column table**. This technique also includes -- similar to the ABC technique described above -- simultaneously occurring emotions and cognitions; however, the second column states the emotion associated with the situation since identification of the emotions is generally easier than that of the cognitions.

Situation	Mood/Emotions	Negative Automatic Thoughts
Call from company during vacation	anxiety, doubt 80%	They want to fire me.
The neighbor did not say hello	depressed, sad 50%	She does not like me; she is angry at me.
Thinking of chores	hopeless, depressed 70%	How can I cope with all this?

Table 3. Three-column table for identification of negative automatic thoughts

http://dx.doi.org/10.5772/54200

8.3.2. Change NATs

After successful identification of NATs based on the description of the problematic situation and the recognition of arduous emotions, the patient should perform a **verification of the degree of reality** of the NATs together with the therapist in order to correct any cognitive distortions. Objectivity of the patient during the assessment of the problem can be augmented by **reattribution, alternative conceptualization** and **changes of perspective**. Reattribution will be particularly beneficial if the patient holds his or her presumable personal deficits responsible for any negative experiences. In this case the patient should write down the situation resulting in the self-criticism and analyze it together with the therapist. Alternative conceptualization refers to the process when the patient gathers alternative solutions in order to explain problematic situations.

Example 1.

The 15-year old son of a female patient is told that he is failing one of his courses.

Patient: *"It is my fault that my son is getting a bad grade in school, because I am a bad mother."*

Cognitive restructuring can be reached by Socratic interviewing performed empathically and carefully within the scope of a collaborative relationship that leads the patient to self-awareness [126]. In this particular case the patient should ask herself if one should really be responsible for everything, and then she should recognize that events usually have multiple causes (reattribution).

Depressed individuals measure themselves and the rest of the world with distorted criteria; they are significantly stricter with themselves than with others. Thus, patients must learn that there are other principles of self-control in addition to their first-person observation focused on self-denunciation, e.g. self-reinforcement.

Change of perspective during role play as well as imagination exercises can be used to give the patient more objectivity concerning her views.

Therapist: *"Please imagine that the sons of Ms. M. and Ms. G. are also told that they are failing school. What do you think about these women as mothers? Are they really bad mothers?"* or:

Therapist: *"Do you know other mothers whose children are failing a class? What do you think about these women? How would you describe these women as mothers?"* or:

Therapist: *"Put yourself in the place of a friend. Which qualities would he or she attribute to you in this situation?" The following questions can also be useful in broadening the patient's horizon: "Is it possible that there is another reason for why your son is getting bad grades?"* or *"Do you think that your opinion about being a bad mother is helpful in feeling the way you want to feel?"* (hedonistic approach).

The following questions could also be helpful: *"Do you have evidence that supports your negative thoughts?"* (verification of the degree of reality). Often it is relatively easy to answer this question because depressed individuals are usually highly convinced of the validity of their negative thoughts. They usually tend to remember negative events and often assess pleasant or neutral events as being negative. Thus, their assumptions are not based on reality [127].

Therapist: *"Imagine how you would evaluate this problem in ten years"*.

Or: "*Can you please describe the characteristics of a bad mother in detail?*"

The degree of reality of this statement is verified using a 7-column table [128], where any cognitive distortions can be analyzed. In the thoughts diary, the above described 'three-column technique' which includes the problematic situation, the correspondingly connected emotional state as well as the NATs, is complemented with arguments FOR and AGAINST the distorted assumption of the patient. The patient should reassess his or her assumption to find other alternatives for different explanations of the situation; then, the alternative hypothesis should be used to reassess the original emotion.

Situation	Emotions	NAT	Pros	Cons	Alternative thought	New emotion
Call from company during vacation	anxiety, doubt 80%	They want to fire me.	none	I recently got a pay raise.	Maybe they need me to fill in for a sick co-worker.	0%
The neighbour did not say hello.	depressed 50%	She is angry with me.	none	Two days ago we had coffee together.	She did not see me.	10%
I think of chores.	depressed 90%	Nobody needs me, I am good for nothing.	My daughter lives her own life.	She asked for my advice yesterday.	Could do something every day.	30%

Table 4. Seven-column table: Examples for verification of degree of reality of distorted perception and corresponding corrections

The last step of cognitive restructuring is **testing of the alternative thoughts** in real life. In the behavioral experiment, the depressed patient who came up with new thoughts with the seven-column table ("*I know that my family needs me even though they do not tell me all the time.*") recognizes the indirect clues implying that she is important to her family [126].

However, it is also possible that the gathered 'evidence' actually supports the negative assumption of the patient *("I was fired.")*. In this case, the therapist should focus on the patient coping with this new situation. Here the following questions could be helpful: *"If so, what could be the worst consequence of this situation?" or "Have you ever been in a seemingly unsolvable situation? How did you solve the problem? What helped?"*

The seven-column technique helps patients discover cognitive defects that represent the actual basis of their depressed mood. Burns [129] lists 10 cognitive distortions:

dichotomous thinking ("*This cake did not turn out good. I'm a lousy baker.*")

over-generalization ("*Things always go wrong.*")

negative filter ("*... that is why I screwed everything up.*")

non-consideration of positive experiences (patient devaluate good grades in school by saying that the test was easy)

jumping to conclusions ("*I will never succeed with this.*")

exaggeration/understatement ("*I am completely incapable.*")

emotional reasoning ("*I think everyone hates me. It has to be this way.*")

labelling ("*I am a bad mother.*")

personalization ("*It is my fault that my children get bad grades.*")

"should" statements ("*I 'should' know better.*")

Correction of dysfunctional attitudes

If symptom improvement can be observed, the next step in therapy is to introduce the exploration of dysfunctional attitudes in order to increase the susceptibility to depression [41,130].

Automatic thoughts and dysfunctional attitudes are similar since both are acquired by learning processes; both contain exaggerated and distorted basic principles, they are self-sustaining, and their correction requires special techniques [128].

Dysfunctional basic assumptions are characterized by defective logic and imbalance; their stable attitudes, rules and beliefs form part of our personality. They are organized mainly around topics such as performance, acceptance/rejection and control. Realizing dysfunctional attitudes is not easy, as they are stored in the deeper, hardly accessible layers of our cognitive hierarchy as compared to automatic thoughts, which are usually linked to a situation. However, these basic assumptions can be reduced by applying Socratic questions, using the dysfunctional attitudes scale [131] or by deviation of the cognitive process through cognitive hierarchies as demonstrated by the technique of a vertical arrow pointing down. During the application of this technique the therapist can tackle the problematic situation using the question *"Why is this important to you?"*, thus exploring progressively deeper elements of the cognitive hierarchy while revealing any dysfunctional attitudes.

Patient: "*My daughter doesn't mind me.*"

Therapist: "*What is so bad about that?*"

Patient: "*A child this age should mind her mother.*"

Therapist: "*How does that apply to you?*"

Patient: "*... that I am doing something wrong.*"

Therapist: "*What do you mean by that?*"

Patient: "*I guess I'm saying that I'm a bad mother.*" [126]

The following intervention techniques are used for modification of dysfunctional attitudes:

1. Analysis of benefits/disadvantages of the basic belief. Dysfunctional basic assumptions that are highly affect-related tend to reflect personal values. Thus, change of these basic beliefs is not easy because the individual often recognizes the benefits and positive aspects of his or her own assumptions. When recording benefits and disadvantages, the patient is often surprised about the small number of benefits that can be recalled.

2. Provide counter-arguments using Socratic interviewing:

Dysfunctional basic belief: "*If I need someone's help that means I am a weak person.*"

Correction: "*When I need and accept help, this means that I have good problem-solving abilities.*"

3. Dysfunctional beliefs can also be corrected by a change in perspective.

Example: The patient only considers people to be valuable and useful except when they perform work. The therapist asks her to name people from her circle of acquaintances that she considers to be valuable; then she assesses the amount of work that these individuals do according to her opinion in order to see whether these two parameters are related to each other. After a comprehensive analysis it is shown that this is not the case. Someone who works less can be very valuable because of personal qualities such as kindness, helpfulness, intelligence etc., and a person who works more can be less valuable by being an exhausted and complaining perfectionist who is always dissatisfied [126].

Dysfunctional attitude: "*If I don't work I am of no worth. That is why I am a loser.*"

Modified belief: "*Although I cannot work at the moment, I am a good person. It is not only work that makes a person valuable.*"

8.4. Completion of therapy, relapse prophylaxis

The final module of the CBT, which usually comprises 2-3 sessions, focuses on making any positive changes achieved during therapy become permanent by conscious comprehension. Therapy success is evaluated together with the patient. During the evaluation the patient rates any subjective changes experienced during the progress of the therapy and compares them to the level of depression recorded at the beginning of therapy. Improvement is measured by comparing the patient's advance on the 10-degree-scale described above. In addition, the patient verbally summarizes the experienced positive changes and identifies the elements of the treatment that contributed most to the healing process. This summary has two purposes: First, it is extremely important to make patients understand that the most important factor of their improvement is their self-efficacy; and second, the therapist should emphasize the necessity of continuous employment of coping strategies after the completion of therapy to prevent relapse. Moreover, with the help of the therapist the patient summarizes the strategies that are pivotal in recognizing the early signs of depression (e.g. sleep disturbances, agitation, mood swings) that can be utilized to prevent relapse. In order to stabilize positive cognitions the therapist should emphasize the importance of self-efficacy tools including cognitive restructuring, maintaining and enhancing social relationships, utilization of 'happiness diaries' as described above, etc. It is equally important to make patients aware of their future goals and to help them engage in positive experiences they enjoy.

Despite their improvement some patients may require a prolonged support of his or her therapist. In this case it is recommended that control sessions be scheduled after the first, third and sixth months; these sessions also offer an excellent opportunity to monitor the patient's status during an extended period.

Author details

Irene Lehner-Adam[1] and Bertalan Dudas[2]

1 Department of Psychiatry and Psychotherapy, Christian Doppler University Clinic Salzburg, Austria

2 Neuroendocrine Organization Laboratory, Lake Erie College of Osteopathic Medicine, Erie, PA, USA

References

[1]

[2] Bauer, M., Berghöfer, A., Adli, M. (Hrsg.). Akute und therapieresistente Depressionen. Pharmakotherapie, Psychotherapie, Innovationen. 2. Aufl. Berlin, Heidelberg, New York: Springer.2005.

[3] Rush, A.J., Zimmerman, M., Wisniewski, S.R., Fava, M., Hollon, S.D., Warden, D., Biggs, M.M., Shores-Wilson, K., Sheltob, R.C., Luther, J.F, Thomas, B. & Trivedi, M.H. Comorbid psychiatric disorders in depressed outpatients: Demographic and clinical features. Journal of Affective Disorders. 2005;871:43-55.

[4] Rush, A.J. Algorithmusgestützte Behandlung. In M. Bauer, A. Berghöfer, M. Adli, (Ed.). Therapieresistente Depressionen. Heidelberg, Berlin, New York: Springer.2005.

[5] Murray, C.J.L. & Lopez, A.D. Global mortality, disability and the contribution of risk factors: Global burden of disease study. Lancet.1997; 349, 1436-1352.

[6] Üstün, T.B., Ayuso-Mateos, J.L., et al.Global burden of depressive disorders in the year 2000. Br. J. Psychiatry. 2004;184:386-392.

[7] Angst, J. Depression and Anxiety: A Review of Studies in the Community and in Primary Health Care. In N. Sartorius, D. Goldberg, G. de Girolamo, J. Costa e Silva, Y.Lecrubier and U. Wittchen (Eds.). Psychological Disorders in General Medical Settings (pp. 60-68). Toronto, Lewiston, New York, Bern, Göttingen, Stuttgart: Hogrefe & Huber Publishers. 1990.

[8] Wittchen, H.-U. & Jacobi, F. Size and Burden of Mental Disorders in Europe – A critical review and appraisal of 27 studies. European Neuropsychopharmacology. 2005;15 (4),357-376.

[9] Greenberg, P.E., Kessler, R.C., et al. The economic burden of depression in the United States: how did it change between 1990 and 2000? Journal of Clinical Psychiatry. 2003;64:1465-1475.

[10] Thomas, C.M., Morris, S. Cost of depression among adults in England in 2000. British Journal of Psychiatry. 2003;183,514-519.

[11] Wittchen, H.-U., Jönsson, B. & Olesen, J. Editorial: Towards a better understanding of the size and burden and cost of brain disorders in Europe. Eur. Neuropsychopharmacol. 2005;15(4):355-356.

[12] Rosenbaum, J.F., Hylan, T.R. Costs of depressive disorders: a review. Depressive Disorders. 1999;21:401-449.

[13] Sturm, R. & Wells, B. How can Depression become more cost-effective? JAMA, 1995;273, 51-58.

[14] Bolton, J.M. et al. A population-based Longitudinal Study of Risk Factors for Suicide Attempts in Major Depression Disorders. J Psychiatr Res 2010 Okt;44(13):817-26.

[15] Judd, L. L., Akiskal, H. S., Maser, J.D. et al. A prospective 12-year study of subsyndromal and syndromal depressive symptoms in unipolar major depressive disorders. Archives of General Psychiatr. 1998;55, 694– 700.

[16] Möller, H.J. Therapieresistenz auf Antidepressiva: Definition, Häufigkeit, Prädiktoren und Interventionsmöglichkeiten. Nervenarzt. 2004;75:499-517.

[17] Hegerl, U., Hautzinger, M. et al. (2010). Effects of pharmacotherapy and psychotherapy in depressed primay-care patients: a randomized, controlled trial including a patient´s choice arm. Int J Neuropsychopharmacol. Feb;13(1):31-44.

[18] Sudak, D.M. Cognitive behavorial therapy for depression. Psychiatr Clin North Am. 2012 Mar; 35(1):99-110.

[19] Ravindran, A.V. et al. Treatment of primary dysthymia with group cognitive therapy and pharmacotherapy: clinical symptoms and functional impairments. Am J Psychiatry. 1999 Oct;156(19): 1608-17.

[20] Teasdale, J.D., Segal, ZV. et al. Prevention of relapse/recurrence in major depression by mindfulness-based cognitive therapy. Journal of Counseling and Clinical Psychology.2000; 68(4):615-623.

[21] Dirmaier, J. et al. Non-pharmacological treatment of depressive disorders: a review of evidence-based treatment options. Rev Recent Clin Trials 2012 May;7(2):141-9.

[22] Burrows, G.D. et al. Definition and differential diagnosis of treatment-resistant depression. Int Clin Psychopharmacol; 1994;9 (suppl.2):5-10

[23] Paykel, E.S., Freeling, P., Hollyman J.A. Are tricyclic antidepressants useful for mild depression? A placebo controlled trial. Pharmacopsychiatry 1988;21:15-18.

[24] Bschor, T., Baethge, C. Wechsel des Antidepressivums. In: T. Bschor (Ed.). Behandlungsmanual therapieresistenter Depression. Pharmakotherapie-Somatische Therapie-Psychotherapie. Stuttgart: Kohlhammer.2008.

[25] Faramarzi, M., Alipor, A., Esmaelzadeh, S. et al. Treatment of depression and anxiety in infertilde women: cognitive behavioral therapy versus fluoxetine. J Affect Disord. 2008May;108(1-2):159-64.

[26] Watkins, K.E., Hunter, S., Hepner, K., Paddock, S., Zhou, A., de la Cruz, E. Group cognitive-behavioral therapy for clients with major depression in residential substance abuse treatment. Psychiatr Serv 2012; Jun 1;63(6):608-11.

[27] Austin, M.P et al. Brief antenatal cognitive behavioral therapy group intervention for the prevention of postnatal depression and anxiety: a randomized controlled trial. J. Affect Disord. 2008 Jan;105(1-3):35-44.

[28] Nardi, B. et al. Is the cognitive behavioral therapy an effective strategy also in the prevention of postpartum depression. Riv Psychiatr. 2012 May-Jun;47(3):205-13.

[29] Arch, J.J. et al. Is exposure-based cognitive behavioral therapy safe during pregnancy? Arch Womens Ment Healt 2012 Sept16.

[30] Pieh, C. et al. Gender differences in Responses to cognitive behavioural therapy-oriented Multimodal treatment in Depressed Patients with chronic pain. Psychiatric Prox 2012. Sept; 39(6):280-5.

[31] Sherril, J.T. & Kovacs,M. Nonsomatic treatment of depression. Child Adolesc Psychiatr Clin N Am 2002 Jul; 11(3):379-93

[32] Beck, A.T., Rush, J., Shaw, B., Emery, G. Cognitive Therapy of Depression. New York, The Guilford Press. 1979.

[33] Rush, A.J., Beck, A.A., Kovacs,M.&Hollon, S.D. Comparative efficacy of cognitive therapy and pharmacotherapy in the treatment of depressed outpatients. Cognitive Therapy and Research. 1977; 1: 17-37.

[34] Bellack, A.S., Hersen, M.& Himmelhoch, J. Social skills training compared with pharmacotherapy and psychotherapy in the treatment of unipolar depression. American Journal of Psychiatry, 1981;138:1562-1567.

[35] Kovacs, M., Rush, A.J., Beck, A.T., Hollon, S.D. Depressed outpatients treated with cognitive therapy or pharmacotherapy. Archives of General Psychiatry, 1981;38, 33-39.

[36] Hautzinger, M. & de Yong- Meyer, R. Depression. Zeitschrift für Klinische Psychologie, 1996;25: 79-160.

[37] Hollon, S.D., DeRubeis, R.J., Shelton, S.C. et al. Prevention of relapse following cognitive therapy vs. medications in moderate to severe depression. Archives of General Psychiatry. 2005;62(4):417-422.

[38] Krebs, G. et al. Cognitive behavioural therapy for adults with body dysmorphic disorders: a case series. Behav Cogn Psychother 2012 Jul;40(4):452-61.

[39] Hesser, H. et al. A systematic review and meta-analysis of randomized controlled trials of cognitive behavioural therapy for tinnitus distress. Clin psychol Rev 2011 Jun; 31(4):545-53.

[40] Öst, L.G., Karlstedt, A., Widén, S. (2012): The effects of cognitive behavior therapy delivered by students in a psychologist training program: an effectiveness study. Behav Ther. 2012. Ma;43(1):160-73.

[41] Sunderland, M., Wong, N., et al. Investigating trajectories of change in psychological distress amongst patients with depression and generalised anxiety disorder treated with internet cognitive behavioural therapy. Behav Res Ther. 2012 Jul;50(1):374-80.

[42] Hautzinger, M. Kognitive Verhaltenstherapie bei Depressionen. 2003.

[43] Weishaar, M. Aaron T. Beck. London, Sage Publications.1993.

[44] David-Ferdon, C., Kaslow, N.J. Evidence-based psychosocial treatments for child and adolescent depression. J Clin Child Adolesc Psychol. 2008;37(1):62-104.

[45] Gallagher-Thomson, D., Thomson, L.W. Treating Late-Life Depression. A cognitive-behavioral therapy approach. Oxford: University Press. 2010.

[46] Serfaty, M.A et al. Clinical effectiveness of individual cognitive behavioural therapy for depressed older people in primary care: a randomized controlled trial. Arch Gen Psychiatry 2009 Dec;66(12):1332-40.

[47] Wilcon, K.C et al. Psychotherapeutic treatments for older depressed people Cochrane Database Syst Rev. 2008 Jan.23;(1).

[48] Mayer, J.D. How Mood Influences Cognition. In N.E. Sharkey (Ed.), Advances in Cognitive Science (pp. 290 -314). Chichester: Ellis Horwood. 1986.

[49] Simon, H.A. Comments. In M.S. Clark & S.T. Fiske (Eds.). Affect and cognition (pp. 333 - 342). Hillsdale, NJ: Erlbaum. 1982.

[50] Petty, R.E., Gleicher, F. & Baker, S.M. Multiple Roles for Affect in Persuasion. In J.P. Forgas (Ed.), Emotion and Social Judgments (pp. 181 - 200). Oxford: Pergamon Press. 1991.

[51] Weissman, M.M., Bland, R.C., Canino,. G.J. et al. Cross-national epidemiology of major depression and bipolar disorder. JAMA.1996;276:293-299

[52] Weissman, M.M., Wolk, S., Goldstein, R.B. et al. Depressed adolescents grown up. Journal of the American Medical Association. 1999;281(18):1707-1713.

[53] Blazer, D. G., Kessler, R. C., McGonagle, K. A., et al. The prevalence and distribution of major depression in a national community sample. American Journal of Psychiatr. 1994;151:979-986.

[54] Carta, M.G., Carpiniello, B. et al. Lifetime prevalence of major depression and dysthymia: results of a community survey in Sardinia. Eur Neuropharmacol. 1995;(5 Suppl):103-107.

[55] Kruijshaar, M.F., Barendreat, I., Vos, T. et al. Lifetime prevalence estimates of major depression: an indirect estimation method and a quantification of recall bias. European Journal of Epidemiology. 2005;20,103-111.

[56] Bijl R.V., Ravelli, A. & van Zessen, G. Prevalence of psychiatric disorder in the general population: Results of the Netherlands Mental Health an Incidence +study. Social Psychiatrc Epidemiology, 1998;33, 587-595

[57] Andrews, G., Poulton, R., Skoog, I. Lifetime risk of depression: restricted to minority or waiting most? The British Journal of Psychiatry. 2005;187:495-496

[58] Weissman, M.M., Bland, R.,et al. Sex differences in rates of depression: cross-national perspectives. Journal of Affective Disorders. 1993;29 (2-3): 77-84.

[59] Benett, D.S., Ambrosini, et al. Gender differences in adolescent depression: do symptoms differ for boys and girls? J Affect Disord. 2005;Dec 89(1-3):35-44

[60] Paykel, CRT MG; Carpiniello B. et al. Lifetime prevalence of major depression and dysthymia: results of a community survey in Sardinia. Eur. Neuropsychopharmacol. 1995;195 (5 Suppl):103-107.

[61] Hankin, B.L., Abramson, L.Y. Development of gender differences in depression: description and possible explanations. Ann Med. 1999 Dec;31(6)372-9.

[62] Goldman, S. Developmental epidemiology of depressive disorders. Child Adolesc Psychiatr Clin N Am 2012 Apr;21(2):217-35.

[63] J. Costello, E., Erkanli, A., Angold, A. Is there an epidemic of child or adolescent depression? Journal of Child Psychology and Psychiatry. 2006;47(12):1263-1271.

[64] Alghamdi, S. & Manassis, K. Characteristic, correlates and outcomes of childhood and adolescent depressive disorders. Dialogues Clin Neuroscie 2009;11(1):45-62.

[65] Lehtinen, V., Youkamaa, M. Epidemiology of depression: prevalence, risk factors and treatment situation. Acta Psychiatr Scand Suppl. 1994;377:7-10.

[66] Paykel, E.S. Depression in women. Br. J Psychiatry Suppl. 1991;May;(10):22-9.

[67] Picinelli, M., Wilkinson, G. Gender differences in depression. Br J Psychiatry. 2000;177:486-92.

[68] Angold, A., Costello, E.J. Depressive comorbidity in children and adolescents: empirical, theoretical and methodological issues. Am J Psychiatry. 1993 Dec;150(12): 1779-91.

[69] Yorbik, O., Birmaher, B., et al. Clinical characteristics of depressive symptoms in children and adolescents with major depressive disorders. J Clin Psychiatry. 2004 Dec; 65(12):1654-9.

[70] Harrington, R., Fudge, H., Rutter, M., Pickles, A., Hill, J. Adult outcomes of childhood and adolescent depression. I. Psychiatric status. Archives of general Psychiatry. 1990;47 (5):465-473.

[71] Weller, E.B.& Weller, R.A. Depression in adolescents growing pains or true morbidity? Journal of Affective Disorders. 2000;61 (supp. 1.): 9-13.

[72] Jamison, K.R. Suicide and bipolar disorder. Journal of Clinical Psychiatry. 2000;61 Suppl 9:47-51.

[73] Lönnqvist, K. Psychiatric aspects of suicidal behaviour: Depression. In: K. Hawton, K. van Heeringen (ed.) Suicide and attempted suicide. Sussex: John Wiley& Sons, Ltd. 2000;pp.107-120.

[74] American Psychiatric Association. Diagnostic and Statistical Manual of Mental Disorders, Fourth ed. Washington, D.C: American Psychiatric Association. 1994.

[75] Dilling, H., Mombour, W.& Schmidt,M.H. International Classification of Disease (ICD-10). Kap. V. (F). Bern: Huber. 1993.

[76] Schulte, D. Therapieplanung. Göttingen: Hogrefe. 1996.

[77] Adler, A. Understanding human nature. New York: Garden City.1927.

[78] Beck, A.T. Cognitive Therapy and the emotional Disorders. New York, International University Press.1975.

[79] Edelmann, W. Lernpsychologie. Weinheim: Psychologie-Verlags-Union. 1995.

[80] Watson J. B. Psychology as the behaviorist views it. Psychological Review, 1913;20:158-177.

[81] Hearst, E. The classical-instrumental distinction: Reflexes, voluntary behavior and categories of associtative learning. In: W.K. Estes (Ed.) Handbook of learning and cognitive processes. Vol.2. Conditioning and behavior theory. Hillsdale, N.J.: L. Erlbaum. 1975.

[82] Mowrer, O.H. On the dual theory nature of learning a reinterpretation of conditioning and problem-solving. Harvard Educational Review 1947. 17, 102-148.

[83] Dollard, J., Miller, N.E. Personality and psychotherapy. New York, McGraw-Hill. 1950.

[84] Schachter, S.& Singer, J. Cognitive, social and physiological determinations of emotional state.1962.

[85] Ellis, A.& Grieger, R. (Ed.). Praxis der Rational-Emotive-Therapie. München: Urban&Schwarzenberg. 1979.

[86] Linahan, M. Dialectic Behavioral Approach to Parasuicide. J Pers Disord, 1987, 1, 328-33.

[87] Hayes, S.C & Strosahl, K.D. (eds.). A practical guide to acceptance and commitment therapy. New York: Springer. 2004.

[88] McCullogh, M.C. Treatment for chronic depression: Cognitive Behavioral Analysis System of Psychotherapy (CBASP). New York: Guilford Press. 2000.

[89] Segal, Z; Teasdale, J.; Williams, M. Mindfulness-Based Cognitive Therapy for Depression. Guilford Press. 2002

[90] Seligman, M. Flourish, wie Menschen aufblühen. München: Kösel. 2012

[91] Young, J.E.;Klosko, J.S.;Weishaar, M.E Schematherapie. Paderborn: Junfermann. 2008

[92] Mischel, W. Personality and assessment. New York: Wiley. 1968.

[93] Beck, A.T & Steer, R.A. BDI-Manual. San Antonio: The psychological Corporation. 1987.

[94] Hamilton, M. The Hamilton rating scale for depression. In Sartorius &T.A. Ban (Eds.), Assessment of depression (pp.278-296). Berlin: Springer. 1986.

[95] Montgomery, S. A. & Asberg, M. A new depression scale designed to be sensitive to change. British Journal of Psychiatry, 1979;134,382-389.

[96] WHO, Composite International Diagnostic Interview. (CIDI, Version 1.0). Geneva: WHO, 1990.

[97] First, M.B. et al. User´s Guide for the Structured Clinical Interview for DSM-IV. Axis 1 Disorders. Washington, DC: American Psychiatric Press. 1996.

[98] Brown, T.A et al. Anxiety Disorders Interview Schedule for DSM-IV (ADIS-IV). New York: Graywind Publications Incorporated. 1994.

[99] Hiller, W. et al. Inpatient Multidimensional Psychiatric Scale (IMPS), Manual. Eine multidimensionale Skala zur systematischen Erfassung des psychopathologischen Befundes (Deutsche Version). Weinheim: Beltz-Test. 1986.

[100] Schulte, D. Verhaltenstherapeutische Diagnostik. In H.Reinecker (Ed.): Lehrbuch der Verhaltenstherapie. DGVT: Tübingen.1999.

[101] Schulte, D. Ein Schema für Diagnose und Therapieplanung in der Verhaltenstherapie. In: D. Schulte (Ed.), Diagnostik in der Verhaltenstherapie (S. 75-104). München: Urban&Schwarzenberg. 1974.

[102] Kanfer, F.H., Reinecker, H., Schmelzer, D. Selbstmanagement-Therapie. 3. Aufl. Berlin, Heidelberg, New York: Springer. 2000.

[103] Kanfer, F.H., Saslow, G. Behavioral analysis: An alternative to diagnostic classification. Archives of general Psychiatry. 1965;12:529-538.

[104] Lindsley, D.R. Direct measurement and prothesis of retarded behavior. Journal of Education,1964;147,62-81.

[105] Kanfer, F.H., Philipps, J.S. Lerntheoretische Grundlagen der Verhaltenstherapie. München: Kindler. 1975.

[106] Parker, G., Kiloh, L., Hayward, Parental representation of neurotic an endogeneous depressives. J. Affect. Disord. 1987;13:75-82.

[107] Tringer, L. A „neurotikus" depresszió. Ideggy.Szeml. 1989;42:193-207.

[108] Ellis, A. Die rationale-emotive Therapie. Das innere Selbstgespräch bei seelischen Problemen und seine Veränderung. München: Pfeiffer. 1977.

[109] Seligman, M. E. P. Erlernte Hilflosigkeit. München, Wien, Baltimore: Urban und Schwarzenberg. 1979.

[110] Lewinsohn, P.M. A behavioral approach to depression. In R.J. Friedman & M.M. Katz (Ed.) The psychology of depression. New York: Wiley. 1974.

[111] Lewinsohn, P.M., Hoberman, H., Teri, L.& Hautzinger, M. An integrative theory of depression. In S. Reiss & R.R. Bootzin (Ed.), Theoretical issues in behavior therapy. New York: Academic Press.1985.

[112] Hautzinger, M. Depression, Göttingen: Hogrefe. 1998

[113] Cautela, J.R., Kastenbaum, R. A reinforcement survey schedule for use in therapy, training and research. Psychol.Rep. 1967;20: 1115-1130.

[114] Gächter, H.P. Projektmanagement. Bern:h.e.p. Verlag AG.2007.

[115] Koppenhöfer, E. Euthyme Behandlungsverfahren in der Verhaltenstherapie. Psychologische Medizin 17(2). 2006, 4-7

[116] Galassi, M.D.& Galassi, J.P. Assertion: A critical review. Psychotherapy. Theory, Research and Practice, 1978;15: 16-28.

[117] Wolpe, J. Psychotherapy by reciprocal inhibition. Stanford, Ca.: Stanford University Press, 1958.

[118] Salter, A. Conditioned reflex therapy. New York: Capricorn, 1949.

[119] Lazarus, A.A. The results of behavior therapy in 126 cases of severe neurosis. Behaviour Research and Therapy, 1963; 1: 69-79.

[120] Ullrich de Muynck, R & Ullrich, R. Standardisierung des Selbstsicherheitstraining für Gruppen. (Assertive-Training-Programm: ATP). In: J.Brengelmann & W.Tunner (Eds): Behavior Therapy – Verhaltenstherapie; München: Urban &Schwarzenberg, 1973; 254-259.

[121] Fliegel, F., Groeger, W. M.,et al. Verhaltenstherapeutische Standardmethoden. 4. Auflage. Beltz: Psychologie Verlags Union: München. 1998.

[122] Lazarus, A.A. Behavior rehearsal vs. Non-directive therapy versus advice in effecting behavior change. Behaviour Research and Therapy, 1966; 4, 209-212.

[123] Hintsch, R. & Pfingsten, U. Gruppentraining sozialer Kompetenz. München: Urban&Sons.1983.

[124] D'Zurilla, T.J.& Goldfried, M.R. Problem solving and behavior modification. Journal of abnormal Psychology, 1971;78:107-126.

[125] Mor, N., Winquist, J. Self-focused Attention and Negative Affect: A Meta-Analysis, Psychological Bulletin, 2002;128, 4:638-662.

[126] Perczel Forintos, D. A kognitív viselkedésterápia néhány gyakorlati kérdése. Integratív hírmondó, 1999. 11., 91-97.

[127] Perczel Forintos, D. A kognitiv viselkedésterápia standard módszerei és hatótényezöi. In D.Perczel Forintos & K. Mórocz (Ed.) Kognitív viselkedésterápia. Budapest: Medicina. 2010.

[128] Clark, D.M., Teasdale,J.D. Diurnal variation in clinical depression and accessibility of memories of positive and negative experiences. 1982.

[129] Padesky, C.& Greenberger, D. A Clinician's Guide to Mind over Mood. London, The Guilford Press. 1995.

[130] Burns, D. The feeling Good Handbook. New York, A Plume Book, Penguin. 1990.

[131] Jarrett, R.B et al. Cognitive reactivity, dysfunctional attitudes and depressive relapse and recurrence in cognitive therapy responders. Behav Res Ther 2012 May;50(5): 280-6.

[132] Weissman, A. Dysfunctional Attitude Scale. 1979.

Chapter 5

Mitochondrial Functions in Mood Disorders

Jana Hroudová, Zdeněk Fišar and Jiří Raboch

Additional information is available at the end of the chapter

http://dx.doi.org/10.5772/53254

1. Introduction

Depression is a serious mental disorder manifested by depressed mood, pessimistic thoughts, feelings of worthlessness, feelings of guilt, tearfulness, reduced or increased sleep, appetite loss or appetite disturbance, weight loss or weight gain, social restlessness, loss of interest, difficulty concentrating. Mania is characterized by abnormally elevated or irritable mood, arousal, and/or energy levels. Bipolar disorder features intermittent episodes of mania or hypomania and depressive episodes; rapid cycling, mixed states, and psychotic symptoms occuring in some cases. Depression and mania are thought to be heterogeneous illnesses that can result from dysfunction of several neurotransmitters or metabolic systems.

The predisposition to the disease is determined by genetic, psychosocial and biological factors; individual sensitivity to depressogenic effects during stressful life events is also a contributing factor. Pathophysiology of mood disorders is not sufficiently elucidated and about 1/3 of patients do not response to pharmacotherapy sufficiently. The exact molecular site and the primary cause of signal transduction disturbance associated with the symptoms of depression or mania are still unknown.

Recently, attention in the research of biological basis of mood disorders has been devoted to an overlapping set of molecular and cellular mechanisms of mood disorders, antidepressant response, neuroplasticity, and chronic stress [1], e.g. to changes in neuroprogression, inflammatory and cell-mediated immune response, antioxidant capacity, oxidative and nitrosative stress, and mitochondrial functions [2]. Therefore, changes in the activities of compounds of these intracellular signalling pathways are studied with the aim of discovering new biological markers of mood disorders or predictors of response to antidepressant treatment [3-4]. Mitochondrial dysfunctions are assuming an increasingly important role in hypotheses of mood disorders, bipolar disorder mainly. Recently discussed biological hypotheses of mood disorders include the neurotrophic and neuroplasticity hypothesis of depression [1,5-8] and the mitochondrial hypothesis [9-11].

It is well-known that mitochondria strongly affect many intracellular processes coupled to signal transduction, neuron survival and plasticity. Impaired mitochondrial functions manifest themselves in various ways, they may be related to many psychiatric and neurodegenerative diseases, including bipolar disorder, major depressive disorder, schizophrenia, psychosis and anxiety [12-16]. Impaired functions of mitochondria can be assessed both in isolated mitochondria and in intact or permeabilized cells. Better insight into molecular mechanisms of cellular respiration, control of oxidative phosphorylation (OXPHOS) and effects of antidepressants and mood stabilizers on these processes is likely to lead to a better understanding of pathophysiology of neuropsychiatric disorders.

2. Mitochondria

Mitochondria are small cellular structures consisting of an outer and inner membrane, an intermembrane space and an intracellular matrix. The outer membrane covers the organelle, the inner membrane folds and forms cristae. This settlement extends the surface and enables plenty of chemical reactions. In the mitochondrial matrix, the enzymes of the tricarboxylic acid cycle (TCA, also called citric acid cycle or Krebs cycle) are localized. It is the central pathway of metabolism; its main function is oxidation of acetyl-CoA derived from carbohydrates, amino acids and fatty acids (FAs). The TCA is organized into a supramolecular complex that enables interaction with mitochondrial membranes and the electron transport chain (ETC) in OXPHOS [17]. Most of the TCA enzymes provide other additional "moonlighting" functions, e.g. they stabilize the mitochondrial DNA (mtDNA) or are associated with mitochondrial RNA (mtRNA) translation, oxidative stress, iron metabolism and tumour suppression [18].

In addition to their crucial role in generation of adenosine-5'- triphosphate (ATP), mitochondria are involved in other important processes, such as regulation of free radicals, neurotransmitters, calcium, and apoptosis. They are also involved in neuronal development - synaptogenesis, synaptic development and plasticity. Impaired function of mitochondria leads to impaired bioenergetics, decrease of ATP production, impaired calcium homeostasis, increased production of free radicals and oxidative stress [19-20]. Furthermore, monoamine oxidase (MAO), the enzyme responsible for the metabolism of monoamine neurotransmitters, is localized in the outer mitochondrial membrane.

Mitochondrial proteins are encoded by both nuclear and mitochondrial DNA. All 13 polypeptides encoded by mtDNA form subunits of respiratory chain complexes I, III, IV and V [21-22]. Furthermore, the mitochondrial genome encodes transfer RNA (tRNA) and ribosomal RNA (rRNA) used for RNA translation [23]. Complex II is encoded only by nuclear DNA (nDNA). OXPHOS is under the control of the nuclear genome as well as the mitochondrial genome, which is only maternally inherited. Nevertheless, the dominant role in the regulation of mitochondrial activity has a nucleus; nuclear-encoded transcript factors control the activity of the mitochondrial genome and coordinate the expression of nuclear and mitochondrial genes to mitochondrial proteins [23-24].

Genetic defects or stress can cause mitochondrial dysfunctions, which leads to increased oxidative stress and/or altered calcium homeostasis [25]. An excess of glutamate in the synapse [26] leads to an excess of cytosolic calcium, which produces overactivity of calcium-dependent enzymes and an overload of mitochondria by calcium; it leads to cytoskeletal degradation, protein malformation, decrease of ATP production, and increase of oxygen radical generation. These processes can lead to atrophy or death of neurons [27-28]. Different stimuli, such as hypoxia-ischemia, seizure and hypoglycemia, all activate this pathway. Thus, enhancing mitochondrial function may represent a critical component for the optimal treatment of stress-related diseases [11].

Eukaryotes synthetize ATP mainly by glycolysis in the cytosol and by OXPHOS in the mitochondria; i.e. the majority of cellular ATP is generated by glycolytic degradation of glucose to pyruvate in cytosol followed by aerobic cellular respiration. When pyruvate is converted to acetyl coenzyme A (acetyl-CoA), acetyl-CoA enters the TCA cycle and the result of this process is ATP production by OXPHOS in mitochondria [29]. OXPHOS yields about 17 times more ATP than glycolysis. Therefore, it is considered as the main energy source and a key element of bioenergetics [30-31]. Integration of main metabolic pathways coupled to OXPHOS is illustrated in Figure 1.

The highest number of mitochondria is present in organs demanding the most energy - brain, liver and muscles. Neurons usually utilize glucose as a source of energy. Since the brain stores only a very small amount of glycogen, it needs a steady supply of glucose. Neurons are known to have a lower glycolytic rate than astrocytes and when stressed they are unable to upregulate glycolysis. Following inhibition of mitochondrial respiration, neurons die rapidly, whereas astrocytes utilize glycolytically generated ATP. Glucose metabolism in neurons is directed mainly to the pentose phosphate pathway, leading to regeneration of reduced glutathione, which probably supports antioxidant controlled neuron survival [32]. The regulative processes of OXPHOS are tightly related to reactive oxygen species (ROS) production, integrity of mitochondrial membranes, apoptosis, and intramitochondrial Ca^{2+} levels. Although this is known, the control mechanisms have not yet been sufficiently investigated.

2.1. Physiology of oxidative phosphorylation

The respiratory chain is localized in cristae, structures formed by the inner mitochondrial membrane and extending to the surface [34]. ETC consists of complexes with supramolecular organization, where mitochondrial proton pumps (complexes I, III and IV) transport protons and generate a proton gradient [31,35]. Continuously, electrons are transported to complex III and finally complex IV enables the conversion of O_2 to H_2O. Most of the ATP synthesis comes from the electrochemical gradient across the inner membranes of mitochondria by ATP synthase (complex V). The CoQ cofactor is responsible for transferring electrons from complexes I and II to complex III; the second important cofactor is cytochrome *c* (cyt *c*), which transfers electrons from complex III to complex IV [36]. Both cofactors modulate energy and free radical production [37-38]. Processes in the inner mitochondrial membrane are depicted in Figure 2.

Energy saved in ATP is used in synaptic ion homeostasis and phosphorylation reactions. ATP is essential for the excitability and survival of neurons, OXPHOS is involved in synaptic signalling and is related to changes of neuronal structure and function. Therefore, mitochondria are included in neurotransmitter exocytosis, in recovery, and in ion homeostasis, and in presynaptic nerve terminals.

Oxidative phosphorylation enzymes and MAO are key mitochondrial enzymes studied in molecular psychiatry.

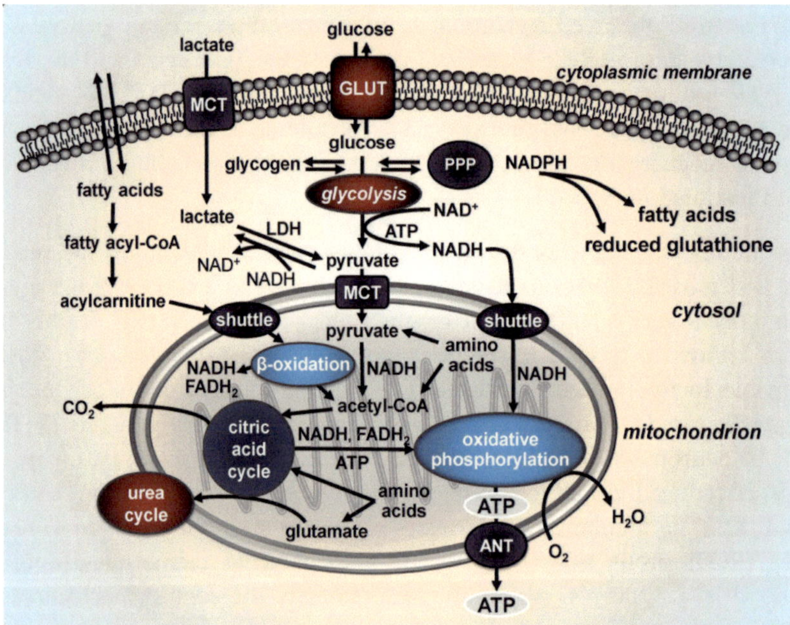

Figure 1. Integration of metabolic pathways. Glucose is transported over a plasma membrane by a glucose transporter (GLUT) and is metabolized to pyruvate by glycolysis. Pyruvate is converted to acetyl-coenzyme A (acetyl-CoA) in the mitochondria, where it is oxidized to CO_2 through the citric acid cycle; redox energy is conserved as reduced nicotinamide adenine dinucleotide (NADH). The mitochondrial respiratory chain couples NADH oxidation to the formation of the electrochemical proton gradient across the inner mitochondrial membrane, which is used to form ATP. ATP produced from OXPHOS is transported from the mitochondrial matrix to the cytoplasm by the adenine nucleotide translocator (ANT). Glucose may be stored as glycogen. Fatty acids and amino acids can also be bioenergetics precursors; however, glucose is considered to be the only metabolic substrate in the brain. Glucose can also be metabolized via the pentose phosphate pathway (PPP), a process that generates pentoses and that is the most important cytosolic source of reduced nicotinamide adenine dinucleotide phosphate (NADPH), a cofactor for biosynthetic reactions and the oxidation-reduction involved in protecting against the oxidative stress, e.g. for fatty acids biosynthesis or regeneration of reduced glutathione. During activation the brain may transiently turn to anaerobic glycolysis occurring in astrocytes, followed by the oxidation of lactate by neurons [32-33]. Monocarboxylate transporters (MCTs) carry lactate or pyruvate across biological membranes; lactate dehydrogenase (LDH) catalyzes the interconversion of pyruvate and lactate with concomitant interconversion of NADH and NAD^+.

http://dx.doi.org/10.5772/53254

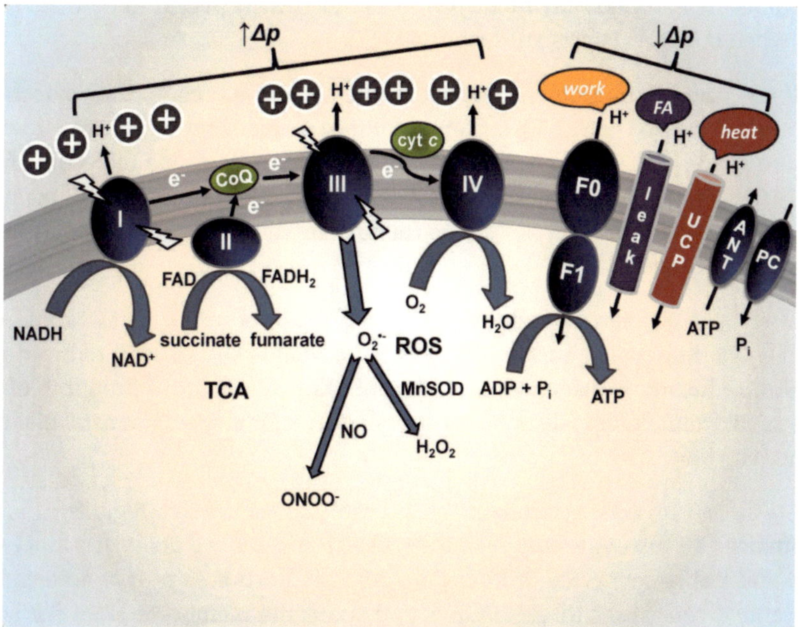

Figure 2. Representation of processes in the inner mitochondrial membrane. ETC consists of I - IV complexes that transfer electrons, pump protons outwardly, and create proton motive force (*Δp*). Complex I catalyses oxidation of nicotinamide adenine dinucleotide (NADH), complex II oxidizes succinate to fumarate. CoQ as a cofactor accepts electrons from complexes I and II, and carries them to complex III; the second mobile carrier cyt *c* move electrons from complex III to complex IV, where O_2 is finally reduced to water. The proton gradient is primarily consumed by F_0F_1 ATP synthase for ATP synthesis from ADP and inorganic phosphate P_i. Secondary consumers causing decreased *Δp* are uncoupling proteins (UCPs), they response to heat production, proton leak is mediated e.g. by FAs. Transport of ADP and ATP across the membrane is enabled by adenine nucleotide translocator (ANT); mitochondrial phosphate carrier protein (PC) catalyses movement of P_i into the mitochondrial matrix. Simultaneously, electron transport is accompanied by generation of reactive oxygen species (ROS), the highest amount of superoxide ($O_2^{\bullet-}$) is formed by complexes I and III. $O_2^{\bullet-}$ can be further transformed by manganese superoxide dismutase (MnSOD) to H_2O_2, or can react with nitric oxide (NO) to form peroxynitrite ($ONOO^-$). $O_2^{\bullet-}$ production leads to increased mitochondrial conductance through UCPs.

2.1.1. *Oxidative phosphorylation enzymes*

Complex I (EC 1.6.5.3, NADH: ubiquinone oxidoreductase, NADH dehydrogenase, NADH-ubiquinone oxidoreductase) is a crucial point of respiration. It catalyzes oxidation of reduced nicotinamide adenine dinucleotide (NADH), thus, regenerates NAD^+ for the TCA cycle and fatty acids (FAs) oxidation, and reduces coenzyme Q_{10} (ubiquinone, CoQ) to ubiquinol [39]. Four protons are pumped from the matrix into the intermembrane space during electron passing through the complex I. Complex I is also a rate-limiting enzyme for oxygen consumption in the synapses [40].

Complex II (EC 1.3.5.1, succinate:ubiquinone oxidoreductase, succinate dehydrogenase (ubiquinone)) is the side entry into Electron transport chain, directly involved in the TCA cycle. It is a 4 subunit membrane-bound lipoprotein, which couples the oxidation of succinate to the reduction of CoQ [41]. Complex II does not contribute to the proton gradient. Hence, complex II subunits are encoded only by nDNA, complex II is suspected to normalize the activity of ETC, when mtDNA defects are suspected [42].

Complex III (EC 1.10.2.2, ubiquinol:ferricytochrome-c oxidoreductase, CoQ-cytochrome *c* reductase) consists of two centers, Q_i center - facing to matrix; and Q_o center - oriented to intermembrane space [43]. Complex III catalyses the oxidation of one molecule of ubiquinol and the reduction of two molecules of cytochrome *c*. Reaction mechanism of complex III occurs in two steps called the Q cycle [44]. In the process of Q cycle four protons are released into the inter membrane space.

Complex IV (EC 1.9.3.1, ferrocytochrome-*c*:oxygen oxidoreductase, cytochrome *c* oxidase, COX) enables the terminal reduction of O_2 to H_2O, retains all partially reduced intermediates until full reduction is achieved [45]. The complex IV mediates pumping of 4 protons across the membrane. Previously, it was suggested as an endogenous metabolic marker for neuronal activity [46].

Complex V (EC 3.6.3.14, ATP synthase, F_oF_1-ATPase) consists of two regions: 1. F_1 portion is soluble domain with three nucleotide binding sites, it is localized above the inner side of the membrane and stably connected with F_o domain; 2. F_o portion is proton pore embedded in the membrane, it consists of three subunits and spans the membrane from the inner to the outer side [47-48]. This formation enables the conversion of electrochemical potential energy to chemical energy - a portion of the F_o rotates as the protons pass through the membrane and forces F_1 as motor to synthetize ATP [47,49].

2.1.2. *Monoamine oxidase*

Monoamine oxidase (MAO, EC 1.4.3.4) is located in the outer mitochondrial membrane and catalyses the oxidative deamination of amine neurotransmitters as well as xenobiotic amines. It regulates the metabolic degradation of catecholamines and serotonin (5-hydroxytryptamin, 5-HT) in neural and other target tissues. A major physiological role of intraneuronal MAO is to keep cytosolic monoamine concentrations very low. This membrane-bound enzyme is a flavoprotein, which use FAD as cofactor. The cofactor was identified as the site, where irreversible inhibitors of MAO are covalently linked [50-51]. It exists in two isoforms MAO-A and MAO-B, they differ in substrate preference, inhibitory specificity, tissue and cell distribution, and in immunological properties [52]. MAO-A metabolizes 5-HT and is sensitive to inhibition by low concentrations of clorgyline, whereas MAO-B prefers benzylamine or 2-phenylethylamine (PEA) as substrate and is sensitive to inhibition by low concentrations of *l*-deprenyl. Tyramine, tryptamine, dopamine, norepinephrine (NE) and epinephrine are equally well oxidized by both isoforms of MAO [50]. The high levels of both forms are found in the brain; MAO-B is found in dopamine-secreting neurons in the brain.

Monoamine metabolism by MAO involves oxidative deamination to corresponding aldehyde and free amine. Catalysis in MAO depends on the transfer of electrons to FAD, and mechanism-based inhibitors, such as the irreversible antidepressants, modify flavin [53]. The aldehyde is rapidly metabolized by aldehyde dehydrogenase to acidic metabolites. Metabolism of monoamines by MAO is a major source of hydrogen peroxide (H_2O_2) in the brain. Normally the H_2O_2 is then inactivated by glutathione peroxidase but it can be converted, chemically, by Fe^{2+} ions (Fenton reaction) into the highly reactive hydroxyl radical. This radical has widespread deleterious effects which can cause neuronal damage and death and may account for associated health-related problems [51,54].

MAOs have important role in brain development and function, and MAO inhibitors (MAOIs) have a range of potential therapeutic uses [53]. Generally, selective inhibitors of MAO-A and nonselective MAOIs seem to be effective in the treatment of patients with depression, panic disorder, and other anxiety disorders [55]. It is supposed that MAO-B inhibition may slow the course of various neurodegenerative disorders; so, selective inhibitors of MAO-B may be efficacious in treating of Parkinson's disease [56] and possibly Alzheimer's disease [57]. MAO-B is the sole type in human platelets and the amino acid sequences of MAO-B in both platelets and brain are identical [58]; thus, platelet MAO can be adopted as a useful surrogate model for the study of aspects of central neuronal function related to monoaminergic neurotransmission [3].

2.2. Regulation of OXPHOS

There are five levels of OXPHOS regulation: 1. direct modulation of ETC kinetic parameters, 2. regulation of intrinsic efficiency of OXPHOS (by changes in proton conductance, in the P/O ratio or in the channelling of ECT intermediate substrates), 3. mitochondrial network dynamics (fusion, fission, motility, membrane lipid composition, swelling), 4. mitochondrial biogenesis and degradation, 5. cellular and mitochondrial microenvironment [59].

OXPHOS efficiency is dependent on delivery of reducing equivalents into ETC and on activities of participating enzymes or enzyme complexes. The optimal efficiency and flow ratios are determined by control of complex I (reflects integrated cellular pathway) and complex II (TCA cycle precedes) [60]. Depletion of TCA cycle intermediates plays an important role in the OXPHOS flux control. In respirometry assays, supplies of complex I as well as complex II are required. Convergent electron input and reconstitution of the TCA cycle are needed to achieve maximal respiration [30]. It is controlled also by the availability of adenosine 5′-diphosphate (ADP) for the adenine nucleotide transporter in the inner mitochondrial membrane [61].

Complex I is suggested to be responsible for adaptive changes and physiological set up of OXPHOS efficiency [62]. The stoichiometric efficiency of OXPHOS is defined by the P/O ratio, or the amount of inorganic phosphate (P_i) incorporated into ATP per amount of consumed oxygen. P/O ratio was analysed in rat brain, liver and heart mitochondria. There were found tissue-specific differences and dependency of the P/O ratio on the respiratory rates with complex I, but not with complex II substrates [62]. Metabolic control analysis, which compared ETC activities and oxygen consumption rates, determined the role of complex I in rat brain synaptosomes. Results of the study suggest complex I as rate-limiting for oxygen consumption and responsible for high level of control over mitochondrial bioenergetics [40].

As mentioned above, mitochondria exhibit transmembrane potential across the inner membrane that is necessary for OXPHOS. Protons are transported outwardly and create proton motive force (Δp), which consists of electrical part $\Delta\psi_m$ (negative inside) and chemical part ΔpH [63-64]. In mitochondria, the Δp is made up of the $\Delta\psi_m$ mainly. The $\Delta\psi_m$ controls the ability of the mitochondria to generate ATP, generate ROS and sequester Ca^{2+} entering the cell. The $\Delta\psi_m$ and ATP synthesis express a degree of coupling; optimal ATP synthesis requires $\Delta\psi_m$ values between the range -100 mV and -150 mV. These values are reached primarily by $\Delta\psi_m$, which maintain at higher values (about -200 mV) and by secondary control mechanisms, which decrease the $\Delta\psi_m$ to lower levels [49]. Changes of $\Delta\psi_m$ influence permeability of biological membranes and ROS production, more negative $\Delta\psi_m$ (< -150 mV) leads to exponentially increased permeability as well as $O_2^{\bullet-}$ and H_2O_2 production [31]. Similarly, mitochondrial membranes increase exponentially their permeability for protons [49]. On the other hand, lower mitochondrial Δp and $\Delta\psi_m$ (e.g. caused by inhibition of respiratory chain) can result in hydrolysis of cytoplasmic ATP and slightly lower potential than that generated by the respiratory chain [65]. Therefore, $\Delta\psi_m$ is precisely controlled and can be regulated by various parameters.

ATP production is controlled by different mechanisms, depending on energy demands, thermogenesis, etc. [49]. First mechanism of OXPHOS control has been called as "respiratory control", and is based on feedback mechanisms controlling the rate of ATP synthesis, first of all by Δp and $\Delta\psi_m$. Higher levels of ADP in mitochondria lead to stimulation of ATP synthase together with decrease of Δp. Originally, pilot studies of OXPHOS dynamics used the terminology of respiratory steady states, described by Chance and Williams. Respiration was characterized by respiratory states (Table 1), by active state 3 (ADP stimulated) and followed by controlled state 4 (decrease after conversion of ADP to ATP) [66-67]. Decreased P/O ratio (caused mostly by increased Δp) leads to energy waste - proton leak (slip in COX), the decrease in the coupling, and increased thermogenesis [68]. However, conception of states had limited applicability in intact cells and in isolated mitochondria, did not include for instance COX, adenine nucleotide transporter, and extramitochondrial ATP/ADP ratio.

Recently, primary control has been implemented by secondary control mechanisms that are Δp independent [49,70]. Mitochondrial Ca^{2+} levels have been included [31]. Ca^{2+} transport was presumed to be important only in buffering of cytosolic Ca^{2+} by acting as sink under conditions of Ca^{2+} overload. When the cytoplasmic Ca^{2+} level was overloaded, Ca^{2+} accumulated in mitochondrial matrix and utilized $\Delta\psi_m$ [65,72-73]. Nowadays it is considered that Ca^{2+} regulates of activities of dehydrogenases via phosphorylation; ATP synthesis is switched on by cAMP-dependent phosphorylation and switched-off by calcium induced dephosphorylation [29,74].

In the TCA cycle, glycerophosphate dehydrogenase, pyruvate dehydrogenase, isocitrate dehydrogenase, and α-ketoglutarate dehydrogenase are influenced by Ca^{2+} levels and their phosphorylation lead to increased ATP production, production of glycogen, and glucose oxidation [73]. Reversible phosphorylation of pyruvate dehydrogenase complex mediated by calcium partly regulates the supply of reducing equivalents ($NADH/NAD^+$ ratio). Activation of the TCA cycle enhances the NADH production that triggers movement of electrons down complexes I through to complex IV by initially donating of complex I [75].

	ADP level	Substrate level	Respiration rate	Rate-limiting component	Relevance
State 1	Low	Low-endogenous	Slow	Phosphate acceptor	Initial activity of the sample
State 2	High	Approaching zero	Slow	Substrate	1. Exhaustion of endogenous substrate utilized in OXPHOS of ADP 2. Residual oxygen consumption (ROX)
State 3	High	High	Fast	Respiratory chain	1. OXPHOS capacity at saturating ADP (State P) 2. Electron transfer system capacity at optimum uncoupler concentration (State 3u)
State 4	Low	High	Slow	Phosphate acceptor	1. Exhaustion of added ADP 2. LEAK respiration (resting state when oxygen flux is maintained mainly to compensate for the proton leak after inhibition of ATP synthesis) (State 4o, L)
State 5	High	High	Zero	Oxygen	1. Anoxia 2. Antimycin A treatment

Table 1. Characterization of respiratory states [30,69]

Regulation of complex I and COX subunits via specific protein kinases and protein phosphatases was observed. cAMP-dependent protein kinase catalyses phosphorylation of complex I subunit and stimulates ETC [76]. At low Ca^{2+} levels, protein phosphatase dephosphorylates and inactivates complex I. It is presumed that COX is regulated by allosteric inhibition of ATP at high ATP/ADP ratios [31]. Extramitochondrial ATP/ADP ratios regulate COX activity by binding to the cytosolic subunit of COX, whereas high mitochondrial ATP/ADP ratios cause exchange of ATP by ADP at COX and induce allosteric inhibition [77]. Similarly, increased intracellular Ca^{2+} levels are suggested to activate mitochondrial phosphatase, which dephosphorylates COX and turns off the allosteric inhibition [78]. This respiratory control by phosphorylated enzyme is assumed to keep the Δp low as prevention of increased Δp, which leads to the slip of protons in COX and decreased H^+/e^- stoichiometry [79-80]. However, in isolated mitochondria high $\Delta\psi_m$ was measured even with high ATP/ADP ratios. The decrease was measured after addition of phosphoenolpyruvate and pyruvate kinase and could be explained as reversal of gluconeogenetic enzymes [61]. Under the physiological conditions, allosteric inhibition is modulated by increased Ca^{2+} levels, high substrate concentrations, and thyroid hormones. Ca^{2+} dependent dephosphorylation induced by hormones results in loss of respiratory control by the ATP/ADP ratio and associated with the increased Δp and respiration [79].

Thyroid hormone, mainly triiodothyronine (T3) and diiodothyronine (T2), has important effects on mitochondrial energetics and mitochondrial genome [81]. Mechanism of allosteric inhibition of COX has been closely linked to regulation by thyroid hormones. 3,5-diiodothyronine (T2) mediates short term effects of thyroid hormones and increases immediately basal metabolic rate. T2 is formed by intracellular deiodination of T3 and binds to specific T2 binding sites, which were identified in the inner mitochondrial membrane [82]. This binding to subunit Va of COX abolishes the allosteric inhibition of respiration by ATP [83] that could result in partial uncoupling of OXPHOS via increased $\Delta\psi_m$, and continue to intrinsic uncoupling of COX by higher membrane potentials [49]. Therefore, thyroid hormones enhance the proton permeability; hyperthyroidism stimulated mitochondrial proton leak and ATP turnover in rat hepatocytes, where non-mitochondrial oxygen consumption remained unchanged [84-85]. Oppositely, in rat hypothyroid cells significant decrease of non-mitochondrial oxygen consumption and proton leak were observed, ATP turnover was unaffected [86].

2.3. Proton permeability of membranes

OXPHOS in cells is not fully efficient. Decrease of the proton gradient across the inner mitochondrial membrane by "proton leak" causes uncoupling of fuel oxidation from ATP generation, and some energy is lost as heat. The mechanism of the basal proton conductance of mitochondria (insensitive to known activators and inhibitors) is not understood. There is correlation between mitochondrial proton conductance and composition of inner membrane: phospholipid fatty acyl polyunsaturation correlates positively and monounsaturation correlates negatively with proton conductance [87].

Uncoupling proteins (UCPs) and adenine nucleotide translocator (ANT) are two types of mitochondrial carrier, which cause inhibitor-sensitive inducible proton conductance. UCPs themselves do not contribute to the basal proton conductance of mitochondria; however, they are important metabolic regulators in permitting fat oxidation and in attenuating free radical production [88]. The amount of ANT present in the mitochondrial inner membrane strongly affects the basal proton conductance of the membrane and suggests that ANT is a major catalyst of the basal FA-independent proton leak in mitochondria [89].

2.3.1. Fatty acids

Long-chain fatty acids (FAs) are weak acids that can cross the membrane in both protonated and deprotonated forms. Effects of FAs are interrelated to 1. increase uncoupling, 2. increase ROS production, 3. opening mitochondrial permeability transition pores (MPTP) [90]. Further, they can modulate effects of thyroid hormones as well as sex steroid hormones [84]. FAs can act as like classic OXPHOS uncouplers with protonophoric action on the inner mitochondrial membrane and/or interactions of FAs with ADP carrier, COX and ATP synthase are presumed [91]. Recent study suggests that FAs are not only inducers of uncoupling, but they also regulate this process. It supposes that transport of FA anions participates in both ADP/ATP antiport and aspartate/glutamate antiport, at the same time [92]. On the other hand, studies using lipid membranes suppose that FAs are capable of spontaneous flip-flop [93]. Since FAs move across the membrane spontaneously and rapidly, no protein transporters are necessary. Further, coupling/uncoupling effects depend on their concentrations pH gradient across the membranes [94-95].

2.3.2. Uncoupling proteins

Uncoupling diverts a significant proportion of energy to thermogenesis. UCPs are mitochondrial carriers catalysing a regulated proton leak across the inner membrane [96-97]. There are five types of UCP in mammals. UCP1 is presented exclusively in the inner mitochondrial membrane of brown adipose tissue, and its main function is to catalyse adaptive thermogenesis [98]. It can be stimulated by FA and has synergic action of norepinephrine and thyroid hormones [49,99]. Concentrations of UCP2 and UCP3 in tissues are much lower than of UCP1, and their functions are not exactly known. They probably minimally contribute to basal metabolic rate, control of adaptive thermogenesis, preventive action against oxidative stress and ROS control, control of cellular energy balance, regulation of Ca^{2+} homeostasis, regulation of FA oxidation and ATP synthesis [100-103]. UCP2, UCP4 and UCP5 are present in the central nervous system (CNS); they have been suggested to have effects protecting neurons from the Ca^{2+} overload and/or oxidative stress [104-105].

UCP activities can be positively or negatively regulated by different factors. UCP are stimulated by FA and by ROS, generated by as a side reaction between CoQ and oxygen [106]. UCP mediate the FA dependent proton influx that leads to uncoupled ATP synthesis and heat production [107]. It is supposed that UCP and FA decrease $\Delta\psi_m$ if it is sufficiently high.

2.4. Reactive oxygen species production

Reduction of O_2 to water by aerobic respiration is accompanied by reactive intermediate formation. Generally, complex I and complex III are considered as the major $O_2^{\bullet-}$ sources [108].

Complex I releases $O_2^{\bullet-}$ to matrix, complex III can release $O_2^{\bullet-}$ to both sides of the inner mitochondrial membrane [109]. Additionally, other ROS sources, e.g. MAO, present in the outer mitochondrial membrane, and α-ketoglutarate dehydrogenase (α-KGDH), the TCA cycle enzyme complex, are able to generate H_2O_2. MAO catalyses the oxidative deamination of biogenic and xenobiotic monoamines and increases the amount of ROS in mitochondria. H_2O_2 production by α-KGDH is dependent on $NADH/NAD^+$ ratio. Higher NADH leads to higher H_2O_2 production, therefore, α-KGDH could significantly contribute to oxidative stress in mitochondria [110].

Physiologically generated H_2O_2 and $O_2^{\bullet-}$ from ETC are dependent on the magnitude of Δp and the respiratory state of mitochondria [111]. State 4 is characterized with high rate of ROS production, contrary to state 3 with high rate of oxygen uptake and slow ROS production. State 5, described as anoxic, with limited oxygen supply and lack of respiration produce minimum ROS [98,112]. In isolated rat liver mitochondria ROS production and $\Delta\psi_m$ were studied in state 3 and state 4. These states attenuate $\Delta\psi_m$ and ROS, correlation of ROS with $\Delta\psi_m$ was observed [113]. However, this correlation with respiratory states was not observed in the study using isolated mitochondria, ROS production correlated directly with $\Delta\psi_m$ [114].

Complex I is considered to be the primary source of ROS in brain under physiological conditions, as well as in pathological processes (e.g. neurodegenerative disorders). ROS seem to be the key factors in brain aging processes and mitochondrial respiration with ROS production significantly contributes to functional changes in brain during aging. Study in isolated rat mitochondria found significantly increased H_2O_2 production and 30 % reduction of complex I activity in aged rats [115]. Defective mitochondria release large amounts of ROS, similarly, decline of antioxidative enzyme activities (e.g. in elderly) enhances ROS production [116]. Negative results of ROS can affect respiratory chain: complexes I, III and IV seem to be the most affected, whereas function of complex II appears to be unchanged [117].

2.5. Apoptosis

Mitochondrial dysfunctions may accompany the clinical picture of neuropsychiatric disorders and contribute to neural apoptosis [118]; mitochondria play a pivotal role in intrinsic pathway of apoptosis [38]. Several interrelated mitochondrial pathways facilitate cell death: mitochondrial permeability transition (MPT) and the release of apoptotic cell death promoting factors, cytochrome *c* release by proapoptotic members of the Bcl-2 (B-cell lymphoma 2) family of proteins, disruption of ATP production, and alteration of the cell's redox status and overproduction of ROS [114]. If they are activated, change their conformations and induce formation of oligomers to form mitochondrial outer membrane pores, resulting to MPT. In apoptotic cells rapid loss of mitochondrial $\Delta\psi_m$ is accompanied by ROS production. Consequently, other proapoptotic proteins cytochrome *c* and Smac are released and trigger the caspase cascade leading to apoptosis [119]. Released cytochrome *c* in cytosol binds to apoptotic protease-activating factor-1 (Apaf-1) and induces formation of apoptosome [120]. MPT means alteration of permeability properties of membranes, originally was defined as increase of the inner mitochondrial membrane permeability to solutes of molecular mass less than 1500 Da [121]. Decreased MPT and activities of respiratory chain complexes, and increased ROS production were observed in cultured fibroblasts obtained from patients with CoQ deficiency [37]. MPT results from formation and opening of a channel known as MPTP. MPTP is dynamic multiprotein complex that span both the outer and inner mitochondrial membrane and contain the adenine nucleotide translocator (ANT) in the inner membrane, and the voltage-dependent anion channels (VDAC) in the outer membrane and cyclophilin D in the matrix [122]. Once open, MPTP allows the release of pro-apoptotic factors, such as cyt *c* and apoptosis inducing factor (AIF), into the cytoplasm.

2.6. Specific inhibitors of complexes of ETC

Rotenone is a specific complex I inhibitor, thenoyltrifluoroacetone (TTFA) specifically inhibits complex II. Both substances induce $O_2^{\bullet -}$ production that may result to major ROS production [45,123-124]. Pyrrolnitrin inhibits both complex I as well as complex II. It affects electron transport among NADH, CoQ and succinate, whereas COX remains unaffected [125].

Complex III inhibitors antimycin, myxothiazol and stigmatellin differ in their mechanism of action. Antimycin A inhibits the transfer of electrons from cytochrome *b* to CoQ, blocks the Q_i side of complex III. Oppositely, myxothiazol or stigmatellin block electron transfer from reduced CoQ at Q_o side [75]. Stigmatellin inhibits transfer of electrons and recycling of CoQ; myxothiazol inhibits electron transfer from reduced CoQ to cytochrome *c* [126].

http://dx.doi.org/10.5772/53254

Complex IV inhibitors KCN and sodium azide decrease COX activity [127]. Azide specifically blocks crossover between cytochrome *a* and cytochrome a_3. Further, it inhibits succinate oxidase activity specific for active respiration (state 3), but without any significant inhibition of state 4 [128]. Inhibition of COX by KCN is reversible, cyanide inhibits both electron and proton transport of COX [129]. Complex V is inhibited by oligomycin, which blocks its proton channel (F_o subunit). This inhibitor increases $\Delta\psi_m$ and is used to prevent state 3 of respiration. Oligomycin induces artificially state 4, i.e. state of respiration independent of ADP phosphorylation or resting state (LEAK) [130].

During the oxidation of complex I substrates (pyruvate, malate, glutamate), rotenone inhibition did not increase H_2O_2; contrary, oxidation of complex I and II substrates in the presence of antimycin A increased H_2O_2. Both myxothiazol and stigmatellin inhibited $O_2^{\bullet-}$ production and/or should inhibit the effect of antimycin [126,131]. The maximum of $O_2^{\bullet-}$ production has been observed in human skin fibroblasts with the prolonged treatment of rotenone, but not with antimycin A [132]. Interestingly, rotenone prevented antimycin A to induce ROS production in complex I, but not in complex II [43]. Q_o side of complex III was found as the source of increased $O_2^{\bullet-}$ after transient exposure to hydrogen peroxide [75]. KCN and sodium azide increase ROS formation [126]. Oligomycin induces hyperpolarization of inner mitochondrial membrane and can increase $O_2^{\bullet-}$ levels [133].

2.7. Mitochondria and neuroplasticity

Mitochondrial distribution and activity are key factors in neuronal morphogenesis - synaptogenesis, developmental and synaptic plasticity and axogenesis. During the development, neuronal stem cells proliferate and differentiate into neurons; subsequently axons and dendrites form synapses [134-135]. The role of mitochondria in neuroplasticity is illustrated in Figure 3 [20]. Due to ATP production and importance of mitochondria in synaptic ion homeostasis and phosphorylation reactions, mitochondria would be accumulated at sites where ATP consumption and Ca^{2+} concentration are higher. It was reported that mitochondria are more abundant in the regions of growing axons than in the non-growing axons. Mitochondrial net movement is anterograde in growing axons and is retrograde in non-growing axons. Shortly before axogenesis mitochondria congregate at the base of the neurite that is destined to become the axon. Nerve growth factor (NGF) was found as one of the signals inducing accumulation of mitochondria in the active growing cone [136]. Interestingly, when the ATP production is impaired and cells provide alternative source of energy, axogenesis is abolished although growth of dendrites remains relatively unaffected [134].

There are changes in mitochondrial energy metabolism occurring in brain cells during CNS development. During embryonic and early postnatal development fats are primarily used, later on, glucose becomes as fuel. This fact supports the role of mitochondria in biochemical requirements of highly proliferative neuronal stem cells and post-mitotic neurons. During neuronal differentiation the number of mitochondria per cell increases, but the velocity at which individual mitochondria move decreases as neurite outgrowth slows and synaptogenesis occurs [20,137].

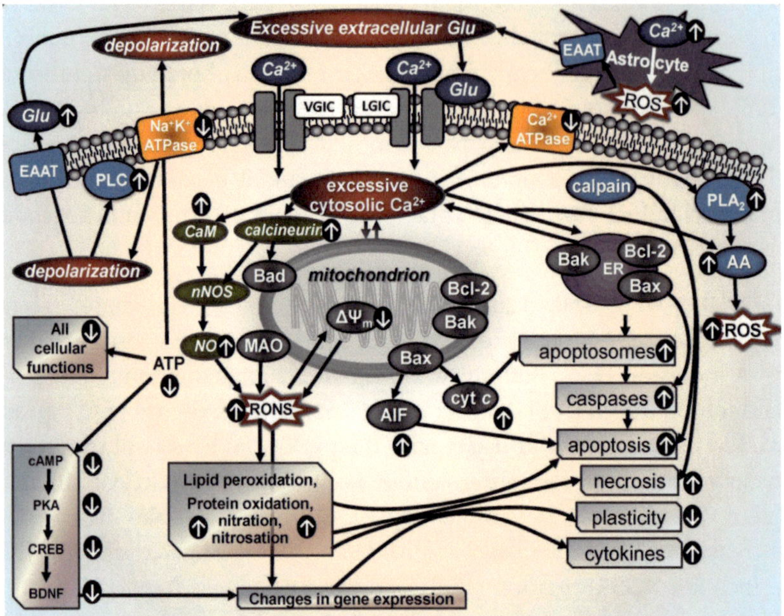

Figure 3. The role of mitochondria in neuroplasticity [20]. Principal mechanisms leading to neuronal impairment and cell death are composed of decreased ATP production, increased production of reactive oxygen and nitrogen species (RONS), initiation of apoptotic processes and impaired calcium homeostasis. Exhaustion of energy supplies and decreased ATP production lead to impairment of ATP dependent processes and therefore to changed cellular functions. Insufficient function of Na^+/K^+- ATPases leads to disturbances of ion transmembrane gradients, efflux of K^+, and influx of Na^+, Cl^- and Ca^{2+}. Increased extracellular concentrations of K^+ mediate depolarisation of membranes and change the functions of amino acids transporters. Voltage gated ion channels (VGIC) and ligand dependent calcium channels (LGIC) are activated and mediate increased cytosolic calcium concentrations. Intracellular calcium causes functional changes of amino acid transporters and enhances the increased extracellular concentrations of excitatory amino acids, glutamate especially, and extends neurotoxicity. Increased levels of synaptic glutamate can be mediated by release of glutamate from astrocytes. Following bound of glutamate to NMDA and AMPA receptors causes higher Ca^{2+} influx into cell, calcium activates phospholipases, proteases, and endonucleases, which degrade membranes, proteins and nucleic acid. E.g. activation of phospholipase A_2 (PLA_2) by calcium releases membrane arachidonic acid (AA), which induces production of superoxide. High intracellular calcium levels cause overload of mitochondrial calcium, increase ROS production, and inhibit ATP production. Activation of calcium dependent protein phosphatases (e.g. calcineurin) causes translocation of proapoptotic factor Bad into the mitochondria and triggers apoptosis by sequestration of anti-apoptotic factors Bcl-2 and Bcl-xL. Release of cytochrome c and other proapoptotic factors from the intermembrane space of mitochondria induce the formation of apoptosome, and consequently trigger activation of caspases and apoptosis. Apoptosis inducing factor (AIF) is another factor released by mitochondria. Disengaged AIF is transported into nucleus and trigger caspases-independent apoptosis. Mitochondria in brain are also a target of nitric oxide (NO) action; AA - arachidonic acid; AIF - apoptosis inducing factor; Bax, Bad, Bad - proapoptotic factors of Bcl-2 family; Bcl-2 - antiapoptotic factor of Bcl-2 family; BDNF - brain-derived neurotrophic factor; CaM - calmoduline; cAMP - cyclic adenosine monophosphate; CREB - cAMP response element-binding protein; cyt *c* - cytochrome *c*; $\Delta\psi_m$ - potential on the inner mitochondrial membrane; EAAT - excitatory amino acid transporter; ER - endoplasmic reticulum; Glu - glutamate; MAO - monoamine oxidase; nNOS - neuronal nitric oxide synthase; NO - nitric oxide; PKA - protein kinase A; PLA_2 - phospholipase A_2; PLC - phospholipase C; LGIC - ligand-gated ion channel; RONS, reactive oxygen and nitrogen species; ROS - reactive oxygen species; RNS - reactive nitrogen species; VGIC - voltage-gated ion channel

It was demonstrated that neuronal activity is influenced by the mitochondrial functions, defective trafficking and dysfunction of mitochondria from axon terminals is implicated in the pathogenesis of axonal degeneration [138-140]. In addition, dendritic mitochondria are essential in the morphogenesis and plasticity of spines and synapses [141]. Recent findings suggest roles for mitochondria as mediators of at least some effects of glutamate and BDNF on synaptic plasticity [136]. BDNF promotes synaptic plasticity, in part, by enhancing mitochondrial energy production. It increases glucose utilization and increases mitochondrial respiratory coupling at complex [62,142].

Mitochondria are dynamic organelles; their function is modulated by fission, fusion and moving within the axons and dendrites [38]. Their structure, functions and properties differ in axons and dendrites [141,143]. Transport and positioning of mitochondria are essential for neuronal homeostasis and the mitochondrial movement is a part of regulation by intracellular signals.

3. Advances in biological hypotheses of mood disorders

Findings about intracellular processes associated with mood disorders and long-term effects of antidepressants demonstrate an important role of signalling pathways primarily regulated by monoamine neurotransmitters; this was settled as the basis of many biochemical hypotheses [144-145]. While dysfunctions within monoaminergic neurotransmitter systems are likely to play an important role in pathophysiology of mood disorders, it probably represents the downstream effects of more primary abnormalities in signal transduction. Thus, new theories about the pathophysiology of depression and the action of antidepressant treatment proposes that mood disorders are caused by structural or functional changes in particular molecules and signalling pathways in the brain, and that antidepressants function by counteracting these molecular changes. It is supposed that structural and functional brain abnormalities in patients with depressive disorder may be associated with low levels of brain-derived neurotrophic factor (BDNF), abnormal function of hypothalamic-pituitary-adrenal (HPA) axis, glutamatergic toxicity, activation of inflammatory and cell-mediated immune response, decreased antioxidant capacity and increased oxidative and nitrosative stress, disturbed chronobiological rythms, and mitochondrial dysfunctions [2,146-148].

Research on the biological basis of mood disorders emphasises the changes of neural networks and synaptic plasticity. Evidence exists for impairment of neuroplasticity in major depression. Chronic stress is known to contribute both to development of major depression in vulnerable persons and to reduction of synaptic plasticity, induction of structural changes in dendrites, and impairment of neurogenesis [1]. Mitochondria may be primary regulators of these processes, as they regulate not only neuronal survival and death, but also plasticity. There is mounting evidence for the role of mitochondrial dysfunction in the pathophysiology and treatment of bipolar disorder [11].

3.1. Monoamine hypothesis

Discovery of the first effective antidepressants, MAOIs and tricyclic antidepressants, implied hypothesis about significant role for the biogenic amine, particularly NE and 5-HT in the ethiopathogenesis of affective disorders. Classic monoamine hypothesis is an early milestone in the field of depression. It proposed that depression might be produced by a 5-HT or NE deficiency at functionally important receptor sites in the brain, i.e. that brain monoamine systems have a primary direct role in depression [149-150]. Soon it became evident that the monoamine hypothesis in its original form could not explain all of the effects of antidepressants [151-152]. In order to test this hypothesis, a series of studies was conducted to evaluate effects of monoamine depletion on depressive symptoms in depressed patients and in healthy controls. Relapse to 5-HT depletion or to catecholamine depletion was found to be specific to the type of antidepressant treatment and type of depletion. 5-HT or NE/dopamine depletion did not decrease mood in healthy controls and slightly lowered mood in healthy controls with a family history of major depressive disorder. In drug-free patients with major depressive disorder in remission, a moderate mood decrease was found for acute tryptophan depletion only. However, acute tryptophan depletion induced relapse in patients in remission who used serotonergic antidepressants [153]. Depletion studies failed to demonstrate a causal relation between 5-HT and NE with depressive disorder [154-155]. The effects of acute tryptophan depletion on cognition in non-vulnerable participants are independent of mood changes [155]. Even simultaneous disruption of 5-HT and catecholamine systems didn't significantly alter mood in unmedicated depressed subjects [156]. These findings forced a major revision of the classic monoamine hypothesis of depression. According to this revised monoamine theory of depression [148,157] monoamine systems are only modulating other brain neurobiological systems that have more primary role in depression.

3.2. Neurotrophic hypothesis

The neurotrophic hypothesis of depression [5-6,8] supposed that vulnerability to depression can arise as a result of neuronal damage, e.g. after chronic stress, long-term increased levels of glucocorticoids, hypoglycemia, ischemia, effects of neurotoxins or certain viral infections, etc. The therapeutic effects of antidepressants consist in the increased function of the noradrenergic or serotonergic system, leading to increased activity of transcription factor CREB (cAMP response element binding protein), higher expression of neurotrophin BDNF and its receptor trkB, and consequently to increased neuronal plasticity and resumption of cellular functions.

According to neurogenic hypothesis [158-159], depression may develop due to the decreased neurogenesis in hippocampus, and antidepressants takes effect through the stimulation of neurogenesis. Hypothesis of cellular plasticity [160] relate the neurotrophic and the neurogenic hypothesis to the statement that depression can be generally caused by damaged cellular plasticity leading to inadequate relations between structure and function. Molecular mechanisms leading to a disturbance of neuroplasticity are not known. The bioenergetic and neurochemical model of bipolar disorder attempts to identify these mechanisms and focuses attention on mitochondrial dysfunctions [9,161].

3.3. Inflammatory and neurodegenerative hypothesis

The central nervous system, endocrine and immune systems use neurotransmitters, cytokines and hormones to communicate among them [162]. Now there is evidence that the activation of the immune system is associated with the symptoms of depression [163-164]. The inflammatory and neurodegenerative hypothesis of depression [165] supposes that depression is associated with both inflammatory processes, as well as with neurodegeneration and reduced neurogenesis. According to this hypothesis, enhanced neurodegeneration and impaired neurogenesis in depression are caused by inflammatory processes, related to the production of oxidative and nitrosative stress, tryptophan catabolites along the indoleamine-2,3-dioxygenase pathway, proinflammatory cytokines and lowered ω-3 polyunsaturated fatty acid status. Anti-inflammatory compounds should be able to counteract at least partly the enhanced neurodegeneration and decreased neurogenesis.

3.4. Mitochondrial hypothesis

Mitochondrial dysfunctions (leading to decreased ATP production, oxidative stress, and induction of apoptosis) occur in the early stages of different neurodegenerative diseases, associated often with mood disorders.

The role of mitochondrial dysfunction during bipolar disorder is supported both by observation of the changes of brain metabolism and by effects of mood stabilizers (lithium and valproate) on mitochondrial functions. Metabolic changes in brain were observed in bipolar disorder by magnetic resonance spectroscopy (MRS). It suggests the presumptions that mitochondrial dysfunctions include impaired OXPHOS, final shift to glycolytic production of energy, general decrease of energy (decreased ATP production), changed concentrations of phosphomonoesters and changed lipid metabolism [9].

mtDNA mutations in the brain, associations of mtDNA polymorphisms and bipolar disorder and changes in gene expression related to mitochondria in the brain were observed [10,166]. Mitochondrial dysfunction hypothesis of bipolar disorder is based on these observations. According to this hypothesis, mtDNA polymorphisms/mutations or mtRNA deletions caused by nuclear gene mutations can cause mitochondrial dysregulation of calcium leading to symptoms of bipolar disorder [10,161,167]. Mitochondrial hypothesis corresponds to, above mentioned, neurotrophic hypothesis because of an important role of calcium signalling pathway in synaptic plasticity regulation.

3.5. Biological markers of mood disorders

Biological markers are defined as a characteristic that is objectively measured and evaluated as an indicator of normal biologic processes, pathogenic processes, or pharmacologic responses to a therapeutic intervention. In medicine, a biomarker is an indicator of a particular disease state or a particular state of an organism.

Identification of biologic markers of mood disorders and factors capable of predicting the response to treatment with antidepressants has not been sufficiently successful [3,168-169].

In accordance to actual neurochemical hypotheses of mood disorders, biological markers have been primarily found at the level of neurotransmitter concentrations, their metabolites or precursors. Subsequently, attention was shifted to the receptor systems, and since the 1990′s, intracellular processes have become main interest. The chance to find sensitive and specific biological predictors of antidepressant treatment has been increased, because of introduction of new methods of molecular biology. These methods enable us better observation of cellular processes connected with the transduction of nervous signals in the brain. The choice of parameters, which should be studied as perspective biological markers of mood disorders, have been derived first of all from new findings of signalling pathways involved in neurotransmission and from above mentioned neurochemical hypotheses of mood disorders. From the view of intracellular processes, energetic metabolism, activities of PKC, CREB, BDNF, Bcl-2, glycogen synthase kinase-3, caspases or calcium could play a principal role in findings of biological markers of mood disorders. According to the complexity and connectivity of signalling pathways involved in etiopathogenesis of mood disorders, number of chosen parameters is not final.

4. Antidepressants, mood stabilizers and mitochondrial functions

Antidepressants are used mainly to alleviate mood disorders, such as major depression and dysthymia and anxiety disorders. Mood stabilizers are psychiatric medication used in treatment of mood disorders, which are characterized by intense and sustained mood shifts (e.g. bipolar disorder).

The antidepressant activity of the first generation of antidepressants, tricyclic antidepressants and MAOIs, was explained by their effects on availability of monoamine neurotransmitters. The next generations of antidepressants included selective serotonin reuptake inhibitors (SSRIs), norepinephrine reuptake inhibitors (NRIs), serotonin-norepinephrine reuptake inhibitors (SNRI), noradrenergic and specific serotonergic antidepressants (NaSSAs), norepinephrine-dopamine reuptake inhibitors (NDRIs), serotonin antagonist and reuptake inhibitors (SARIs), selective serotonin reuptake enhancer (SSRE), melatonergic agonists (MASSA), sigma receptor agonists etc. The therapeutic response to antidepressants occurs after long-term treatment; therefore, effects of antidepressants are linked to cellular adaptations including density and/or sensitivity of neurotransmitter receptors and transporters, regulation of signal transduction cascades, and changes in gene expression [170].

Most of mood stabilizers are anticonvulsants (valproate, carbamazepine, and lamotrigine), with an important exception of lithium, which is the oldest and the best known mood stabilizing drug. Some atypical antipsychotics (olanzapine, quetiapine, aripiprazole, risperidone, ziprasidone) have mood stabilizing effects, as well.

Although a wide range of pharmacologically different antidepressants and mood stabilizers is available, molecular mechanisms of their therapeutic effects haven't yet been sufficiently clarified. Relatively little information is known about the association among therapeutic and/or adverse effects of drugs and mitochondrial enzyme activities. Incomplete data exist on the effect of pharmacologically selective antidepressants and mood stabilizers on MAO activity. Measurement of both mitochondrial respiration and membrane potential during action of appropriate endogenous and exogenous substances enables the identification of the primary sites of effectors and the distribution of control, allowing deeper quantitative analyses [171].

4.1. Inhibition of MAO

MAO inhibition is the best known direct action of some antidepressants on mitochondrial enzymes. The antidepressant effect of MAOIs has been established more than 50 years ago. Iproniazid became the first MAO inhibitor to be used successfully in the treatment of depression; it is an irreversible and nonselective MAO inhibitor [172]. It is known to act as a pro-drug and can be converted into isopropyl hydrazine which binds covalently to MAO [173]. Clorgyline is an irreversible inhibitor preferential for MAO-A, structurally related to pargyline (MAO-B inhibitor). It has antidepressant activity, and may potentially be useful in the treatment of Parkinson's disease. Selegiline (l-deprenyl) is an irreversible inhibitor preferential for MAO-B; it is used for the treatment of Parkinson's disease, depression and senile dementia. Inhibitors of MAO lose its selectivity at high doses. Moreover, there are feedbacks and interconnections of intracellular signalling pathways which lead to mutual interactions of monoaminergic and other systems [4]. So, inhibiting of MAO-B should influence processes mediated primarily by substrates for MAO-A, and vice versa. The major disadvantage was the incidence of the cheese reaction with those early inhibitors [51].

The selective reversible MAO-A inhibitors such as moclobemide increase the content of 5-HT, NE and dopamine in the brain [174] but did not provoke the cheese reaction. Moclobemide has been extensively evaluated in the treatment of a wide spectrum of depressive disorders and social phobia. Overall, moclobemide appears to be safe and devoid of major side effects, although it is considered as a mild antidepressant, better tolerated by older patients [175-181]. Moclobemide undergoes extensive metabolism with less than 1 % of the dose being excreted unchanged. Metabolic pathways of moclobemide include mainly oxidative attack on the morpholine moiety [182]. However, major metabolites in plasma were found to be less effective MAO-A inhibitors than moclobemide or pharmacologically inactive [183-184].

MAO inhibitors were developed as antidepressants but many drugs, including the oxazolidinone antibacterial agents, share similar molecular properties and have MAO inhibitory activity. These compounds were of interest as potential antidepressants because they could be selective inhibitors of either the A or B isoforms and were usually reversible [53].

Antidepressants which act primarily as 5-HT and/or NE reuptake inhibitors show inhibitory activity towards MAO also. It has been suggested that tricyclic antidepressants exert some of their therapeutic effect by inhibiting MAO [185]. They are able to inhibit MAO-B both *in vitro* [186-187] and *in vivo* [188-189]. However, *in vivo* inhibition of the human platelet MAO-B in the patients taking tricyclic antidepressants was not confirmed by others [190-191]. Five tricyclic antidepressants, amitriptyline, clomipramine, desipramine, imipramine and iprindole, have comparable potencies as inhibitors of MAO in rodent brain and liver [192]. These antidepressants have been shown to partially protect mouse brain MAO *in vivo* from the irreversible enzyme inhibition produced by subsequent injection of phenelzine [193]. Concentrations of tricyclic antidepressants, which showed a pronounced inhibitory effect on the MAOs activity, were significantly higher than plasma levels of the drug found under therapeutic conditions [194-195]. MAO activity was inhibited after long-term administration of viloxazine, nomifensine, zimelidine, maprotiline, imipramine, amitriptyline, and nortriptyline in systematic studies of Egashira [196-197]. Competitive inhibition of MAO-A and noncompetitive inhibition of MAO-B was found for these drugs. Similar results were obtained when different tricyclic antidepressants and SSRIs were examined with isolated rat brain mitochondria [198]. Fluoxetine and norfluoxetine showed affinities both for MAO-A [199] and MAO-B [200]. Fluoxetine and norfluoxetine also significantly inhibited the binding of the specific radioligands to MAO *in vivo*. These results support a potential role of MAO inhibition in the therapeutic effects of fluoxetine.

4.2. Effects of antidepressants on mitochondrial functions

There is relatively little data about effects of antidepressants on mitochondrial functions as summarized in the Table 2. *In vitro* study examined influence of pharmacologically different antidepressants and mood stabilizers on activity both mitochondrial MAO [201] and respiratory chain complexes; imipramine, desipramine, amitriptyline, citalopram, and mirtazapine were found as complex I inhibitors in isolated pig brain mitochondria [202]. In isolated rat liver mitochondria effects of imipramine and clomipramine were compared to classic uncouplers, drugs enhanced ATP synthase activity, hindered ATP synthesis and released respiratory control [203]. In isolated rat liver mitochondria, nefazodone was found as inhibitor of mitochondrial complexes I and IV; buspirone inhibited complex I but had no effect on complex IV. Trazodone did not affect on both complex I and complex IV [204], but decreased oxygen consumption and reduced Na^+, K^+-ATPase activity. Trazodone acts also as uncoupler of OXPHOS [205].

Effects of antidepressants on apoptotic markers, e.g. cytochrome *c* release and DNA fragmentation, seem to be different. Various antidepressants exhibited potential anticancer properties and caused cytotoxic effects. Paroxetine, fluoxetine and clomipramine increased levels of apoptotic markers leading to apoptosis in glioma and neuroblastoma cells, whereas imipramine and mianserin do not [206]. Desipramine induced apoptosis in rat glioma cells by activation of caspases, without any change of mitochondrial membrane potential $\Delta\psi_m$ [207]. Fluoxetine and amitriptyline protected PC12 cells from cell death induced by hydrogen peroxide [208]. Amitriptyline and tranylcypromine prevented the loss of mitochondrial $\Delta\psi_m$, over expression of Bax, reduction in Bcl-2 level, cytochrome *c* release, caspase-3 activation, and formation of ROS. In contrast, fluoxetine seemed to have additive toxic effect to 1-methyl-4-phenylpyridinium (MPP^+) against neuronal cell damage by increasing mitochondrial damage and oxidative stress [209]. Nortriptyline was identified as strong inhibitor of MPT and was observed as potential inhibitor of neuronal cell death; it protected isolated mitochondria against programmed cell death, inhibited release of apoptotic mitochondrial factors and caspases, increased Ca^{2+} retention in mitochondria and delayed the Ca^{2+} induced loss of $\Delta\psi_m$, further leading to neuronal cell death [210-211].

4.3. Effects of mood stabilizers on mitochondrial functions

Mood stabilizers affect multiple sites in intracellular signalling pathways [4]. Main targets of mood stabilizers are neurotrophin BDNF, ERK pathway, and pathways modulated by GSK-3 or Bcl-2 [8,226-227]. Molecular and cellular targets of mood stabilizers include enzymes inhibited by lithium (inositol monophosphatase, inositol polyphosphate 1-phosphatase, GSK-3, fructose 1,6-bisphosphatase, bisphosphate nucleotidase, phosphoglucomutase), enzymes inhibited by valproate (succinate semialdehyde dehydrogenase, succinate semialdehyde reductase, histone deacetylase), targets of carbamazepine (sodium channels, adenosine receptors, adenylate cyclase), and components of signalling pathways regulated by multiple drugs (PKC, cAMP, arachidonic acid) [228]. Furthermore, lithium and valproate reduce transport of myo-inositol into the cells, which leads to reduced PKC activity. Lithium and valproate increase Bcl-2 concentrations [229] and inhibit GSK-3 activity (lithium directly, valproate indirectly). Valproate activates MAPK signalling pathway and regulates stress proteins of ER [230]. Through the effects on Bcl-2 and p53 (proapoptotic protein), lithium affects mitochondria by stabilization of membrane integrity and prevention of MPTPs opening; i.e. by regulating the key process in cell death leading to at least temporary loss of $\Delta\psi_m$, input of water into matrix and equilibration of ions concentrations. Both lithium and valproate have neuroprotective effects based on protection from glutamatergic neurotoxicity by inactivation of NMDA receptors, on activation of cell survival factors such as phosphoinositide 3-kinase/protein kinase B pathway, and on induction of neurotrophic and neuroprotective proteins. Lithium protects against DNA damage, caspases activation, and apoptosis of neurons [231]. Increased concentrations of N-acetyl aspartate (NAA, marker of neuronal viability and functionality) in grey matter after the chronic lithium administration support its strong neuroprotective and neurotrophic effects in humans.

Effects of mood stabilizers on monoaminergic activity have been studied; majority of data is about the effects of lithium. Lithium enhances the antidepressant effect both of MAOIs and inhibitors of the reuptake of 5-HT and/or NE [232-234]. The mode of action for the lithium augmentation of antidepressants is partly mediated by an increase of 5-HT neurotransmission [235-237]. However, lithium could not either inhibit MAO-A or MAO-B in the brain mitochondrial [195,201]. Unipolar and bipolar depressive patients showed significantly higher platelet MAO activity than controls, but there was no significant change in activity after the institution of lithium treatment [191].

Antidepressant	Biological model	Affected mitochondrial function	Reference
Imipramine	Isolated rat liver mitochondria Beef heart submitochondrial particles	Uncoupling effects on OXPHOS (release of respiratory control, hindered ATP synthesis, enhanced ATP synthase activity) Inhibition NADH oxidation, inhibition of ATP synthase	[203]
Imipramine	Rat brain mitochondria	Increased state 3 and state 4 respiratory rates	[212]
Imipramine	Rat liver mitochondria	Increased state 3 and state 4 respiratory rates	[213]

Antidepressant	Biological model	Affected mitochondrial function	Reference
Imipramine, clomipramine, citalopram	Human peripheral lymphocytes and lymphoblasts	Dose-dependent induction of apoptosis	[214,215]
Imipramine, clomipramine, citalopram	Human acute myeloid leukaemia HL-60 cells	Loss in cell viability, increased ROS production, loss of $\Delta\psi_m$	[216]
Clomipramine, desipramine, norfluoxetine, Tianeptine	Rat heart isolated mitochondria and CHO cells	Reductions of $\Delta\psi_m$, decrease in state 3 respiration, inhibition of activities of complexes I, II/III and IV Insignificant change of $\Delta\psi_m$, decrease in state 3 respiration, inhibition of complex I activity	[217]
Tianeptine	Rat liver mitochondria	Inhibited beta-oxidation and TCA cycle	[218]
Fluoxetine	Rat liver mitochondria	Inhibition of state 3 respiration, stimulation of state 4 respiration, decrease of RCR and uncoupling effects on OXPHOS	[219]
Fluoxetine	Rat brain mitochondria	Inhibition of OXPHOS, decreased activity of ATP synthase	[220]
Amitriptyline, fluoxetine	Differentiated rat pheocytochroma PC12 cells	Prevention of the loss of $\Delta\psi_m$, cyt *c* release, formation of ROS induced by MPP^+	[209]
Amitriptyline, fluoxetine	Rat pheocytochroma cells	Attenuation of H_2O_2 neurotoxic effects, upregulation of superoxide dismutase	[208]
Nortriptyline	*ALS mouse	Strong inhibitor of MPT	[210]
Nortriptyline	Mouse model of ischemia	Inhibition of $\Delta\psi_m$, inhibited release of mitochondrial factors and caspase 3 activation	[211]
Nortriptyline	Rat brain mitochondria	Inhibitor of MPT, inhibition of ETC, mild uncoupling	[221]
Fluoxetine and/or Olanzapine	Rat brain homogenates	Increased citrate synthase activity after acute, but not chronic treatment	[222]
Nefazodone Trazodone	Isolated rat liver mitochondria	Severe inhibition of oxygen consumption, inhibition complexes I and IV Modest inhibition of oxygen consumption, inhibition of complex I	[204]
Nefazodone Trazodone	Isolated rat liver mitochondria	Complex I and complex IV inhibitor No effects	[205]
Fluoxetine	Hippocampal synaptic plasma membranes	Increased ATP synthase activity	[223]

http://dx.doi.org/10.5772/53254

Antidepressant	Biological model	Affected mitochondrial function	Reference
Sertraline	Isolated rat liver mitochondria	Uncoupling effects on OXPHOS, inhibition of complex I and complex V activities, induction of Ca^{2+} mediated MPT	[224]
Venlafaxine, paroxetine, nortriptiline	Rat brain homogenates (after 15 days of drug administration)	Differences in brain areas: increased or unchanged citrate synthase and SDH activities	[225]
Paroxetine, fluoxetine, klomipramine	Rat glioma and human neuroblastoma cell lines	Increased cyt *c* release, caspase-3-like activity, induction of apoptosis	[206]
Desipramine	Rat glioma cells	Activation of caspases 3 and 9, no changes of $\Delta\psi_m$	[207]
ALS mouse – model of neurodegeneration			

Table 2. Effects of antidepressants on mitochondrial functions

Studies have shown effects of mood stabilizing drugs on mitochondria. In isolated brain mitochondria lithium caused desensitisation to calcium, antagonized permeability transition, and diminished cytochrome *c* release [238]. In isolated rat liver mitochondria valproate inhibited OXPHOS [239]. In isolated pig brain mitochondria both lithium and valproate inhibited respiratory chain complexes I and IV [202]. According to study performed in rats [240], valproate reversed the decreased activity of citrate synthase caused by amphetamine and lithium prevented the inhibition. The cytoprotective effect of lithium and valproate was observed after 7 days, of pre-treatment of human neuroblastoma (SH-SY5Y) cells against cytotoxicity resulting from oxidative stress evoked by rotenone and H_2O_2. This effect was not observed after one day of pre-treatment [241]. Chronic treatment of SH-SY5Y cells prevents reduction of methamphetamine-induced reduction of cytochrome *c*, mitochondrial antiapoptotic Bcl-2/Bax ratio and mitochondrial COX activity [242]. Interestingly, long-term lithium and valproate did not protect SH-SY5Y cells against endoplasmic reticulum stress-induced cytotoxicity [241]. Lithium and carbamazepine could facilitate activation of CREB, valproate and lamotrigine did not affect BDNF-mediated signalling [243]. Thus, these mood stabilizers likely decrease the vulnerability of mitochondrial functions caused by oxidative stress and have neuroprotective effects [241].

Chronic treatment with lithium, valproate and carbamazepine protects against NMDA-mediated toxicity [244]. Interestingly, recent study performed with epileptic children examined the influence of carbamazepine and lamotrigine on mitochondrial functions - both drugs influenced respiratory chain complexes and significantly affected ATP production, carbamazepine decreased the production, oppositely to stimulatory effect of lamotrigine [245]. Carbamazepine interferes in adenylate cyclase pathway: inhibits adenylate cyclase and the synthesis of cAMP [246]. Lamotrigine prevented the toxicity caused by rotenone and MPP^+ in rat PC12 cells by suppressing the MPT formation, which leads to cytochrome *c* release and subsequent apoptosis. Though, lamotrigine seems to have neuroprotective effect due to the mitochondrial respiratory complex I inhibition [247].

Effects of mood stabilizers on mitochondrial functions are summarized in the Table 3.

Mood stabilizer	Biological model	Affected mitochondrial function	Reference
Valproate	Rat liver mitochondrial fractions	Inhibition of oxygen consumption rate, sequestration of intramitochondrial CoA	[248]
Valproate	Isolated rat liver mitochondria	State 3 rates of oxygen consumption inhibited	[239]
Valproate	Isolated beef brain α-KGDH	Inactivation of α-KGDH complex	[249]
Valproic acid	Isolated rat hepatocytes	CoA, acetyl-CoA and long chain acyl-CoA fractions decreased (accumulation of valproyl-CoA; without any evidence of this metabolite in brain tissue)	[250]
Valproate and its metabolites	Submitochondrial particles from rat liver	Inhibition of pyruvate uptake	[251]
Valproate	Rat liver mitochondria. Digitonin permeabilized rat hepatocytes	Inhibition of pyruvate-driven OXPHOS. Inhibition of the rate of ATP synthesis (pyruvate as substrate used, no inhibitory effects caused by succinate and glutamate as substrates)	[252]
Valproate and lithium	Rat brain tissue obtained from animals pretreated by d-amphetamine	No modification of complex I, II, III and IV activities after the treatment with valproate and lithium in controls	[253]
Valproate and lithium	Rat brain tissue obtained from animals pretreated by d-amphetamine	Treated animals with lithium and valproate prevented inhibition caused by d-amphetamine	[240]
Valproate and lithium	Rat brain tissue obtained from animals pretreated by d-amphetamine	Reversed ATP synthase activity (increased after d-amphetamine) after lithium and valproate treatment	[254]
Valproate and lithium	Human neuroblastoma and glioma cells	Protective effects against H_2O_2 or rotenone induced cytotoxicity in neuroblastoma cells	[241]
Valproate and lithium	Human neuroblastoma cells	Reduction of methamphetamine-induced reduction of cyt *c*, antiapoptotic Bcl-2/Bax ratio and COX activity	[242]
Lithium	Plasma synaptic membrane from rat brain	Impaired function of ATP synthase was modulated (reversed by lithium, and prevented by lithium pretreatment)	[255]
Lithium	Isolated brain mitochondria	Desensitisation to calcium, antagonized MPT, diminished cytochrome *c* release	[238]

Mood stabilizer	Biological model	Affected mitochondrial function	Reference
Lithium	Postmortem human brain cortex	Dose-depedent increased activities of complexes I+III, II+III and succinate dehydrogenase	[256]
Lithium	Human neuroblastoma SH-SY5Y cells	Attenuation of rotenone-induced caspase-3 activation	[257]
Carbamazepine	Rat liver mitochondria	Decreased state 3 respiration, RCR, ATP synthesis, $\Delta\psi_m$	[258]
Carbamazepine	Rat brain mitochondria	Protection against rotenone induced complex I inhibition	[259]
Carbamazepine, lamotrigine	Human white blood cells	Carbamazepine decreased ATP production, stimulatory effect on production by lamotrigine	[245]
Lamotrigine	Human neuroblastoma SH-SY5Y cells	Suppression of MPT formation, attenuation of rotenone-toxicity, inhibition of ROS production	[247]

Table 3. Effects of mood stabilizers on mitochondrial functions

5. Conclusions

Biological markers of depression, predictors of the response to the drug administration and molecular targets of new antidepressants are searched on the basis of recently known hypotheses of affective disorders. We come out mostly from stimuli of neurotrophic hypothesis and mitochondrial hypothesis. According to these hypotheses, the leading role in the pathophysiology of mood disorders and therapeutic effects of antidepressants has mitochondria, which are destined for changes in energetic metabolism of cells. Mitochondrial dysfunctions and thereby impaired neuronal metabolism can lead to disturbances in neuronal function, plasticity and brain circuitry. Impaired functions of mitochondria contribute to a wide range of diseases; the role of mitochondria in the pathophysiology of schizophrenia, bipolar disorder, and major depressive disorder is supported by studies investigating genomic differences, changes of energy metabolism and mitochondrial changes included.

Acknowledgment

This. research was supported by grant no. 41310 given by Grant Agency of Charles University in Prague, by project MSM0021620849 given by Ministry of Education, Youth and Sports and by project PRVOUK-P26/LF1/4 given by Charles University in Prague, Czech Republic.

Author details

Jana Hroudová, Zdeněk Fišar and Jiří Raboch

*Address all correspondence to: hroudova.jana@gmail.com

Department of Psychiatry, First Faculty of Medicine, Charles University in Prague and General University Hospital in Prague, Prague, Czech Republic

References

[1] Pittenger C, Duman RS. Stress, depression, and neuroplasticity: a convergence of mechanisms. Neuropsychopharmacology 2008;33(1): 88-109.

[2] Maes M, Fišar Z, Medina M, Scapagnini G, Nowak G, Berk M. New drug targets in depression: inflammatory, cell-mediated immune, oxidative and nitrosative stress, mitochondrial, antioxidant, and neuroprogressive pathways. And new drug candidates-Nrf2 activators and GSK-3 inhibitors. Inflammopharmacology 2012;20(3): 127-150.

[3] Fišar Z, Raboch J. Depression, antidepressants, and peripheral blood components. Neuro Endocrinol Lett 2008;29(1): 17-28.

[4] Fišar Z, Hroudová J. Intracellular signalling pathways and mood disorders. Folia Biol 2010b;56(4): 135-148.

[5] Duman RS, Heninger GR, Nestler, EJ. A molecular and cellular theory of depression. Arch Gen Psychiatry 1997;54(7): 597-606.

[6] Duman RS. Synaptic plasticity and mood disorders. Mol Psychiatry 2002;7(Suppl 1): S29-S34.

[7] Zarate CA Jr, Singh J, Manji HK. Cellular plasticity cascades: targets for the development of novel therapeutics for bipolar disorder. Biol Psychiatry 2006;59(11): 1006-1020.

[8] Einat, H, Manji HK. Cellular plasticity cascades: genes-to-behavior pathways in animal models of bipolar disorder. Biol Psychiatry 2006;59(12): 1160-1171.

[9] Stork C, Renshaw RF. Mitochondrial dysfunction in bipolar disorder: evidence from magnetic resonance spectroscopy research. Mol Psychiatry 2005;10(10): 900-919.

[10] Kato T. Role of mitochondrial DNA in calcium signaling abnormality in bipolar disorder. Cell Calcium 2008;44(1): 92-102.

[11] Quiroz JA, Gray NA, Kato T, Manji HK. Mitochondrially mediated plasticity in the pathophysiology and treatment of bipolar disorder. Neuropsychopharmacology 2008;33(11): 2551-2565.

[12] Shao L, Martin MV, Watson SJ, Schatzberg A, Akil H, Myers RM, Jones EG, Bunney WE, Vawter MP. Mitochondrial involvement in psychiatric disorders. Ann Med 2008;40(4): 281-295.

[13] Rezin GT, Amboni G, Zugno AI, Quevedo J, Streck EL. Mitochondrial dysfunction and psychiatric disorders. Neurochem Res 2009;34(6): 1021-1029.

[14] Jou SH, Chiu NY, Liu CS. Mitochondrial dysfunction and psychiatric disorders. Chang Gung Med J 2009;32(4): 370-379.

[15] Orth M, Schapira AH. Mitochondria and degenerative disorders. Am J Med Genet 2001;106(1): 27-36.

[16] Schapira AHV. Mitochondrial diseases. Lancet 2012;379(9828): 1825-1834.

[17] Vélot C, Srere PA. Reversible transdominant inhibition of a metabolic pathway. In vivo evidence of interaction between two sequential tricarboxylic acid cycle enzymes in yeast. J Biol Chem 2000;275(17): 12926-12933.

[18] Sriram G, Martinez JA, McCabe ER, Liao JC, Dipple KM. Single-gene disorders: what role could moonlighting enzymes play? Am J Hum Genet 2005;76(6): 911-924.

[19] Fišar Z, Hroudová J. Common aspects of neuroplasticity, mood disorders and mitochondrial functions. Act Nerv Super Rediviva 2010a;52(1): 3-20.

[20] Hroudova J, Fisar Z. Connectivity between mitochondrial functions and psychiatric disorders. Psychiatry Clin Neurosci 2011;65(2): 130-141.

[21] Scheffler IE. Molecular genetics of succinate: quinone oxidoreductase in eukaryotes. Prog Nucleic Acid Res Mol Biol 1998;60: 267-315.

[22] Müller U, Troidl C, Niemann S. SDHC mutations in hederitary paraganglioma/pheochromocytoma. Fam Cancer 2005;4(1): 9-12.

[23] Reinecke F, Smeitink JA, van der Westhuizen FH. OXPHOS gene expression and control in mitochondrial disorders. Biochim Biophys Acta 2009;1792(12): 1113-1121.

[24] Cannino G, Di Liegro CM, Rinaldi AM. Nuclear-mitochondrial interaction. Mitochondrion 2007;7(6): 359-366.

[25] Hovatta I, Juhila J, Donner J. Oxidative stress in anxiety and comorbid disorders. Neurosci Res 2010;68(4): 261-275.

[26] Moghaddam B. Stress activation of glutamate neurotransmission in the prefrontal cortex: implications for dopamine-associated psychiatric disorders. Biol Psychiatry 2002;51(10): 775-787.

[27] Atlante A, Calissano P, Bobba A, Giannattasio S, Marra E, Passarella S. Glutamate neurotoxicity, oxidative stress and mitochondria. FEBS Lett 2001;497(1): 1-5.

[28] Lipton P. Ischemic cell death in brain neurons. Physiol Rev 1999;79(4): 1431-1568.

[29] Ludwig B, Bender E, Arnold S, Hüttemann M, Lee I, Kadenbach B. Cytochrome C oxidase and the regulation of oxidative phosphorylation. Chembiochem 2001;2(6): 392-403.

[30] Gnaiger E. Capacity of oxidative phosphorylation in human skeletal muscle: new perspectives of mitochondrial physiology. Int J Biochem Cell Biol 2009;41(10): 1837-1845.

[31] Kadenbach B, Ramzan R, Wen L, Vogt S. New extension of the Mitchell Theory for oxidative phosphorylation in mitochondria of living organisms. Biochim Biophys Acta 2010;1800(3): 205-212.

[32] Bolaños JP, Almeida A, Moncada S. Glycolysis: a bioenergetic or a survival pathway? Trends Biochem Sci 2010;35(3): 145-149.

[33] Magistretti PJ, Pellerin L. Cellular mechanisms of brain energy metabolism and their relevance to functional brain imaging. Philos Trans R Soc Lond B Biol Sci 1999;354(1387): 1155-1163.

[34] Vonck J, Schäfer E. Supramolecular organization of protein complexes in the mitochondrial inner membrane. Biochim Biophys Acta 2009;1793(1): 117-124.

[35] Bunoust O, Devin A, Avéret N, Camougrand N, Rigoulet M. Competition of electrons to enter the respiratory chain: a new regulatory mechanism of oxidative metabolism in Saccharomyces cerevisiae. J Biol Chem 2005;280(5): 3407-3413.

[36] Solmaz SR, Hunte C. Structure of complex III with bound cytochrome c in reduced state and definition of a minimal core interface for electron transfer. J Biol Chem 2008;283(25): 17542-17549.

[37] Rodríguez-Hernández A, Cordero MD, Salviati L, Artuch R, Pineda M, Briones P, Gómez Izquierdo L, Cotán D, Navas P, Sánchez-Alcázar JA. Coenzyme Q deficiency triggers mitochondria degradation by mitophagy. Autophagy 2009;5(1): 19-32.

[38] Mattson MP, Gleichmann M, Cheng A. Mitochondria in neuroplasticity and neurological disorders. Neuron 2008;60(5): 748-766.

[39] Hirst J. Towards the molecular mechanism of respiratory complex I. Biochem J 2009;425(2): 327-339.

[40] Telford JE, Kilbride SM, Davey GP. Complex I is rate-limiting for oxygen consumption in the nerve terminal. J Biol Chem 2009;284(14): 9109-9114.

[41] Tomitsuka E, Kita K, Esumi H. Regulation of succinate-ubiquinone reductase and fumarate reductase activities in human complex II by phosphorylation of its flavoprotein subunit. Proc Jpn Acad Ser B Phys Biol Sci 2009;85(7): 258-265.

[42] Saada A, Shaag A, Mandel H, Nevo Y, Eriksson S, Elpeleg O. Mutant mitochondrial thymidine kinase in mitochondrial DNA depletion myopathy. Nat Genet 2001;29(3): 342-344.

[43] Chen Q, Vazquez EJ, Moghaddas S, Hoppel CL, Lesnefsky EJ. Production of reactive oxygen species by mitochondria. Central role of complex III. J Biol Chem 2003;278(38): 36027-36031.

[44] Trumpower BL. The protonmotive Q cycle. Energy transduction by coupling of proton translocation to electron transfer by the cytochrome bc_1 complex. J Biol Chem 1990;265(20): 11409-11412.

[45] Turrens JF. Mitochondrial formation of reactive oxygen species. J Physiol 2003;552(Pt 2): 335-344.

[46] Wong-Riley MT. Cytochrome oxidase: an endogenous metabolic marker for neuronal activity. Trends Neurosci 1989;12(3): 94-101.

[47] Noji H, Yoshida M. The rotary machine in the cell, ATP synthase.J Biol Chem 2001;276(3): 1665-1668.

[48] Zanotti F, Gnoni A, Mangiullo R, Papa S. Effect of the ATPase inhibitor protein IF_1 on H^+ translocation in the mitochondrial ATP synthase complex. Biochem Biophys Res Commun 2009;384(1): 43-48.

[49] Kadenbach B. Intrinsic and extrinsic uncoupling of oxidative phosphorylation. Biochim Biophys Acta 2003;1604(2): 77-94.

[50] Youdim MB, Bakhle YS. Monoamine oxidase: isoforms and inhibitors in Parkinson's disease and depressive illness. Br J Pharmacol 2006;147(Suppl 1): S287-S296.

[51] Youdim MB, Edmondson D, Tipton KF. The therapeutic potential of monoamine oxidase inhibitors. Nat Rev Neurosci 2006;7(4): 295-309.

[52] Bach AWJ, Lan NC, Johnson DL, Abell CW, Bembenek ME, Kwan S-W, Seeburg PH, Shih JC. cDNA cloning of human liver monoamine oxidase A and B: molecular basis of differences in enzymatic properties. Proc Natl Acad Sci U S A 1988;85(13): 4934-4938.

[53] Ramsay RR, Gravestock MB. Monoamine oxidases: to inhibit or not to inhibit. Mini Rev Med Chem 2003;3(2): 129-136.

[54] Naoi M, Maruyama W, Akao Y, Yi H, Yamaoka Y. Involvement of type A monoamine oxidase in neurodegeneration: regulation of mitochondrial signaling leading to cell death or neuroprotection. J Neural Transm Suppl 2006;(71): 67-77.

[55] Stahl SM, Felker A. Monoamine oxidase inhibitors: a modern guide to an unrequited class of antidepressants. CNS Spectr 2008;13(10): 855-870.

[56] Horstink M, Tolosa E, Bonuccelli U, Deuschl G, Friedman A, Kanovsky P, Larsen JP, Lees A, Oertel W, Poewe W, Rascol O, Sampaio C, European Federation of Neurological Societies, Movement Disorder Society-European Section. Review of the therapeutic management of Parkinson's disease. Report of a joint task force of the European Federation of Neurological Societies and the Movement Disorder Society-European

Section. Part I: early (uncomplicated) Parkinson's disease. Eur J Neurol 2006;13(11): 1170-1185.

[57] Riederer P, Danielczyk W, Grünblatt E. Monoamine oxidase-B inhibition in Alzheimer's disease. NeuroToxicology 2004;25(1-2): 271-277.

[58] Chen K, Wu HF, Shih JC. The deduced amino acid sequences of human platelet and frontal cortex monoamine oxidase B are identical. J Neurochem 1993;61(1): 187-190.

[59] Benard G, Bellance N, Jose C, Melser S, Nouette-Gaulain K, Rossignol R. Multi-site control and regulation of mitochondrial energy production. Biochim Biophys Acta 2010;1797(6-7): 698-709.

[60] Cairns CB, Walther J, Harken AH, Banerjee A. Mitochondrial oxidative phosphorylation thermodynamic efficiencies reflect physiological organ roles. Am J Physiol 1998;274(5 Pt 2): R1376-R1383.

[61] Ramzan R, Staniek K, Kadenbach B, Vogt S. Mitochondrial respiration and membrane potential are regulated by the allosteric ATP-inhibition of cytochrome c oxidase. Biochim Biophys Acta 2010;1797(9): 1672-1680.

[62] Cocco T, Pacelli C, Sgobbo P, Villani G. Control of OXPHOS efficiency by complex I in brain mitochondria. Neurobiol Aging 2009;30(4): 622-629.

[63] Mitchell P. Coupling of phosphorylation to electron and hydrogen transfer by a chemi-osmotic type of mechanism. Nature 1961;191: 144-148.

[64] Mitchell P. Chemiosmotic coupling in oxidative and photosynthetic phosphorylation, Biol Rev Camb Philos Soc 1966;41(3): 445-502.

[65] Nicholls DG, Vesce S, Kirk L, Chalmers S. Interactions between mitochondrial bioenergetics and cytoplasmic calcium in cultured cerebellar granule cells. Cell Calcium 2003;34(4-5): 407-424.

[66] Chance B, Willams GR. The respiratory chain and oxidative phosphorylation. Adv Enzymol Relat Subj Biochem 1956;17: 65-134.

[67] Tager JM, Wanders RJ, Groen AK, Kunz W, Bohnensack R, Küster U, Letko G, Böhme G, Duszynski J, Wojtczak L. Control of mitochondrial respiration. FEBS Lett 1983;151(1): 1-9.

[68] Mourier A, Devin A, Rigoulet M. Active proton leak in mitochondria: a new way to regulate substrate oxidation. Biochim Biophys Acta 2010;1797:255-261.

[69] Chance B, Williams GR. Respiratory enzymes in oxidative phosphorylation. III. The steady state. J Biol Chem 1955;217(1): 409-427.

[70] Walsh C, Barrow S, Voronina S, Chvanov M, Petersen OH, Tepikin A. Modulation of calcium signalling by mitochondria. Biochim Biophys Acta 2009;1787(11): 1374-1382.

[71] Kadenbach B, Hüttemann M, Arnold S, Lee I, Bender E. Mitochondrial energy metabolism is regulated via nuclear-coded subunits of cytochrome c oxidase. Free Radic Biol Med 2000;29(3-4): 211-221.

[72] McCormack JG, Halestrap AP, Denton RM. Role of calcium ions in regulation of mammalian intramitochondrial metabolism. Physiol Rev 1990;70(2): 391-425.

[73] Rizzuto R, Bernardi P, Pozzan T. Mitochondria as all-round players of the calcium game. J Physiol 2000;529 Pt 1:37-47.

[74] Lee I, Bender E, Arnold S, Kadenbach B. New control of mitochondrial membrane potential and ROS formation--a hypothesis. Biol Chem 2001;382(12): 1629-1636.

[75] Viola HM, Hool LC. Qo site of mitochondrial complex III is the source of increased superoxide after transient exposure to hydrogen peroxide. J Mol Cell Cardiol 2010;49(5): 875-885.

[76] Papa S, Scacco S, Sardanelli AM, Petruzzella V, Vergari R, Signorile A, Technikova-Dobrovova Z. Complex I and the cAMP cascade in human physiopathology. Biosci Rep 2002;22(1): 3-16.

[77] Napiwotzki J, Kadenbach B: Extramitochondrial ATP/ADP-ratios regulate cytochrome c oxidase activity via binding to the cytosolic domain of subunit IV. Biol Chem 1998;379(3): 335-339.

[78] Lee I, Bender E, Kadenbach B. Control of mitochondrial membrane potential and ROS formation by reversible phosphorylation of cytochrome c oxidase. Mol Cell Biochem 2002;234-235(1-2): 63-70.

[79] Bender E, Kadenbach B. The allosteric ATP-inhibition of cytochrome c oxidase activity is reversibly switched on by cAMP-dependent phosphorylation. FEBS Lett 2000;466(1):130-134.

[80] Arnold S, Kadenbach B. Cell respiration is controlled by ATP, an allosteric inhibitor of cytochrome-c oxidase. Eur J Biochem 1997;249(1): 350-354.

[81] Cheng SY, Leonard JL, Davis PJ. Molecular aspects of thyroid hormone actions. Endocr Rev 2010;31(2): 139-170.

[82] Goglia F, Moreno M, Lanni A. Action of thyroid hormones at the cellular level: the mitochondrial target. FEBS Lett 1999;452(3): 115-120.

[83] Arnold S, Goglia F, Kadenbach B. 3,5-Diiodothyronine binds to subunit Va of cytochrome-c oxidase and abolishes the allosteric inhibition of respiration by ATP. Eur J Biochem 1998;252(2): 325-330.

[84] Starkov AA. "Mild" uncoupling of mitochondria. Biosci Rep 1997;17(3): 273-279.

[85] Harper ME, Brand MD. Hyperthyroidism stimulates mitochondrial proton leak and ATP turnover in rat hepatocytes but does not change the overall kinetics of substrate oxidation reactions. Can J Physiol Pharmacol 1994;72(8): 899-908.

[86] Harper ME, Brand MD. The quantitative contributions of mitochondrial proton leak and ATP turnover reactions to the changed respiration rates of hepatocytes from rats of different thyroid status. J Biol Chem 1993;268(20): 14850-14860.

[87] Brand MD, Turner N, Ocloo A, Else PL, Hulbert AJ. Proton conductance and fatty acyl composition of liver mitochondria correlates with body mass in birds. Biochem J 2003;376(Pt 3): 741-748.

[88] Azzu V, Jastroch M, Divakaruni AS, Brand MD. The regulation and turnover of mitochondrial uncoupling proteins. Biochim Biophys Acta 2010;1797(6-7): 785-791.

[89] Brand MD, Pakay JL, Ocloo A, Kokoszka J, Wallace DC, Brookes PS, Cornwall EJ. The basal proton conductance of mitochondria depends on adenine nucleotide translocase content. Biochem J 2005;392(Pt 2): 353-362.

[90] Rial E, Rodríguez-Sánchez L, Gallardo-Vara E, Zaragoza P, Moyano E, González-Barroso MM. Lipotoxicity, fatty acid uncoupling and mitochondrial carrier function. Biochim Biophys Acta 2010;1797(6-7): 800-806.

[91] Wojtczak L, Schönfeld P. Effect of fatty acids on energy coupling processes in mitochondria. Biochim Biophys Acta 1993;1183(1): 41-57.

[92] Samartsev VN, Marchik EI, Shamagulova LV. Free fatty acids as inducers and regulators of uncoupling of oxidative phosphorylation in liver mitochondria with participation of ADP/ATP- and aspartate/glutamate-antiporter. Biochemistry (Mosc) 2011;76(2): 217-224.

[93] Kleinfeld AM, Chu P, Romero C. Transport of long-chain native fatty acids across lipid bilayer membranes indicates that transbilayer flip-flop is rate limiting. Biochemistry 1997;36(46): 14146-14158.

[94] Di Paola M, Lorusso M. Interaction of free fatty acids with mitochondria: coupling, uncoupling and permeability transition. Biochim Biophys Acta 2006;1757(9-10): 1330-1337.

[95] Kamp F, Hamilton JA. pH gradients across phospholipid membranes caused by fast flip-flop of un-ionized fatty acids. Proc Natl Acad Sci U S A 1992;89(23): 11367-11370.

[96] Hagen T, Vidal-Puig A. Mitochondrial uncoupling proteins in human physiology and disease. Minerva Med 2002;93(1): 41-57.

[97] Echtay KS, Roussel D, St-Pierre J, Jekabsons MB, Cadenas S, Stuart JA, Harper JA, Roebuck SJ, Morrison A, Pickering S, Clapham JC, Brand MD. Superoxide activates mitochondrial uncoupling proteins. Nature 2002;415(6867): 96-99.

[98] Brand MD, Affourtit C, Esteves TC, Green K, Lambert AJ, Miwa S, Pakay JL, Parker N. Mitochondrial superoxide: production, biological effects, and activation of uncoupling proteins. Free Radic Biol Med 2004;37(6): 755-767.

[99] Zaninovich AA. Role of uncoupling proteins UCP1, UCP2 and UCP3 in energy balance, type 2 diabetes and obesity. Synergism with the thyroid]. Medicina (B Aires) 2005;65(2): 163-169.

[100] Douette P, Sluse FE. Mitochondrial uncoupling proteins: new insights from functional and proteomic studies. Free Radic Biol Med 2006;40(7): 1097-1107.

[101] Boss O, Hagen T, Lowell BB. Uncoupling proteins 2 and 3: potential regulators of mitochondrial energy metabolism. Diabetes 2000;49(2): 143-156.

[102] Trenker M, Malli R, Fertschai I, Levak-Frank S, Graier WF. Uncoupling proteins 2 and 3 are fundamental for mitochondrial Ca^{2+} uniport. Nat Cell Biol 2007;9(4): 445-452.

[103] De Marchi U, Castelbou C, Demaurex N. Uncoupling protein 3 (UCP3) modulates the activity of Sarco/endoplasmic reticulum Ca^{2+}-ATPase (SERCA) by decreasing mitochondrial ATP production. J Biol Chem 2011;286(37): 32533-32541.

[104] Liu D, Chan SL, de Souza-Pinto NC, Slevin JR, Wersto RP, Zhan M, Mustafa K, de Cabo R, Mattson MP. Mitochondrial UCP4 mediates an adaptive shift in energy metabolism and increases the resistance of neurons to metabolic and oxidative stress. Neuromolecular Med 2006;8(3): 389-414.

[105] Kwok KH, Ho PW, Chu AC, Ho JW, Liu HF, Yiu DC, Chan KH, Kung MH, Ramsden DB, Ho SL. Mitochondrial UCP5 is neuroprotective by preserving mitochondrial membrane potential, ATP levels, and reducing oxidative stress in MPP+ and dopamine toxicity. Free Radic Biol Med 2010;49(6): 1023-1035.

[106] Wolkow CA, Iser WB. Uncoupling protein homologs may provide a link between mitochondria, metabolism and lifespan. Ageing Res Rev 2006;5(2): 196-208.

[107] Beck V, Jabůrek M, Demina T, Rupprecht A, Porter RK, Jezek P, Pohl EE. Polyunsaturated fatty acids activate human uncoupling proteins 1 and 2 in planar lipid bilayers. FASEB J 2007;21(4): 1137-1144.

[108] Ježek P, Hlavatá L. Mitochondria in homeostasis of reactive oxygen species in cell, tissues, and organism. Int J Biochem Cell Biol 2005;37(12): 2478-2503.

[109] Muller FL, Liu Y, Van Remmen H. Complex III releases superoxide to both sides of the inner mitochondrial membrane. J Biol Chem 2004;279(47): 49064-49073.

[110] Tretter L, Adam-Vizi V. Generation of reactive oxygen species in the reaction catalyzed by alpha-ketoglutarate dehydrogenase. J Neurosci 2004;24(36): 7771-7778.

[111] Murphy MP. How mitochondria produce reactive oxygen species. Biochem J 2009;417(1): 1-13.

[112] Cadenas E, Davies KL. Mitochondrial free radical generation, oxidative stress, and aging. Free Radic Biol Med 2000;29: 222-230.

[113] Tirosh O, Aronis A, Melendez JA. Mitochondrial state 3 to 4 respiration transition during Fas-mediated apoptosis controls cellular redox balance and rate of cell death. Biochem Pharmacol 2003;66(8): 1331-1334.

[114] Aronis A, Melendez JA, Golan O, Shilo S, Dicter N, Tirosh O. Potentiation of Fas-mediated apoptosis by attenuated production of mitochondria-derived reactive oxygen species. Cell Death Differ 2003;10(3): 335-344.

[115] Petrosillo G, Matera M, Casanova G, Ruggiero FM, Paradies G. Mitochondrial dysfunction in rat brain with aging Involvement of complex I, reactive oxygen species and cardiolipin. Neurochem Int 2008;53(5): 126-131.

[116] Schönfeld P, Wojtczak L. Fatty acids as modulators of the cellular production of reactive oxygen species. Free Radic Biol Med 2008;45(3): 231-241.

[117] Boffoli D, Scacco SC, Vergari R, Solarino G, Santacroce G, Papa S. Decline with age of the respiratory chain activity in human skeletal muscle. Biochim Biophys Acta 1994;1226(1): 73-82.

[118] Marazziti D, Baroni S, Picchetti M, Landi P, Silvestri S, Vatteroni E, Catena Dell'Osso M. Psychiatric disorders and mitochondrial dysfunctions. Eur Rev Med Pharmacol Sci 2012;16(2): 270-275.

[119] Bolaños JP, Moro MA, Lizasoain I, Almeida A. Mitochondria and reactive oxygen and nitrogen species in neurological disorders and stroke: Therapeutic implications. Adv Drug Deliv Rev 2009;61(14): 1299-1315.

[120] Jiang X, Wang X. Cytochrome c promotes caspase-9 activation by inducing nucleotide binding to Apaf-1. J Biol Chem 2000;275(40): 31199-31203.

[121] Tsujimoto Y, Shimizu S. Role of the mitochondrial membrane permeability transition in cell death. Apoptosis 2007;12(5): 835-840.

[122] Baines CP, Kaiser RA, Sheiko T, Craigen WJ, Molkentin JD. Voltage-dependent anion channels are dispensable for mitochondrial-dependent cell death. Nat Cell Biol 2007;9(5): 550-555.

[123] Chen Y, McMillan-Ward E, Kong J, Israels SJ, Gibson SB. Mitochondrial electron-transport-chain inhibitors of complexes I and II induce autophagic cell death mediated by reactive oxygen species. J Cell Sci 2007;120(Pt 23): 4155-4166.

[124] Foster KA, Galeffi F, Gerich FJ, Turner DA, Müller M. Optical and pharmacological tools to investigate the role of mitochondria during oxidative stress and neurodegeneration. Prog Neurobiol 2006;79(3): 136-171.

[125] Wong DT, Horng JS, Gordee RS. Respiratory chain of a pathogenic fungus, Microsporum gypseum: effect of the antifungal agent pyrrolnitrin. J Bacteriol 1971;106(1): 168-73.

[126] Raha S, McEachern GE, Myint AT, Robinson BH. Superoxides from mitochondrial complex III: the role of manganese superoxide dismutase. Free Radic Biol Med 2000;29(2): 170-180.

[127] Ferguson M, Mockett RJ, Shen Y, Orr WC, Sohal RS. Age-associated decline in mitochondrial respiration and electron transport in Drosophila melanogaster. Biochem J 2005;390(Pt 2): 501-511.

[128] Wilson DF, Chance B. Azide inhibition of mitochondrial electron transport. I. The aerobic steady state of succinate oxidation. Biochim Biophys Acta 1967;131(3): 421-430.

[129] Nůsková H, Vrbacký M, Drahota Z, Houštěk J. Cyanide inhibition and pyruvate-induced recovery of cytochrome c oxidase. J Bioenerg Biomembr 2010;42(5): 395-403.

[130] Sjövall F, Morota S, Hansson MJ, Friberg H, Gnaiger E, Elmér E. Temporal increase of platelet mitochondrial respiration is negatively associated with clinical outcome in patients with sepsis. Crit Care 2010;14(6): R214.

[131] Konstantinov AA, Peskin AV, Popova EYu, Khomutov GB, Ruuge EK. Superoxide generation by the respiratory chain of tumor mitochondria. Biochim Biophys Acta 1987;894(1): 1-10.

[132] Koopman WJ, Nijtmans LG, Dieteren CE, Roestenberg P, Valsecchi F, Smeitink JA, Willems PH. Mammalian mitochondrial complex I: biogenesis, regulation, and reactive oxygen species generation. Antioxid Redox Signal 2010;12(12): 1431-1470.

[133] Kirkland RA, Franklin JL. Bax affects production of reactive oxygen by the mitochondria of non-apoptotic neurons. Exp Neurol 2007;204(1): 458-461.

[134] Mattson MP, Partin J. Evidence for mitochondrial control of neuronal polarity. J Neurosci Res 1999;56(1): 8-20.

[135] Erecinska M, Cherian S, Silver IA. Energy metabolism in mammalian brain during development. Prog Neurobiol 2004;73(6): 397-445.

[136] Chada SR, Hollenberck PJ. Nerve growth factor signaling regulates motility and docking of axonal mitochondria. Curr Biol 2004;14(14): 1272-1276.

[137] Chang DT, Reynolds IJ. Differences in mitochondrial movement and morphology in young and mature primary cortical neurons in culture. Neuroscience 2006;141(2): 727-736.

[138] Cai Q, Sheng ZH. Mitochondrial transport and docking in axons. Exp Neurol 2009;218(2): 257-267.

[139] Stamer K, Vogel R, Thies E, Mandelkow E, Mandelkow EM. Tau blocks traffic of organelles, neurofilaments, and APP vesicles in neurons and enhances oxidative stress. J Cell Biol 2002;156(6): 1051-1063.

[140] Konradi C, Eaton M, MacDonald ML, Walsh J, Benes FM, Heckers S. Molecular evidence for mitochondrial dysfunction in bipolar disorder. Arch Gen Psychiatry 2004;61(3): 300-308.

[141] Overly CC, Rieff HI, Hollenberck PJ. Organelle motility and metabolism in axons vs dendrites of cultured hippocampal neurons. J Cell Sci 1996;109(Pt 5): 971-980.

[142] Markham A, Cameron I, Franklin P, Spedding M. BDNF increases rat brain mitochondrial respiratory coupling at complex I, but not complex II. Eur. J Neurosci 2004;20(5): 1189-1196.

[143] Ruthel G, Hollenberck PJ. Response of mitochondrial traffic to axon determination and differential branch growth. J Neurosci 2003;23(24): 8618-8624.

[144] Fišar Z, Jirák R, Bob P, Papežová H. Vybrané kapitoly z biologické psychiatrie. Praha: Grada Publishing, a.s.; 2009.

[145] Fišar Z. Biochemické hypotézy afektivních poruch. Praha: Galén; 1998.

[146] Krishnan V, Nestler EJ. The molecular neurobiology of depression. Nature 2008;455(7215): 894-902.

[147] Mathew SJ, Manji HK, Charney DS. Novel drugs and therapeutic targets for severe mood disorders. Neuropsychopharmacology 2008;33(9): 2080-2092.

[148] aan het Rot M, Mathew SJ, Charney DS. Neurobiological mechanisms in major depressive disorder. CMAJ 2009;180(3): 305-313.

[149] Coppen A. The biochemistry of affective disorders. Br J Psychiatry 1967;113(504): 1237-1264.

[150] Schildkraut JJ. The catecholamine hypothesis of affective disorders: a review of supporting evidence. Am J Psychiatry 1965;122(5): 509-522.

[151] Nestler EJ, Barrot M, DiLeone RJ, Eisch AJ, Gold SJ, Monteggia LM. Neurobiology of depression. Neuron 2002;34(1): 13-25.

[152] Delgado PL, Miller HL, Salomon RM, Licinio J, Krystal JH, Moreno FA, Heninger GR, Charney DS. Tryptophan-depletion challenge in depressed patients treated with desipramine or fluoxetine: implications for the role of serotonin in the mechanism of antidepressant action. Biol Psychiatry 1999;46(2): 212-220.

[153] Ruhé HG, Mason NS, Schene AH. Mood is indirectly related to serotonin, norepinephrine and dopamine levels in humans: a meta-analysis of monoamine depletion studies. Mol Psychiatry 2007;12(4): 331-359.

[154] Cowen PJ.Serotonin and depression: pathophysiological mechanism or marketing myth? Trends Pharmacol Sci 2008;29(9): 433-436.

[155] Mendelsohn D, Riedel WJ, Sambeth A. Effects of acute tryptophan depletion on memory, attention and executive functions: a systematic review. Neurosci Biobehav Rev 2009;33(6): 926-952.

[156] Berman RM, Sanacora G, Anand A, Roach LM, Fasula MK, Finkelstein CO, Wachen RM, Oren DA, Heninger GR, Charney DS. Monoamine depletion in unmedicated depressed subjects. Biol Psychiatry 2002;51(6): 469-473.

[157] Heninger GR, Delgado PL, Charney DS. The revised monoamine theory of depression: a modulatory role for monoamines, based on new findings from monoamine depletion experiments in humans. Pharmacopsychiatry 1996;29(1): 2-11.

[158] Jacobs BL. Adult brain neurogenesis and depression. Brain Behav Immun 2002;16(5): 602-609

[159] Jacobs BL, van Praag H, Gage FH. Adult brain neurogenesis and psychiatry: a novel theory of depression. Mol Psychiatry 2000;5(3): 262-269.

[160] Kempermann G, Kronenberg G. Depressed new neurons--adult hippocampal neurogenesis and a cellular plasticity hypothesis of major depression. Biol Psychiatry 2003;54(5): 499-503.

[161] Kato T, Kato N. Mitochondrial dysfunction in bipolar disorder. Bipolar Disord 2000;2(3 Pt 1): 180-190.

[162] Haddad JJ, Saadé NE, Safieh-Garabedian B. Cytokines and neuro-immune-endocrine interactions: a role for the hypothalamic-pituitary-adrenal revolving axis. J Neuroimmunol 2002;133(1-2): 1-19.

[163] Leonard BE, Myint A. The psychoneuroimmunology of depression. Hum Psychopharmacol 2009;24(3): 165-175.

[164] Catena-Dell'Osso M, Bellantuono C, Consoli G, Baroni S, Rotella F, Marazziti D. Inflammatory and neurodegenerative pathways in depression: a new avenue for antidepressant development? Curr Med Chem 2011;18(2): 245-255.

[165] Maes M, Yirmyia R, Noraberg J, Brene S, Hibbeln J, Perini G, Kubera M, Bob P, Lerer B, Maj M. The inflammatory & neurodegenerative (I&ND) hypothesis of depression: leads for future research and new drug developments in depression. Metab Brain Dis 2009;24(1): 27-53.

[166] Iwamoto K, Bundo M, Kato T. Altered expression of mitochondria-related genes in postmortem brains of patients with bipolar disorder or schizophrenia, as revealed by large-scale DNA microarray analysis. Hum Mol Genet 2005;14(2): 241-253.

[167] Kato T. Mitochondrial dysfunction as the molecular basis of bipolar disorder: therapeutic implications. CNS Drugs 2007;21(1): 1-11.

[168] Balon R. Biological predictors of antidepressant treatment outcome. Clin Neuropharmacol 1989;12(3): 195-214.

[169] Joyce PR, Paykel ES. Predictors of drug response in depression. Arch Gen Psychiatry 1989;46(1): 89-99.

[170] Duman RS. Depression: a case of neuronal life and death? Biol Psychiatry 2004;56(3): 140-145.

[171] Brand MD, Nicholls DG. Assessing mitochondrial dysfunction in cells. Biochem J 2011;435(2): 297-312.

[172] Fagervall I, Ross SB. Inhibition of monoamine oxidase in monoaminergic neurones in the rat brain by irreversible inhibitors. Biochem Pharmacol 1986;35(8): 1381-1387.

[173] Smith TE, Weisssbach H, Udenfriend S. Studies on monoamine oxidase: the mechanism of inhibition of monoamine oxidase by iproniazid. Biochemistry 1963;2(4): 746-751.

[174] Haefely W, Burkard WP, Cesura AM, Kettler R, Lorez HP, Martin JR, Richards JG, Scherschlicht R, Da Prada M.: Biochemistry and pharmacology of moclobemide, a prototype RIMA. Psychopharmacology (Berl) 1992;106(Suppl): S6-S14.

[175] Lecrubier Y, Guelfi JD. Efficacy of reversible inhibitors of monoamine oxidase-A in various forms of depression. Acta Psychiatr Scand Suppl 1990;360: 18-23.

[176] Lecrubier Y. Risk-benefit assessment of newer versus older monoamine oxidase (MAO) inhibitors. Drug Saf 1994;10(4): 292-300.

[177] Iwersen S, Schmoldt A. Three suicide attempts with moclobemide. J Toxicol Clin Toxicol 1996;34(2): 223-225.

[178] Lotufo-Neto F, Trivedi M, Thase ME. Meta-analysis of the reversible inhibitors of monoamine oxidase type A moclobemide and brofaromine for the treatment of depression. Neuropsychopharmacology 1999;20(3): 226-247.

[179] Magder DM, Aleksic I, Kennedy SH. Tolerability and efficacy of high-dose moclobemide alone and in combination with lithium and trazodone. J Clin Psychopharmacol 2000;20(3): 394-395.

[180] Bonnet U. Moclobemide: therapeutic use and clinical studies. CNS Drug Rev 2003;9(1): 97-140.

[181] Praško J, Dockery C, Horáček J, Houbová P, Kosová J, Klaschka J, Pašková B, Prašková H, Seifertová D, Záleský R, Höschl C. Moclobemide and cognitive behavioral therapy in the treatment of social phobia. A six-month controlled study and 24 months follow up. Neuro Endocrinol Lett 2006;27(4): 473-481.

[182] Jauch R, Griesser E, Oesterhelt G, Arnold W, Meister W, Ziegler WH, Guentert TW. Biotransformation of moclobemide in humans. Acta Psychiatr Scand Suppl 1990;360: 87-90.

[183] Da Prada M, Kettler R, Keller HH, Burkard WP, Muggli-Maniglio D, Haefely WE. Neurochemical profile of moclobemide, a short-acting and reversible inhibitor of monoamine oxidase type A. J Pharmacol Exp Ther 1989;248(1): 400-414.

[184] Baker GB, Urichuk LJ, McKenna KF, Kennedy SH. Metabolism of monoamine oxidase inhibitors. Cell Mol Neurobiol 1999;19(3): 411-426.

[185] Reyes E, Lisansky J. Effects of tricyclic antidepressants on platelet monoamine oxidase activity. Clin Pharmacol Ther 1984;35(4): 531-534.

[186] Roth JA, Gillis CN. Inhibition of lung, liver and brain monoamine oxidase by imipramine and desipramine. Biochem Pharmacol 1974;23(6): 1138-1140.

[187] Edwards DJ, Burns MO. Effects of tricyclic antidepressants upon human platelet monoamine oxidase. Life Sci 1974;15(12): 2045-2058.

[188] Sullivan JL, Dackis C, Stanfield C. In vivo inhibition of platelet MAO activity by tricyclic antidepressants. Am J Psychiatry 1977;134(2): 188-190.

[189] Sullivan JL, Zung WW, Stanfield CN, Cavenar JO Jr. Clinical correlates of tricyclic antidepressant-mediated inhibition of platelet monoamine oxidase. Biol Psychiatry 1978;13(3): 399-407.

[190] Davidson J, Mcleod MN, Linnoila M, Kurland AA, White HL. Platelet MAO inhibition following tricyclic antidepressant therapy. Am J Psychiatry 1978;135(5): 603-605.

[191] Reveley MA, Glover V, Slander M, Coppen A. Absence of platelet monamine oxidase inhibition during amitriptyline or zimelidine treatment. Br J Clin Pharmacol 1979;8(4): 375-378.

[192] Green AL, McGachy HA. The inhibition of monoamine oxidase by tricyclic antidepressants: the influence of the nature of the substrate and the source of the enzyme. J Pharm Pharmacol 1987;39(5): 392-394.

[193] Green AL, O'Grady JE, Vass M. The effect of some tricyclic antidepressants on the inhibition of mouse brain monoamine oxidase in-vivo by phenelzine. J Pharm Pharmacol 1989;41(1): 50-51.

[194] Honecker H, Christ W, Müller-Oerlinghausen B, Coper H. Critical evaluation of measurement of platelet monoamine oxidase in man. J Clin Chem Clin Biochem 1976;14(9): 453-458.

[195] Nag M. Effect of chlorpromazine, imipramine and lithium on MAO-A and MAO-B activity in rat brain mitochondria. Indian J Exp Biol 2004;42(9): 941-944.

[196] Egashira T, Takayama F, Yamanaka Y. Effects of long-term treatment with dicyclic, tricyclic, tetracyclic, and noncyclic antidepressant drugs on monoamine oxidase activity in mouse brain. Gen Pharmacol 1996;27(5): 773-778.

[197] Egashira T, Takayama F, Yamanaka Y. The inhibition of monoamine oxidase activity by various antidepressants: differences found in various mammalian species. Jpn J Pharmacol 1999;81(1): 115-121.

[198] Gnerre C, Kosel M, Baumann P, Carrupt PA, Testa B. Interaction of psychotropic drugs with monoamine oxidase in rat brain. J Pharm Pharmacol 2001;53(8): 1125-1130.

[199] Mukherjee J, Yang Z-Y.: Monoamine oxidase A inhibition by fluoxetine: an in vitro and in vivo study. Synapse 1999;31(4): 285-289.

[200] Mukherjee J, Yang ZY. Evaluation of monoamine oxidase B inhibition by fluoxetine (Prozac): an in vitro and in vivo study. Eur J Pharmacol 1997;337(1): 111-114.

[201] Fišar Z, Hroudová J, Raboch J. Inhibition of monoamine oxidase activity by antidepressants and mood stabilizers. Neuro Endocrinol Lett 2010;31(5): 645-656.

[202] Hroudova J, Fisar Z. Activities of respiratory chain complexes and citrate synthase influenced by pharmacologically different antidepressants and mood stabilizers. Neuro Endocrinol. Lett 2010;31(3): 336-342.

[203] Weinbach EC, Costa JL, Nelson BD, Claggett CE, Hundal T, Bradley D, Morris SJ. Effects of tricyclic antidepressant drugs on energy-linked reactions in mitochondria. Biochem Pharmacol 1986;35(9): 1445-1451.

[204] Dykens JA, Jamieson JD, Marroquin LD, Nadanaciva S, Xu JJ, Dunn MC, Smith AR, Will Y. In vitro assessment of mitochondrial dysfunction and cytotoxicity of nefazodone, trazodone, and buspirone. Toxicol Sci 2008;103(2): 335-345.

[205] Velasco A, González-Calvo V, Alvarez FJ, Dueñas A, García-Roldán JL. Effect of trazodone on oxidative metabolism of rat brain in vitro. Rev Esp Fisiol 1985;41(2): 201-205.

[206] Levkovitz, Y, Gil-Ad I, Zeldich E, Dayag M, Weizman A. Differential induction of apoptosis by antidepressants in glioma and neuroblastoma cell lines: evidence for p-c-Jun, cytochrome c, and caspase-3 involvement. J Mol Neurosci 2005;27(1): 29-42.

[207] Ma J, Qiu Y, Yang L, Peng L, Xia Z, Hou LN, Fang C, Qi H, Chen HZ. Desipramine induces apoptosis in rat glioma cells via endoplasmic reticulum stress-dependent CHOP pathway. J Neurooncol 2010;101(1): 41-48.

[208] Kolla N, Wei Z, Richardson JS, Li XM. Amitriptyline and fluoxetine protect PC12 cells from cell death induced by hydrogen peroxide. J Psychiatry Neurosci 2005;30(3): 196-201.

[209] Han YS, Lee CS. Antidepressants reveal differential effect against 1-methyl-4-phenylpyridinium toxocity in differentiated PC12 cells. Eur J Pharmacol 2009;604(1-3): 36-44.

[210] Wang H, Guan Y, Wang X, Smith K Cormier K, Zhu S, Stavrovskaya IG, Huo C, Ferrante RJ, Kristal BS, Friedlander RM. Nortriptyline delays disease onset in models of chronic neurodegeneration. Eur J Neurosci 2007;26(3): 633-641.

[211] Zhang WH, Wang H, Wang X, Narayanan MV, Stavrovskaya IG, Kristal BS, Friedlander RM. Nortriptyline protects mitochondria and reduces cerebral ischemia/hypoxia injury. Stroke 2008;39(2): 455-462.

[212] Katyare SS, Rajan RR. Effect of long-term in vivo treatment with imipramine on the oxidative energy metabolism in rat brain mitochondria. Comp Biochem Psysiol C Pharmacol Toxicol Endocrinol 1995;112(3): 353-357.

[213] Katyare SS, Rajan RR. Enhanced oxidative phosphorylation in rat liver mitochondria following prolonged in vivo treatment with imipramine. Br J Pharmacol 1988;95(3): 914-922.

[214] Xia Z, Karlsson H, DePierre JW, Nässberger L. Tricyclic antidepressants induce apoptosis in human T lymphocytes. Int J Immunopharmacol 1997;19(11-12): 645-654.

[215] Karlsson H, Gu Y, DePierre J, Nässberger L. Induction of apoptosis in proliferating lymphocytes by tricyclic antidepressants. Apoptosis 1998;3(4): 255-260.

[216] Xia Z, Lundgren B, Bergstrand A, DePierre JW, Nässberger L. Changes in the generation of reactive oxygen species and in mitochondrial membrane potential during apoptosis induced by the antidepressants imipramine, clomipramine, and citalopram and the effects on these changes by Bcl-2 and Bcl-X(L). Biochem Pharmacol 1999;57(10): 1199-1208.

[217] Abdel-Razaq W, Kendall DA, Bates TE. The effects of antidepressants on mitochondrial function in a model cell system and isolated mitochondria. Neurochem Res 2011;36(2): 327-338.

[218] Fromenty B, Freneaux E, Labbe G, Deschamps D, Larrey D, Letteron P, Pessayre D. Tianeptine, a new tricyclic antidepressant metabolized by beta-oxidation of its heptanoic side chain, inhibits the mitochondrial oxidation of medium and short chain fatty acids in mice. Biochem Pharmacol 1989;38(21): 3743-3751.

[219] Souza ME, Polizello AC, Uyemura SA, Castro-Silva O, Curti C. Effect of fluoxetine on rat liver mitochondria. Biochem Pharmacol 1994;48(3): 535-541.

[220] Curti C, Mingatto FE, Polizello AC, Galastri LO, Uyemura SA, Santos AC. Fluoxetine interacts with the lipid bilayer of the inner membrane in isolated rat brain mitochondria, inhibiting electron transport and F1F0-ATPase activity. Mol Cell Biochem 1999;199(1-2): 103-109.

[221] Morota S, Månsson R, Hansson MJ, Kasuya K, Shimazu M, Hasegawa E, Yanagi S, Omi A, Uchino H, Elmér E. Evaluation of putative inhibitors of mitochondrial permeability transition for brain disorders--specificity vs. toxicity. Exp Neurol 2009;218(2): 353-362.

[222] Agostinho FR, Réus GZ, Stringari RB, Ribeiro KF, Ferraro AK, Benedet J, Rochi N, Scaini G, Streck EL, Quevedo J. Treatment with olanzapine, fluoxetine and olanzapine/fluoxetine alters citrate synthase activity in rat brain. Neurosci Lett 2011;487(3): 278-281.

[223] Gamaro GD, Streck EL, Matté C, Prediger ME, Wyse AT, Dalmaz C. Reduction of hippocampal Na+, K+-ATPase activity in rats subjected to an experimental model of depression. Neurochem Res 2003;28(9): 1339-1344.

[224] Li Y, Couch L, Higuchi M, Fang JL, Guo L. Mitochondrial dysfunction induced by sertraline, an antidepressant agent. Toxicol Sci 2012;127(2): 582-591.

[225] Scaini G, Santos PM, Benedet J, Rochi N, Gomes LM, Borges LS, Rezin GT, Pezente DP, Quevedo J, Streck EL. Evaluation of Krebs cycle enzymes in the brain of rats after chronic administration of antidepressants. Brain Res Bull 2010;82(3-4): 224-227.

[226] Gould TD, Manji HK. Glycogen synthase kinase-3: a putative molecular target for lithium mimetic drugs. Neuropsychopharmacology 2005;30(7): 1223-1237.

[227] Shaltiel G, Chen G, Manji HK. Neurotrophic signaling cascades in the pathophysiology and treatment of bipolar disorder. Curr Opin Pharmacol 2007;7(1): 22-26.

[228] Gould TD, Quiroz JA, Singh J, Zarate CA, Manji HK. Emerging experimental therapeutics for bipolar disorder: insights from the molecular and cellular actions of current mood stabilizers. Mol Psychiatry 2004;9(8): 734-755.

[229] Chen G, Zeng WZ, Yuan PX, Huang LD, Jiang YM, Zhao ZH, Manji HK. The mood-stabilizing agents lithium and valproate robustly increase the levels of the neuroprotective protein bcl-2 in the CNS. J Neurochem 1999;72(2): 879-882.

[230] Bown CD, Wang JF, Chen B, Young LT. Regulation of ER stress proteins by valproate: therapeutic implications. Bipolar Disord 2002;4(2): 145-151.

[231] Chuang DM. The antiapoptotic actions of mood stabilizers: molecular mechanisms and therapeutic potentials. Ann N Y Acad Sci 2005;1053: 195-204.

[232] Magder DM, Aleksic I, Kennedy SH. Tolerability and efficacy of high-dose moclobemide alone and in combination with lithium and trazodone. J Clin Psychopharmacol 2000;20(3): 394-395.

[233] Nierenberg AA, Fava M, Trivedi MH, Wisniewski SR, Thase ME, McGrath PJ, Alpert JE, Warden D, Luther JF, Niederehe G, Lebowitz B, Shores-Wilson K, Rush AJ. A comparison of lithium and T_3 augmentation following two failed medication treatments for depression: a STAR*D report. Am J Psychiatry 2006;163(9): 1519-1530.

[234] Kitaichi Y, Inoue T, Nakagawa S, Izumi T, Koyama T. Effect of co-administration of subchronic lithium pretreatment and acute MAO inhibitors on extracellular monoamine levels and the expression of contextual conditioned fear in rats. Eur J Pharmacol 2006;532(3): 236-245.

[235] Redrobe JP, Bourin M. Evidence of the activity of lithium on 5-HT1B receptors in the mouse forced swimming test: comparison with carbamazepine and sodium valproate. Psychopharmacology (Berl) 1999;141(4): 370-377.

[236] Haddjeri N, Szabo ST, de Montigny C, Blier P. Increased tonic activation of rat forebrain 5-HT(1A) receptors by lithium addition to antidepressant treatments Neuropsychopharmacology. 2000;22(4): 346-356.

[237] Muraki I, Inoue T, Hashimoto S, Izumi T, Ito K, Koyama T. Effect of subchronic lithium treatment on citalopram-induced increases in extracellular concentrations of serotonin in the medial prefrontal cortex. J Neurochem 2001;76(2): 490-497.

[238] Shalbuyeva N, Brustovetsky T, Brustovetsky N. Lithium desensitizes brain mitochondria to calcium, antagonizes permeability transition, and diminishes cytochrome C release. J Biol Chem 2007;282(25): 18057-18068.

[239] Haas R, Stumpf DA, Parks JK, Eguren L. Inhibitory effects of sodium valproate on oxidative phosphorylation. Neurology 1981;31(11): 1473-1476.

[240] Corrêa C, Amboni G, Assis LC, Martins MR, Kapczinski F, Streck EL, Quevedo J. Effects of lithium and valproate on hippocampus citrate synthase activity in an animal model of mania. Prog Neuropsychopharmacol Biol Psychiatry 2007;31(4): 887-891.

[241] Lai JS, Zhao C, Warsh JJ, Li PP. Cytoprotection by lithium and valproate varies between cell types and cellular stresses. Eur J Pharmacol 2006;539(1-2): 18-26.

[242] Bachmann RF, Wang Y, Yuan P, Zhou R, Li X, Alesci S, Du J, Manji HK. Common effects of lithium and valproate on mitochondrial functions: protection against methamphetamine-induced mitochondrial damage. Int J Neuropsychopharmacol 2009;12(6): 805-822.

[243] Mai L, Jope RS, Li X. BDNF-mediated signal transduction is modulated by GSK3beta and mood stabilizing agents. J Neurochem 2002;82(1): 75-83.

[244] Bown CD, Wang JF, Young LT. Attenuation of N-methyl-D-aspartate-mediated cytoplasmic vacuolization in primary rat hippocampal neurons by mood stabilizers. Neuroscience 2003;117(4): 949-955.

[245] Berger I, Segal I, Shmueli D, Saada A. The effect of antiepileptic drugs on mitochondrial activity: a pilot study. J Child Neurol 2010;25(5): 541-545.

[246] Chen G, Pan B, Hawver DB, Wright CB, Potter WZ, Manji HK. Attenuation of cyclic AMP production by carbamazepine. J Neurochem 1996;67(5): 2079-2086.

[247] Kim YJ, Ko HH, Han ES, Lee CS. Lamotrigine inhibition of rotenone- or 1-methyl-4-phenylpyridinium-induced mitochondrial damage and cell death. Brain Res Bull 2007;71(6): 633-640.

[248] Ponchaut S, van Hoof F, Veitch K. In vitro effects of valproate and valproate metabolites on mitochondrial oxidations. Relevance of CoA sequestration to the observed inhibitions. Biochem Pharmacol 1992;43(11): 2435-2442.

[249] Luder AS, Parks JK, Frerman F, Parker WD Jr. Inactivation of beef brain alpha-ketoglutarate dehydrogenase complex by valproic acid and valproic acid metabolites. J Clin Invest 1990;86(5): 1574-1581.

[250] Becker CM, Harris RA. Influence of valproic acid on hepatic carbohydrate and lipid metabolism. Arch Biochem Biophys 1983;223(2): 381-392.

[251] Aires CC, Soveral G, Luís PB, ten Brink HJ, de Almeida IT, Duran M, Wanders RJ, Silva MF. Pyruvate uptake is inhibited by valproic acid and metabolites in mitochondrial membranes. FEBS Lett 2008;582(23-24): 3359-3366.

[252] Silva MF, Ruiter JP, Illst L, Jakobs C, Duran M, de Almeida IT, Wanders RJ. Valproate inhibits the mitochondrial pyruvate-driven oxidative phosphorylation in vitro. J Inherit Metab Dis 1997;20(3): 397-400.

[253] Valvassori SS, Rezin GT, Ferreira CL, Moretti M, Gonçalves CL, Cardoso MR, Streck EL, Kapczinski F, Quevedo J. Effects of mood stabilizers on mitochondrial respiratory chain activity in brain of rats treated with d-amphetamine. J Psychiatr Res 2010;44(14): 903-909.

[254] Zugno AI, Valvassori SS, Scherer EB, Mattos C, Matté C, Ferreira CL, Rezin GT, Wyse AT, Quevedo J, Streck EL. Na+,K+-ATPase activity in an animal model of mania. J Neural Transm 2009;116(4): 431-436.

[255] de Vasconcellos AP, Zugno AI, Dos Santos AH, Nietto FB, Crema LM, Gonçalves M, Franzon R, de Souza Wyse AT, da Rocha ER, Dalmaz C. Na+,K(+)-ATPase activity is reduced in hippocampus of rats submitted to an experimental model of depression: effect of chronic lithium treatment and possible involvement in learning deficits. Neurobiol Learn Mem 2005;84(2): 102-110.

[256] Maurer IC, Schippel P, Volz HP. Lithium-induced enhancement of mitochondrial oxidative phosphorylation in human brain tissue. Bipolar Disord 2009;11(5): 515-522.

[257] King TD, Bijur GN, Jope RS. Caspase-3 activation induced by inhibition of mitochondrial complex I is facilitated by glycogen synthase kinase-3beta and attenuated by lithium. Brain Res 2001;919(1): 106-114.

[258] Santos NA, Medina WS, Martins NM, Mingatto FE, Curti C, Santos AC. Aromatic antiepileptic drugs and mitochondrial toxicity: effects on mitochondria isolated from rat liver. Toxicol In Vitro 2008;22(5): 1143-1152.

[259] Costa C, Belcastro V, Tozzi A, Di Filippo M, Tantucci M, Siliquini S, Autuori A, Picconi B, Spillantini MG, Fedele E, Pittaluga A, Raiteri M, Calabresi P. Electrophysiology and pharmacology of striatal neuronal dysfunction induced by mitochondrial complex I inhibition. J Neurosci 2008;28(32): 8040-8052.

Chapter 6

Long-Term Adaptive Changes Induced by Antidepressants: From Conventional to Novel Therapies

Ouissame Mnie-Filali, Erika Abrial,
Laura Lambás-Señas and Nasser Haddjeri

Additional information is available at the end of the chapter

http://dx.doi.org/10.5772/54553

1. Introduction

Major depressive disorder (MDD) is a devastating disease in terms of human suffering, health costs and economic burden to society. As described in the Diagnostic and Statistical Manual of Mental Disorders, various symptoms can be observed in depressed patients including disheartened mood, loss of interest or pleasure (anhedonia), feeling of guilt or worthlessness, disturbed sleep or appetite, low energy, poor concentration and suicidal ideation. The prevalence of MDD in the general population is 4.4% to 5% with an annual incidence of 2.4% to 3.8% [1]. Regional variation in the 12-month prevalence of the major depressive episodes was also noted, ranging from 2.2% in Japan to 10.45% in Brazil with similar averages of 5.5% in developed and 5.9% in developing countries [2]. In the USA, 59% of MDD patients experience severe degree of functional impairment, making depression the largest contributor to work loss [3, 4]. Furthermore, MDD was strongly associated to self-perceived stress, childhood adversity, working status and quality of life [5-7]. According to the estimation results reported in the global burden of disease study (a study measuring disability-adjusted life-years, DALY), MDD will have become the leading cause of disability in developed countries by the year 2030 [8], indicating that the situation is not likely to improve unless something changes. A major contributor to this crisis is the lack of adequate medication to treat a large proportion of patients. Indeed, 20% do not respond to antidepressants (ADs) recommended as "first-line" drugs, 40% do so only partially, and among responders, there is a time lag of several weeks to months before a meaningful clinical effect can be observed. Failure of clinical recovery with the first AD treatment used and high risk of relapses are also common features. A common trait of all conventional ADs is that they have a similar mode of action, which is an enhancement of synaptic transmission of the monoamines serotonin (5-HT) and/or norepinephrine (NE) [9]. In fact, development of AD medications was largely based on the monoaminergic theory of depression that links the pathophysiology of this illness to a deficiency on cerebral 5-HT and/ or NE levels. Hence, first generation of ADs, monoamine oxidase inhibitors (MAOIs) and tricyclic antidepressants (TCAs) inhibit the breakdown of 5-HT, NE and dopamine in presynaptic neurons and block the presynaptic uptake of 5-HT and NE through high-affinity 5-HT (SERT) or NE (NET) transporters, respectively. Although effective, the severe side effects and toxicity of MAOIs and TCAs limited their usefulness. Later, drugs with more novel approaches, including selective 5-HT reuptake inhibitors (SSRIs), NE reuptake inhibitors (NRIs) and combined-action 5-HT/NE reuptake inhibitors (SNRIs) have been introduced, but as well as the prior generation of ADs, they act through the modulation of monoamine transporters, which may explain their suboptimal therapeutic efficacy. A number of emerging ADs that target monoamine transmission attempt to act on existing targets in more synergic ways (combining 5-HT reuptake inhibition with inhibition of autoreceptors) or to broaden the spectrum of monoamine systems targeted (dopamine, melatonin) to either enhance efficacy or speed response.

Nevertheless, the complexity and heterogeneity of symptoms of MDD makes incompatible the association of a disease with a single pathophysiological disturbance. Hence, years of research and efforts gave rise to a multitude of hypotheses trying to explain the different facets of this disorder. For example, studies have associated depression with abnormalities in the hypothalamus-pituitary-adrenal axis activity including elevated concentrations of the corticotropin-releasing hormone in the cerebrospinal fluid, increased volumes of adrenal gland and pituitary and an impairment of corticosteroid receptor signaling [10, 11]. Also, extensive studies reported circadian rhythms deregulations in depressed patients, as well as an AD effect of drugs that are capable to resynchronize this biological rhythm (i.e. agomelatine) [12, 13]. Pro-inflammatory cytokines such as interleukin (IL)-6 and tumor necrosis factors (TNF)-α were also implicated in depressive disorders [14, 15]. Other possible mechanisms that have been suggested to be involved in the etiology and treatment of MDD include deficit in the gamma-aminobutyric acid (GABA) transmission [16], dysfunction of glutamatergic system [17], acetylcholine imbalance [18], estrogens [19, 20] and so many others [21]. In spite of these hypotheses, one of the oldest, "the monoaminergic hypothesis of depression" which assumes that MDD is caused by an imbalance in serotoninergic, norepinephrinergic and possibly dopaminergic functions, is still driving clinical development of ADs since the empirical discovery of MAOIs and TCAs. Although these monoamines are undoubtedly involved, it is now recognized that, following AD administration, changes in the levels of monoamines and subsequent adaptive processes, in particular a change in the sensitivity of some of monoamine receptors, are not sufficient on their own to explain the mechanism of action of ADs. Indeed, it is difficult to correlate the time of the delayed clinical onset of AD action (several weeks) with the increase in synaptic levels of monoamines, as this change occurs already after the initial dose of the drug. In the last decade, investigations focusing on mood disturbances have been extended to brain neuroplasticity, leading to the "neurogenic and neurotrophic hypothesis of depression".

This latter postulates that development of MDD is, at least partially, related to a reduced neuroplasticity and/or depletion of neurotrophic factors which can lead to a structural deformity and functional impairment of the central nervous system.

The monoaminergic hypothesis of depression is still valid today, and intense research keeps focusing on the 5-HT system, its implication in the pathophysiology of depression and in the mode of action of ADs. Extensive data reported a number of cellular and molecular adaptive changes of the 5-HT system both at pre- (i.e. autoreceptor desensitization) and postsynaptic levels (i.e. stimulation of hippocampal neurogenesis and normalization of neurotrophins levels) following long-term treatment with various classes of ADs [22-24]. These neuroadaptations occurred with a time course consistent with the observation of a significant AD action. Naturally, a number of questions has to be asked; how the 5-HT system reacts in case of depression and after AD treatment? Which cellular and molecular actors are implicated in such reaction? Which brain areas are prevalent in these responses? To address these questions and others, the present chapter aims a better understanding of the biological basis of pharmacological treatments of depression. Attention will be paid to the neuroadaptive consequences of combination strategies (i.e. adjunction of antipsychotics) as well as promising targets on AD development (5-HT_7 receptor antagonism, 5-HT_4 agonism).

2. Neuroadaptations according to the monoaminergic hypothesis

2.1. Chronic effects of the first generation of ADs on the 5-HT system

MAOIs and TCAs were the first ADs discovered and they have proven their efficacy for treating MDD, particularly atypical depression, anergic bipolar depression and treatment-resistant depression. However, they are not supported as first-line drugs in clinical use due to life-threatening interactions with a variety of medications and common food as well as lethal cardiac irregularities [25, 26]. Early preclinical studies showed that acute administration of MAOIs (pargyline, tranylcypromine, phenelzine and iproniazid) and TCAs (clomipramine, imipramine, amitriptyline and nortriptyline) suppresses the firing activity of 5-HT neurons in the dorsal raphe nucleus (DRN) [27-29], which is reversed by an injection of the 5-HT_{1A} receptors antagonist, WAY-100635 [28, 30].

A prolonged administration of MAOIs induces a complete recovery of the firing activity of DRN 5-HT neurons, an effect attributable to a desensitization of the somatodendritic 5-HT_{1A} autoreceptors since the reducing effect of 5-HT_{1A} receptors agonists is completely abolished (Figure 1) [31-33]. Accordingly, a reduction of the ability of 8-OH-DPAT to inhibit forskolin-stimulated adenylate cyclase activity [34] and an increase of the ED_{50} for 8-OH-DPAT induced lower lip retraction [35] were reported after chronic treatment with MAOIs (MDL 72394, clorgyline or tranylcypromine) in rats. This desensitization of 5-HT_{1A} autoreceptors seems to occur at the level of receptor-G protein interactions rather than their simple downregulation. In fact, an autoradiographic study showed that the 5-HT_{1A} agonist-stimulated [^{35}S]-GTPγS binding is reduced in rats treated for 21 days with clorgyline [36]. Importantly, such chronic treatment with MAOIs was shown to increase the extracellular concentrations of 5-HT, an effect greater in raphe nuclei than in their projection areas [37]. A microdialysis study measuring the extracellular levels of 5-HT in the frontal cortex of rats reported that chronic administration of the reversible MAOI MDL72394 significantly increased 5-HT amounts, without having any effect on the ability of the 5-HT_{1A} and 5-HT_{1B} agonist RU24969 to reduce these levels [38], suggesting that the sensitivity of these autoreceptors are not affected by chronic treatment with MAOIs. This is supported by data from an electrophysiological study demonstrating that long-term administration of clorgyline increased the efficacy of the stimulation of the 5-HT pathway to suppress the firing activity of CA3 pyramidal neurons of the dorsal hippocampus, whereas the enhancing effect of the antagonist of the terminal 5-HT autoreceptors methiothepin remained unchanged [39]. However, it is for high interest to note that long-term treatment with the reversible MAO-A inhibitor befloxatone resulted in a tonic activation of postsynaptic 5-HT_{1A} receptors located on the dorsal hippocampus CA3 pyramidal neurons since the highly potent and selective antagonist, WAY-100635, markedly increased the firing activity of these neurons (Figure 2] [40]. It is also noteworthy that MAO-A knock-out mice exhibit high extracellular amounts of 5-HT and an overall decrease of 5-HT_{1A} receptors density, including raphe autoreceptors as well as hippocampus and spinal cord postsynaptic receptors [41, 42]. In summary, chronic treatment with MAOIs does desensitize inhibitory 5-HT_{1A} autoreceptors, keep sensitivity of terminal 5-HT autoreceptors unaltered and enhance the tonic activation of postsynaptic 5-HT_{1A} receptors. Similarly to MAOIs, chronic treatment with TCAs (imipramine, iprindole, desipramine and femoxetine) did not change the mean firing rate of the DRN 5-HT neurons in comparison to controls [31]. However, the responsiveness to intravenous injection of the 5-HT agonist LSD or the effectiveness of microiontophoretic application of 5-HT and LSD were not altered by such treatment [31], suggesting that the sensitivity of the 5-HT autoreceptors is not modified. The 5-HT_{1A}/G-protein coupling is usually assessed by measuring [^{35}S]-GTPγS binding induced by 5-HT_{1A} receptor activation [43]. It was reported that chronic treatment with the TCA amitriptyline did not alter the 5-HT_{1A} agonist-stimulated [^{35}S]-GTPγS binding in dorsal and median raphe nuclei [44, 45], further confirming an absence of desensitization of the somatodendritic 5-HT_{1A} autoreceptor following chronic TCAs. In contrast, the same treatments have different effects on postsynaptic levels. Indeed, long-term application of imipramine increased the responsiveness of postsynaptic CA3 hippocampus pyramidal neurons to the microiontophoretic application of 5-HT or 8-OH-DPAT [46]. In accordance, Rossi et al. [45] showed that chronic administration of amitriptyline increased the 5-HT_{1A} receptor-stimulated [^{35}S]-GTPγS binding in the hippocampus, without affecting the binding of [^{3}H]8-OH-DPAT (indicating the number of 5-HT_{1A} receptors in the coupled high-affinity agonist state). These authors suggest that, in absence of an increase in the binding of [^{3}H]8-OH-DPAT, the increased capacity of 5-HT_{1A} receptors to activate G proteins in CA1 and dentate gyrus of the hippocampus may be due to regulatory changes at the level of the G protein, e.g. phosphorylation [45]. In summary, chronic TCA treatment does not desensitize inhibitory 5-HT_{1A} autoreceptors and enhance the sensitivity of postsynaptic 5-HT_{1A} receptors in the hippocampus.

http://dx.doi.org/10.5772/54553

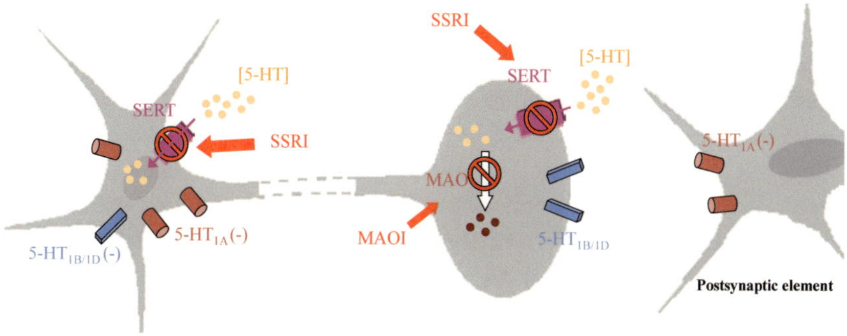

Figure 1. Representation of the effects of the serotoninergic antidepressants on 5-HT neurotransmission. Monoamine oxidase inhibitors (MAOIs) and selective serotonin reuptake inhibitors (SSRIs) act on the 5-HT system, respectively, by inhibiting the 5-HT degradation and by blocking the 5-HT transporter (SERT). Their administration induces the raise of extracellular levels of 5-HT which activate 5-HT receptors. In the raphe nuclei, the somatodendritic 5-HT_{1A} autoreceptors negatively control the firing activity of the 5-HT neurons, while the 5-HT_{1B}/$_{1C}$ autoreceptors control the 5-HT release. Long-term administration of both classes of antidepressants desensitize 5-HT_{1A} autoreceptors. Modified from Faure et al. [22].

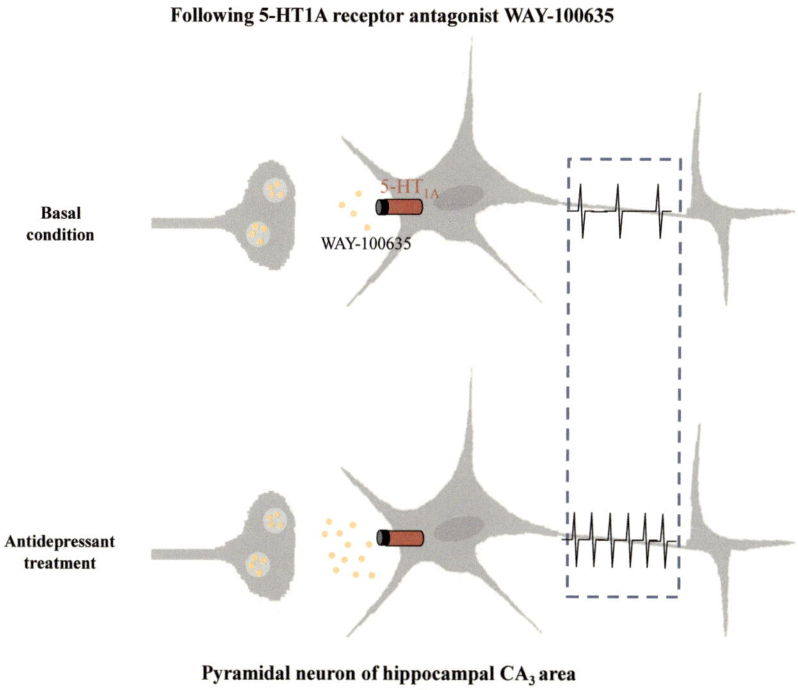

Figure 2. Representation of the effect of antidepressant treatments on hippocampal neurons. The raise of extracellular 5-HT levels decreases the firing activity of hippocampus CA3 pyramidal neuron and this is mediated by postsynaptic 5-HT_{1A} receptors. In control animals, no or low firing activity increase is observed after administration of the antagonist WAY-100635. However, in antidepressant-treated animals, WAY-100635 disinhibits pyramidal cells, suggesting that antidepressants increase 5-HT tone in the hippocampus. Modified from Blier and de Montigny [201].

2.2. Chronic effects of the SSRIs on the 5-HT system

SSRIs represent the first-line ADs in clinical use nowadays, mainly due to their relatively lower burden of adverse effects and safety in overdose. SSRIs include fluoxetine, fluvoxamine, paroxetine, sertraline, citalopram, escitalopram and more recently vilazodone [47, 48]. These drugs are believed to exert their effects by blocking SERT, which induces an increase of 5-HT synaptic levels. In turn, the chronic enhancement of 5-HT bioavailability produces numerous neuroadaptive changes leading to an enhancement of the 5-HT neurotransmission (Figure 1) [22, 40, 49]. In particular, it was widely reported that acute administration of SSRIs inhibits the firing activity of the 5-HT neurons in DRN, resulting from an enhancement of somatodendritic 5-HT release which activates the 5-HT_{1A} autoreceptors [50-55]. However, immunoelectron microscopy studies using specific antibodies showed a significant decrease of the 5-HT_{1A} immunogold labeling of the plasma membrane of the DRN dendrites and an increase in their cytoplasmic labeling after a single injection of the SSRI fluoxetine in animals, indicating an internalization of these autoreceptors under acute conditions [56, 57]. Importantly, a very recent double-blind positron emission tomography study investigated the binding of the 5-HT_{1A} radioligand [^{18}F]MPPF in human volunteers after taking a single tablet of fluoxetine or placebo. This study clearly demonstrated that in DRN, and nowhere else in the brain, a significant decrease in [^{18}F]MPPF binding potential between fluoxetine and placebo [58]. In animals, this autoreceptor internalization seems to be very transient since a microdialysis study reported that administration of a 5-HT_{1A} receptor agonist a few hours after single injection of fluoxetine reverses the SSRI-induced increase in the 5-HT levels [59]. Short-term treatment with SSRIs also reduced the firing activity of the DRN 5-HT neurons [50]. Only chronic (2 to 3 weeks) treatments with these drugs completely recover the 5-HT firing activity, and this is accompanied with a desensitization of the somatodendritic 5-HT_{1A} autoreceptors [50, 51, 60, 61]. Interestingly, when rats chronically treated with fluoxetine were challenged with a single dose of 8-OH-DPAT, there was no internalization of the 5-HT_{1A} autoreceptors in keeping with their desensitized form [62]. In fact, after such treatment, neither the density of the 5-HT_{1A} autoreceptors on the plasma membrane of DRN neurons nor the [^{18}F]MPPF binding were changed [56, 58, 62, 63]. One explanation is that, after repeated internalization and retargeting, functional 5-HT_{1A} autoreceptors are replaced by receptors uncoupled from their G proteins (inactivated form of the receptor) on the plasma membrane of DRN 5-HT neurons [62]. However, controversial results have been reported about the effects of chronic SSRI treatment on the functional status of the 5-HT_{1A} autoreceptors. An attenuation of 8-OH-DPAT-mediated [^{35}S]-GTPγS stimulation has been consistently observed in the DRN by certain groups after chronic fluoxetine [36, 44, 49, 64, 65], while others reported no change in this parameter after chronic sertraline or citalopram [63, 66]. These findings raised the possibility that SSRIs may not be a homogenous class of AD drugs with regard to the mechanism by which the function of somatodendritic 5-HT_{1A} autoreceptors is regulated. Thus, at least in the case of fluoxetine, acute and chronic treatments seem to induce two distinct types of 5-HT_{1A} autoreceptor desensitization: one rapid and reversible (associated with the internalization of the functional pool of membrane-bound receptors), the other being progressive and long-lasting, no longer accompanied with receptor sequestration, but which probably resulted from the reiteration of this process throughout the course of chronic fluoxetine treatment [58]. Another picture can be drawn for the postsynaptic 5-HT_{1A} heteroreceptors. In fact, neither acute nor chronic treatment with SSRIs induced a change in the subcellular distribution of the 5-HT_{1A} receptors in dendrites or in the in vivo binding of the 5-HT_{1A} radioligand [18F]MPPF in projection areas, particularly hippocampus and frontal cortex [56, 62, 63]. Such differences between 5-HT_{1A} receptors in DRN and projection areas were explained by a differential coupling, the autoreceptors being coupled to $G\alpha_{i3}$ while heteroreceptors are coupled to $G\alpha o$ protein [67]. However, agonist-induced [^{35}S]-GTPγS binding data showed an increase [36, 63, 64] or no change [44, 49, 68] after long-term SSRI treatment, further adding complexity to the whole picture. Importantly, long-term application of SSRIs produced an increase in tonic activation of pyramidal neurons, indicated by the disinhibition of firing rate in response to the antagonist WAY-100635 (Figure 2) [40, 51]. This further supports the increase of the efficacy of the 5-HT neurotransmission seen in vivo (enhancing the effectiveness of the stimulation of the 5-HT pathway to suppress the firing activity of CA3 pyramidal neurons) and in vitro (increasing the electrically-evoked release of tritiated 5-HT from preloaded hippocampal slices) [46, 69]. More recent studies noted a decrease in the density of the 5-HT_4 receptor binding in the CA1 field of hippocampus of rats as well as in several areas of the striatum after a 21-day treatment with the SSRI fluoxetine [70]. The activity of these postsynaptic receptors in the hippocampus, measured as the excitatory action of the 5-HT_4 agonist zacopride in pyramidal cells of CA1 evoked by Schaffer collateral stimulation, was attenuated also after such chronic treatment [70]. This suggests a net decrease in the signalisation pathway of 5-HT_4 receptors after chronic SSRI treatment. In addition, desensitization of the 5-HT_7 receptors [71] and downregulation in the 5-HT_7 binding site in the hypothalamus [72] were reported following chronic treatment with fluoxetine.

Another interesting consequence of chronic, but not acute, treatment with SSRIs is a reduction of the surface expression of SERT. In fact, electron microscopy studies reported that long-term administration of fluoxetine induced an internalization of SERT in both cell bodies and axon terminals of 5-HT neurons [58]. Moreover, the total amounts of SERT immunoreactivity is also reduced, suggesting that, rather than a simple internalization, a long-term degradation of this protein happened in the course of the treatment [58].

2.3. Chronic effects of new antidepressant strategies

The suboptimal efficacy and the delayed onset of action of different classes of ADs raises the necessity to find new strategies to treat depression, especially treatment-resistant depression and depressive episodes associated with bipolar disorders. For example, a number of second-generation antipsychotics have been investigated and approved for use as augmentation agents in combination with currently approved first-line ADs such as adjunctive aripiprazole, olanzapine or quetiapine to standard doses of SSRIs [73-75]. The effect of such combination on the 5-HT system is yet not well described in the literature, and only very recent preclinical studies began to investigate their mechanisms of action. For example, Chernoloz et al. [76] showed in rats that long-term administration (14 days) of quetiapine alone or in combination with the SSRI escitalopram led to significant inhibition of the spontaneous firing activity of the DRN 5-HT neurons, while escitalopram alone (as previously described for SSRIs) induced a recovery of this neuronal activity at this time point. Co-administration of quetiapine and escitalopram for 14 days produced an increase in tonic activation of postsynaptic 5-HT$_{1A}$ receptors located on the dorsal hippocampus CA3 pyramidal neurons, but in the same range as that obtained with chronic escitalopram alone [76]. The enhancement in 5-HT transmission produced by this combination was attributable to the attenuated inhibitory function of α_2-adrenergic receptors on 5-HT terminals and possibly to direct 5-HT$_{1A}$ receptor agonism by quetiapine [76]. Similarly, risperidone co-administered with escitalopram for 14 days was shown to prevent the restoration of the 5-HT neuronal firing rate, obtained with the SSRI alone [77]. Therefore, it might be suggested that risperidone co-administrated with the SSRIs increases 5-HT neurotransmission by indirect action on the 5-HT system. Indeed, Marcus et al. [78] reported that adjunctive low-dose of risperidone to escitalopram significantly enhanced both dopamine outflow and NMDA receptor-mediated transmission in the medial prefrontal cortex (PFC) of rats. Taken together, these results pointed out the possibility that, rather than a direct action on the 5-HT system, combining an SSRI and an antipsychotic of second-generation implicate multiple neurotransmitter systems to exert their beneficial effects.

Among novel targets to develop more efficacious and fast-acting ADs, 5-HT$_4$ and 5-HT$_7$ receptors are promising candidates [71, 79]. For example, brain regional changes in the binding of the 5-HT$_4$ receptors were found in murine models of depression-related states including olfactory bulbectomy model, glucocorticoid receptor heterozygous mice and Flinders sensitive line depression model [80, 81]. Lucas et al. [79] showed in rats that a 3-day treatment with the 5-HT$_4$ receptor agonist RS67333 modifies several rat brain parameters considered as key markers of AD action, which are changed only after 2 to 3 weeks with classical ADs. These changes include desensitization of the 5-HT$_{1A}$ autoreceptors and increased tonus on hippocampal postsynaptic 5-HT$_{1A}$ receptors [79]. Accordingly, subchronic (3 days) administration of RS67333, but not acute, increased basal 5-HT levels and decreased its metabolite levels 5-HIAA in the rat ventral hippocampus [82]. Furthermore, a 3-day co-administration of the SSRI citalopram and a 5-HT$_4$ receptor agonist, RS67333 or prucalopride, resulted in an increase of DRN 5-HT neuron mean firing activity, displaying a similar, or even slightly superior, firing amplitude obtained with each agonist alone [83]. At the postsynaptic level, this translated into the manifestation of a tonus on hippocampal postsynaptic 5-HT$_{1A}$ receptors, which was two to three times stronger when the 5-HT$_4$ receptor agonist was combined with citalopram [83]. This suggests an important increase on the 5-HT neurotransmission following adjunction of an SSRI to a 5-HT$_4$ receptor agonist, clearly indicating a rapid AD-like potential of these agonists.

Moreover, antipsychotics (lurasidone, amisulpride), as well as a novel AD-like multimodal 5-HT agent (Lu-AA21004), have been proved to be potent 5-HT$_7$ antagonists [84-88]. Furthermore, genetic deletion of this receptor confers to mice AD-like behaviors including decreased immobility in the forced swim and tail suspension tests as well as shorter and less frequent episodes of rapid eye movement sleep [89], indicating that antagonists might have therapeutic value as ADs. In this context, we showed that a 1-week treatment with the selective 5-HT$_7$ receptor antagonist, SB-269970, did not alter 5-HT firing activity but desensitized somatodendritic 5-HT$_{1A}$ autoreceptors and enhanced the tonic activation of postsynaptic 5-HT_{1A} receptors in the hippocampus [71]. Taken together, these findings show that new AD strategies targeting 5-HT receptor manipulation resulted in similar adaptive changes of the 5-HT system than those produced by classical ADs, except that they took place faster in both pre- and postsynaptic levels.

In summary, a change of 5-HT receptor sensitivity that occurs only after chronic treatment seems to be a common mechanism of AD action, which takes place depending on the delay onset of action of each 5-HT AD. This represents the major argument supporting the 5-HT hypothesis of depression. However, it became obvious that depression involves further modifications besides those at the 5-HT system. Several studies emerged to assess new pharmacological models that may help to better understand the mechanisms and pathophysiological changes leading to a depressive behaviour.

3. Neurogenic and neurotrophic adaptations induced by 5-HT antidepressants

Recent studies indicate that an impairment of cellular and synaptic plasticity in specific areas of the brain, especially the hippocampus and PFC, may be a core factor in the pathophysiology of depression. The abnormal neuronal plasticity including neurogenesis, axon branching, dendritogenesis and synaptogenesis was suggested to be related to alterations in the level of neurotrophic factors, particularly brain-derived neurotrophic factor (BDNF) which plays a central role in the adaptation of neural networks. Numerous studies reported that AD treatments may act by normalizing neurotrophic levels in the brain and enhancing neurogenesis and synaptogenesis, leading to a gain of function in neuronal networks altered by depressive states. In the following paragraphs, we enumerate the chronic effects of the previously cited AD strategies on the cellular and synaptic plasticity, as well as neurotrophin expression. A critical view of the role of each parameter on the etiology of depression and AD action is also described.

3.1. Neurogenesis

The first evidence of newly generated neurons in the adult central nervous system was reported in 1965 when Altman and Das [90] used ^{3}H-thymidine to label proliferating cells in the rat dentate gyrus (DG) of the hippocampus. Subsequent studies confirmed the existence of this hippocampal neurogenesis in adulthood in several species including humans [91, 92], using the new tool bromodeoxyuridine (BrdU), a thymidine analog that labels dividing cells in S-phase [93]. In the hippocampus, progenitor cells are located in the subgranular zone (SGZ) where they divide and a subset of the new cells survive, migrate into granule cell layer and differentiates into neurons. An excellent review of Hanson et al. [94] described the timeline of cell division and maturation as well as markers of cells from different stages of neurogenesis in the SGZ. The subventricular zone (SVZ) was also identified as a highly neurogenic area of the adult brain [95], although other regions retain the potential to generate new neurons [96-98].

The hippocampal neurogenesis was shown to be implicated in the pathophysiology of depression (Table 1). Clinical studies showed that patients suffering from MDD had lower hippocampal volume than healthy subjects [99, 100], that may be linked to increased neuronal atrophy. Only patients who remitted after 8 weeks of AD treatment present larger hippocampal volume in comparison to subjects who did not remit [101]. A more evident correlation came firstly from the preclinical study of Santarelli et al. [102]. In this study, mice treated 28 days with the SSRI fluoxetine exhibited an increase in the number of BrdU-positive cells in the SGZ of DG with a concomitant decrease in the latency to feed in the novelty suppressed-feeding (NSF) paradigm. However, ablation of cell proliferation in the SGZ, but not the SVZ, following X-ray treatment suppressed behavioral responses to chronic fluoxetine [102]. The requirement of hippocampal neurogenesis for therapeutic efficacy of ADs was subsequently confirmed in non-human primates [103]. Consistent with the time course of their therapeutic action, only chronic treatment regimen with MAOIs [104, 105], TCAs [106, 107], SSRIs [61, 102, 105, 108], putative fast-acting AD drugs including 5-HT_4 agonists [79] and 5-HT_7 antagonists [71] and finally adjunctive strategies (olanzapine plus fluoxetine) [108] increased the cell proliferation in the SGZ of the hippocampus at comparable extent. This indicates that upregulation of hippocampal neurogenesis may be a common denominator of the mechanism of action of ADs. Although the function of these newly generated cells in the adult brain is still unclear, it has been suggested that young granule cells constitute a distinct population exhibiting a greater degree of plasticity than mature neurons. In particular, they display a reduced threshold to induction of long-term potentiation (LTP) [109], and can be tonically activated by ambient GABA before being sequentially innervated by GABA- and glutamate-mediated synaptic inputs, leading to marked defects in their synapse formation and dendritic development in vivo [110].

Given the emergence of new data, the initial research cited above suggesting a model of hippocampal degeneration as basis of depression and reversal by ADs through neurogenesis seems to be uncertain. In fact, as chronic ADs, mood stabilizers (lithium) and atypical anti-psychotics induce hippocampal cell proliferation [108, 111-113], but whether these drugs can be used as monotherapy in depression is an area of debate and clinical data failed to support it. It is also noteworthy that, even in the famous study of Santarelli et al. [102], X-ray of hippocampus suppressing neurogenesis in non-treated rats failed to induce a depressive-like behavior. Accordingly, cyclin D2 (a protein involved in the cell cycle regulation) knock-out mice, specifically lacking adult brain neurogenesis, showed normal anxiety levels in the open-field and elevated plus maze [114]. In contrast, increasing hippocampal neurogenesis in mice was not reported to produce anxiolytic or AD-like behavioral effects [115]. These latter reports add complexity to the understanding of the role of altered neurogenesis in the pathology of depression. That is why, some neuroscientists postulate that, beyond a simple increase of hippocampal neurogenesis in response to ADs, insertion of the newly generated neurons (even a small number) in functional neural networks especially through synaptogenesis, may be more relevant for the explanation of their mechanism of action.

In this context, an elegant theory in which neurogenesis is seen as an epiphenomenon of a more widespread alteration in dendritic length and spine number was already proposed [116].

According to this theory, exposure to chronic stress and stressful life events increases excitotoxic glutamatergic neurotransmission in multiple brain areas. To protect neurons from consequent apoptosis, dendrites retract and spine number decreases thus limiting the number of exposed glutamate receptors.

3.2. Synaptic plasticity and synaptogenesis

The regulation of synapse formation or synaptogenesis is a subcellular neuronal alteration that contributes to synaptic plasticity [117, 118], which defines the ability to integrate informations from different neuronal inputs and make the appropriate adaptive responses. An increase in functional synaptogenesis is typically accompanied by an increase in the number of dendritic spines, the physical site of synaptic connections [118, 119]. In recent years, it has become clear that spines are dynamic structures that undergo rapid remodeling important for synapse formation, function and plasticity [120, 121]. In the adulthood, spines continue to remodel in response to a variety of physiological stimuli. For example, synaptic activity that induces LTP, a long-lasting enhancement of synaptic strength, promotes spine enlargement and new spine formation [122], whereas activity that induces long-term depression (LTD), a persistent weakening of synaptic strength, causes spine shrinkage or retraction [123]. The potential role of spines and dendrites in MDD (Table 1] is supported by preclinical studies demonstrating that exposure to chronic stress negatively influence dendritic spine density and morphology in brain areas such as DG, CA1 and CA3 subfields of the hippocampus and PFC [124-126]. This includes a decrease in spine density, dendritic length and branch number [127, 128]. These effects could contribute to the reduction in volume of PFC and hippocampus determined by imaging the brains of depressed patients [100, 101, 129]. In accordance, a recent study revealed lower expression of synaptic function-related genes in the dorsolateral PFC of MDD subjects and a corresponding lower number of synapses [130].

As for neurogenesis, ADs regulate these different forms of synaptic plasticity. Synaptic communication is altered by chronic stress which impairs LTP and facilitates LTD induction in the CA1 of the hippocampus [131-133]. It has been reported that repeated application of the SSRI fluvoxamine (21 days) increased the extent of LTP induction in the CA1 region of rats that experienced chronic mild stress [131]. Using rats neonatally-exposed to clomipramine as an animal model of depression, Bhagya et al. [134] found that these animals displayed a decreased LTP in the hippocampal CA1 and a 14-day treatment with the SSRI escitalopram restored this LTP. Similarly, retrieval of LTP in the CA1 field of hippocampus was obtained in stressed animals after repeated application of other classes of ADs including the SNRI milnacipran and electroconvulsive stimulation (ECS) [132, 135]. In contrast, other groups described an impairment of LTP after chronic SSRI fluoxetine, TCA imipramine, SNRI venlafaxine or ECS, but in non-stressed animals [136-138], indicating a stress-dependent action of the ADs on hippocampal LTP. In the same way, chronic fluoxetine was reported to increase dendritic spine density and arborization of granule cells in the mouse hippocampus [139, 140]. Daily administration of fluoxetine to ovariectomized rats for 5 days was shown to induce a robust increase in pyramidal cell dendritic spine synapse density in the hippocampal CA1 field, with similar changes appearing in CA3 after 2 weeks of treatment [141]. This rapid synaptic remodelling might represent an early step in the fluoxetine-induced cascade of responses that spread across the entire hippocampal circuitry, leading to the restoration of normal function in the hippocampus [141]. In accordance, a recent study using ovariectomized hamsters exposed to diminished light at night displayed depressive-like behaviors and reduced hippocampal CA1 dendritic spine density, but a 2-week treatment with citalopram rescued this behavior and moderately improved the spine density in the CA1 but not fully restored it [142]. Also, chronic treatment with the TCA amitriptyline reversed the bulbectomy-induced reduction in dendritic spine density in CA1, CA3 and dentate gyrus of hippocampus [143]. It has to be noted that single injection of the 5-HT_4 receptor partial agonist SL65.0155 does not promote spine growth in the naive mouse hippocampus [144], and the 5-HT_7 receptor agonist AS-19 increased neurite length and number in primary embryonic hippocampal neurons [145], still the characterization of the in vivo effects of their chronic manipulation is missing. It is obvious that the effects on synaptic plasticity of chronic treatment with different AD strategies will be an important area of further research.

Significant evidence suggests that ADs regulate synaptic plasticity and reorganization through the modulation of cell adhesion protein and synaptic function/structure related genes. In particular, the neural cell adhesion molecule NCAM is necessary for activity-dependent LTP in the hippocampus [146]. Its highly sialylated isoform PSA-NCAM promotes plasticity through the negatively charged PSA, postulated to be a spacer that reduces adhesion forces between cells allowing their dynamic changes [147]. It was reported that chronic treatment with the selective MAO-B inhibitor deprenyl, the TCA imipramine or the SSRI fluoxetine increased the expression of PSA-NCAM in the hippocampus and medial PFC [148-151]. Interestingly, chronic exposure to second-generation antispychotics olanzapine or risperidone enhances PSA-NCAM expression in the PFC, but not in the hippocampus, suggesting that modulation of cell adhesion protein in the hippocampus may be specific to the mechanism of action of ADs [152, 153]. Moreover, an increased expression of synaptophysin, a glycoprotein localized in presynaptic vesicle membranes required for docking and fusion of neurotransmitter-containing synaptic vesicles as well as endocytosis [154], was observed in hippocampus and/or cerebral cortex of rats chronically treated with the MAOI tranylcypromine, the TCA amitriptyline or the SSRI fluoxetine [148, 155, 156]. Also, Arc (Activity-regulated, cytoskeletal-associated protein), a highly expressed protein in dendrites and postsynaptic densities [157] is implicated in LTP and spine size and type [158-160]. Repeated administration (14 days) of the SSRI paroxetine, the TCA desipramine or the MAOI tranylcypromine increased Arc mRNA and the number of Arc-immunoreactive cells in frontal and parietal cortex as well as in the CA1 region of the hippocampus, while acute injection had no effect [161].

How do ADs exert their effect on synaptic plasticity is a matter of discussion. Several putative mechanisms have been proposed in this context. However, the observation that antidepressants increased anti-apoptotic factors and the synthesis of neurotrophic factors raises the possibility that these drugs act via a mechanism of neuroprotection rather than a neuroregeneration [23]. Particular attention was given to neurotrophins such as brain-derived neurotrophic factor (BDNF).

3.3. Neurotrophins modulation by 5-HT antidepressants

Neurotrophins are growth factors with crucial roles in the formation and plasticity of neuronal networks [162], and BDNF is the most studied in this context. The dystrophic action of stress was reported in animal models of depression (Table 1). Animals exposed to chronic stress such as chronic mild stress or social deprivation displayed a decrease in the protein levels of BDNF and an increase of its receptor tyrosine-kinase TrkB in several brain regions including hippocampus (DG, CA1 and CA3), frontal cortex and midbrain [163-168]. BDNF-deficient mice or with specific knockdown of BDNF in the DG also displayed depressive-like behaviors [169, 170]. Accordingly, drug-free MDD patients showed lower serum or plasma BDNF levels in comparison to healthy subjects [171-174]. Moreover, human BDNF gene polymorphism Val66Met was suggested to be related to the pathophysiology of MDD and affect clinical response to AD treatment [175-177].

Studies	Stress type	Neuroplasticity consequence	References
Preclinical			
	Repeated restraint stress paradigm in rats	Reduction on the number and length of apical dendritic branches in mPFC	[127] [126]
		Atrophy of apical dendrites of CA3 pyramidal neurons	[201]
		LTP suppression in DG and CA3 in a site-specific manner	[202]
	Chronic unpredictable stress paradigm in rats	Dendritic atrophy in CA3 region Atrophy in granule and CA1 pyramidal neurons	[125]
		LTP impairment in CA1 area and decrease of synaptophysin density in CA3 region	[131]
		Decrease in BDNF mRNA level in hippocampus and cerebral cortex	[203,204]
	Chronic corticosterone administration in rats	Atrophy in granule and CA1 pyramidal neurons Dendritic atrophy in CA3 area	[125]
		Retraction of apical dendrites in mPFC	[205]
		Decrease in BDNF mRNA level in hippocampus and cerebral cortex	[204]
	Chronic sleep deprivation in rats	Decrease in hippocampal volume	[207]
		Suppression of cell proliferation in the hippocampus	[208]
		Impairment of LTP in the CA1 region	[209]
Clinical			
	Unipolar depression	Lower hippocampal volume	[99, 210]
		Volume reduction in orbitofrontal cortex, frontal cortex, hippocampus, striatum, and cingulate cortex	[128]

Studies	Stress type	Neuroplasticity consequence	References
	Recurrent MDD	Lower hippocampal volume	[211, 212]
		Reduced volume in dorsolateral prefrontal cortex	[213]
		Lower plasma BDNF	[172]
	First-episode depression	Lower hippocampal volume	[214, 215]
		Smaller left hippocampal volume only in males	[216]
		Lower plasma BDNF	[172]
	Late-life depression	Reduction in hippocampal volume	[217, 218]
		Specific reduction in left hippocampus	[219]
		Volume reduction in orbitofrontal cortex, putamen and thalamus	[217]
		Lower plasma BDNF	[220]
	Familial recurrent MDD	Smaller volume of the right hippocampus	[221, 222]
	Cumulative adversity (recurrent stressful life events)	Smaller volume in medial prefrontal cortex, insular cortex and subgenual anterior cingulate regions)	[223]

Table 1. Effects of chronic stress and depression on different neuroplasticity actors in the brain. mPFC: median prefrontal cortex. DG: dentate gyrus. LTP: long-term potentiation. BDNF: Brain-derived neurotrophic factor. MDD: major depressive disorder.

Intracortical infusion of BDNF in the adult rat was shown to produce a robust sprouting of 5-HT nerve terminals and accelerated the regrowth of 5-HT axons in basal conditions or following their destruction [178, 179]. AD treatments could oppose or reverse the actions of stress on the 5-HT system via a positive action on cerebral BDNF. Indeed, several studies showed that long-term AD treatments including SSRIs (fluoxetine) and MAOIs (tranylcypromine, phenelzine) increase BDNF levels in the brain [168, 180-182], although a time-dependent modulation seems to occur. Indeed, De Foubert et al. [182] demonstrated in rat hippocampus that a 4-day administration of the SSRI fluoxetine decreased BDNF mRNA levels, a 7-day treatment had no effect, but a 14-day treatment increased it. One explanation of this biphasic change in BDNF gene expression could be a differential transcript regulation, since the rat BDNF gene expresses four mRNA isoforms which can be modulated by different signaling cascades. In fact, a recent study demonstrated that acute injection of fluoxetine or tranylcypromine decreased total BDNF mRNA (exon V) as well as exon IV mRNA with no significant changes on exon I or III mRNAs [183]. In contrast, chronic administration of these two drugs enhanced expression of exon V and exon I mRNAs with no changes for exon III or IV [183]. It is of high interest to note that ADs, besides regulating BDNF levels in naive animals, normalize it under stress conditions. Hence, chronic treatment with fluoxetine increased the BDNF protein till control levels in the hippocampus of rats experiencing chronic mild stress [184], indicating that AD treatment can oppose the dystrophic actions of stress. Accordingly, clinical studies reported that untreated depressed patients showed a decrease of serum or platelet

BDNF levels before treatment, and a normalization of this parameter following several weeks of SSRI (escitalopram or paroxetine) administration accompanied with an improvement in depressive symptoms [185, 186]. Unfortunately, very few studies were conducted in this field using novel ADs targeting the 5-HT system. For example, subchronic administration (3 injections in 24h) of the 5-HT_4 receptor partial agonist SL65.0155, but not citalopram or clomipramine, was reported to enhance hippocampal BDNF protein levels in rats, further supporting a fast-acting AD profile of 5-HT_4 receptor agonists [187]. Also, Agostinho et al. [188] reported that combinatory treatment for 28 days with olanzapine and fluoxetine had no effect on BDNF protein levels but enhanced specifically in the PFC the protein levels of NT-3, a neurotrophin implicated in the pathophysiology of MDD [189]. However, these authors reported also that 28 days of fluoxetine administration did not increase BDNF proteins levels neither in the hippocampus nor in the PFC, even at high doses [188], raising some concern about this study. Obviously, more investigations are needed to characterize the exact effects on BDNF of these new treatment strategies.

4. Conclusion

The study of MDD is a real challenge for those who want to reveal the pathophysiological basis of this disease. The monoaminergic and neurotrophic/neurogenic hypotheses cited in this review give only a partial explanation of this basis. In the former, the function of a number of 5-HT receptors is still not yet elucidated and growing data implicate each receptor in a different way in the AD mechanism of action. In the latter, the role of new-added neurons in the hippocampus is still under investigation, although their integration in functional networks may confer additional plasticity to rescue stress effects. These hypotheses can be considered complementary as the activation of monoamine receptors may modulate the expression of intracellular proteins and neurotrophic factors, permitting the re-organization of complex neuronal networks involved in depression. Hence, ADs, particularly those targeting the 5-HT system, were shown to induce changes at the level of 5-HT autoreceptors localized in the raphe nuclei as well as the activation of neurotrophic factors expression and induction of cellular proliferation within projecting areas such as the hippocampus. Yet, combining these two hypotheses is not sufficient to fully explain the pathophysiology of depression, since conventional ADs were shown to modulate each factor (5-HT sensitivity, hippocampal cell proliferation, neurotrophic expression), but still displaying moderate efficacy to alleviate depression symptoms. Thus, the re-construction of a new and more convincing model is an urgent necessity.

While there has been a major emphasis on the co-incidental changes in neurotransmitters and the related receptors, neurogenesis and neurotrophic factors, less attention has been paid to changes in glia. These non-neuronal cells, particularly astrocytes, were long considered to have simple supportive role for neurons providing structure and adequate environmental conditions for neuronal functions. However, recent discoveries changed this view and led to a reconceptualization of neuronal signaling with astrocytes forming an integral part of the "tripartite synapse" along with the pre- and postsynaptic neurons [190]. In fact, glia was shown to use variations in cytoplasmic calcium as a form of cellular excitability allowing signaling to other glia, neurons and blood vessels [191]. The astrocytes excitability can be triggered by various neurotransmitters receptors expressed on glia and, in turn, these cells can release a wide variety of gliotransmitters including glutamate, adenosine triphosphate and D-serine, which regulate synaptic transmission and plasticity [191] [192]. Strikingly, reductions in the density and ultrastructure of glial cells were detected in fronto-limbic regions in major depression [193, 194], indicating the relevance of studying these cells in the pathophysiological basis of MDD. Also, glial cells seem to play a central role in inflammation that contributes to the main symptom of depression [195, 196], while fluoxetine requires microglia to exert its neuroprotective action [184].

Being a heterogeneous condition, depression is unlikely to be explained by a single pathophysiological disturbance, hence, it is not expected that a single mechanism of drug action can be uniformly effective. A new vision in which neurons and glial cells are involved side by side will be more adequate to explain the heterogeneity of MDD. In the basis of very recent researches, a "network hypothesis", in which information processing implicating neurons and glia within particular brain networks is altered in MDD and can be improved by AD treatment, can be proposed. Hence, Sheline et al. [197] reported, in depressed subjects, a dramatic increase in connectivity of three different brain networks: the cognitive control network, default mode network and affective network, with the "dorsal nexus", a bilateral region of the dorsal medial PFC. Recent reports using subpsychomimetic doses of ketamine, an ionotropic glutamatergic N-methyl-D-aspartate (NMDA) receptor antagonist, showed a rapid AD response in MDD subjects [198], which is hypothesized to be mediated by i) lower Glx/glutamate ratio in the PFC associated with reductions in glial cells in the same region [199] and, ii) decreased functional connectivity of the default mode network to the dorsal nexus [200]. More investigations are needed to define how brain networks can respond faster to this novel antidepressant, how neurons and glia are implicating in such process and how the involved mechanism can be used to the discovery of new treatment strategies in MDD.

Author details

Ouissame Mnie-Filali[1], Erika Abrial[2,3], Laura Lambás-Señas[2,3] and Nasser Haddjeri[2,3*]

*Address all correspondence to: nasser.haddjeri@univ-lyon1.fr

1 Département de Pathologie et Biologie cellulaire, Université de Montréal, Montréal, Québec, Canada

2 Institut Cellule Souche et Cerveau, INSERM U, Université de Lyon, F-69373, Lyon, France

3 Université Lyon , Equipe Neuropsychopharmacologie des troubles affectifs, Lyon, France

References

[1] Ferrari AJ, Somerville AJ, Baxter AJ, Norman R, Patten SB, Vos T, et al. Global variation in the prevalence and incidence of major depressive disorder: a systematic review of the epidemiological literature. Psychological medicine. 2012:1-11. Epub 2012/07/27.

[2] Bromet E, Andrade LH, Hwang I, Sampson NA, Alonso J, de Girolamo G, et al. Cross-national epidemiology of DSM-IV major depressive episode. BMC medicine. 2011;9:90. Epub 2011/07/28.

[3] Kessler RC, Akiskal HS, Ames M, Birnbaum H, Greenberg P, Hirschfeld RM, et al. Prevalence and effects of mood disorders on work performance in a nationally representative sample of U.S. workers. The American journal of psychiatry. 2006;163(9): 1561-8. Epub 2006/09/02.

[4] Wang PS, Beck A, Berglund P, Leutzinger JA, Pronk N, Richling D, et al. Chronic medical conditions and work performance in the health and work performance questionnaire calibration surveys. Journal of occupational and environmental medicine / American College of Occupational and Environmental Medicine. 2003;45(12): 1303-11. Epub 2003/12/11.

[5] Fisher HL, Cohen-Woods S, Hosang GM, Korszun A, Owen M, Craddock N, et al. Interaction between specific forms of childhood maltreatment and the serotonin transporter gene (5-HTT) in recurrent depressive disorder. Journal of affective disorders. 2012. Epub 2012/07/31.

[6] McIntyre RS, Soczynska JK, Liauw SS, Woldeyohannes HO, Brietzke E, Nathanson J, et al. The association between childhood adversity and components of metabolic syndrome in adults with mood disorders: results from the international mood disorders collaborative project. International journal of psychiatry in medicine. 2012;43(2):165-77. Epub 2012/08/02.

[7] Rusli BN, Edimansyah BA, Naing L. Working conditions, self-perceived stress, anxiety, depression and quality of life: a structural equation modelling approach. BMC public health. 2008;8:48. Epub 2008/02/08.

[8] Organization WH. The Global Burden of Disease: 2004 Update. WHO Press [Internet]. 2008; Geneva, Switzerland 2008.

[9] Jayanthi LD, Ramamoorthy S. Regulation of monoamine transporters: influence of psychostimulants and therapeutic antidepressants. The AAPS journal. 2005;7(3):E728-38. Epub 2005/12/16.

[10] Holsboer F. The corticosteroid receptor hypothesis of depression. Neuropsychopharmacology : official publication of the American College of Neuropsychopharmacology. 2000;23(5):477-501. Epub 2000/10/12.

[11] Kunugi H, Hori H, Adachi N, Numakawa T. Interface between hypothalamic-pituitary-adrenal axis and brain-derived neurotrophic factor in depression. Psychiatry and clinical neurosciences. 2010;64(5):447-59. Epub 2010/10/07.

[12] Carney RM, Shelton RC. Agomelatine for the treatment of major depressive disorder. Expert opinion on pharmacotherapy. 2011;12(15):2411-9. Epub 2011/09/16.

[13] Kasper S, Hamon M. Beyond the monoaminergic hypothesis: agomelatine, a new antidepressant with an innovative mechanism of action. The world journal of biological psychiatry : the official journal of the World Federation of Societies of Biological Psychiatry. 2009;10(2):117-26. Epub 2009/03/04.

[14] Dantzer R, O'Connor JC, Freund GG, Johnson RW, Kelley KW. From inflammation to sickness and depression: when the immune system subjugates the brain. Nature reviews Neuroscience. 2008;9(1):46-56. Epub 2007/12/13.

[15] Dowlati Y, Herrmann N, Swardfager W, Liu H, Sham L, Reim EK, et al. A meta-analysis of cytokines in major depression. Biological psychiatry. 2010;67(5):446-57. Epub 2009/12/18.

[16] Luscher B, Shen Q, Sahir N. The GABAergic deficit hypothesis of major depressive disorder. Molecular psychiatry. 2011;16(4):383-406. Epub 2010/11/17.

[17] Sanacora G, Treccani G, Popoli M. Towards a glutamate hypothesis of depression: an emerging frontier of neuropsychopharmacology for mood disorders. Neuropharmacology. 2012;62(1):63-77. Epub 2011/08/11.

[18] Mineur YS, Picciotto MR. Nicotine receptors and depression: revisiting and revising the cholinergic hypothesis. Trends in pharmacological sciences. 2010;31(12):580-6. Epub 2010/10/23.

[19] Craig MC, Murphy DG. Estrogen: effects on normal brain function and neuropsychiatric disorders. Climacteric : the journal of the International Menopause Society. 2007;10 Suppl 2:97-104. Epub 2007/10/27.

[20] Estrada-Camarena E, Lopez-Rubalcava C, Vega-Rivera N, Recamier-Carballo S, Fernandez-Guasti A. Antidepressant effects of estrogens: a basic approximation. Behavioural pharmacology. 2010;21(5-6):451-64. Epub 2010/08/12.

[21] Maes M, Fisar Z, Medina M, Scapagnini G, Nowak G, Berk M. New drug targets in depression: inflammatory, cell-mediated immune, oxidative and nitrosative stress, mitochondrial, antioxidant, and neuroprogressive pathways. And new drug candidates--Nrf2 activators and GSK-3 inhibitors. Inflammopharmacology. 2012;20(3): 127-50. Epub 2012/01/25.

[22] Faure C, Mnie-Filali O, Haddjeri N. Long-term adaptive changes induced by serotonergic antidepressant drugs. Expert review of neurotherapeutics. 2006;6(2):235-45. Epub 2006/02/10.

[23] Neto FL, Borges G, Torres-Sanchez S, Mico JA, Berrocoso E. Neurotrophins role in depression neurobiology: a review of basic and clinical evidence. Current neuropharmacology. 2011;9(4):530-52. Epub 2012/06/02.

[24] Paizanis E, Hamon M, Lanfumey L. Hippocampal neurogenesis, depressive disorders, and antidepressant therapy. Neural plasticity. 2007;2007:73754. Epub 2007/07/21.

[25] Grady MM, Stahl SM. Practical guide for prescribing MAOIs: debunking myths and removing barriers. CNS spectrums. 2012;17(1):2-10. Epub 2012/07/14.

[26] Miller J. Managing antidepression overdoses. Emergency medical services. 2004;33(10): 113-9. Epub 2004/11/24.

[27] Aghajanian GK, Graham AW, Sheard MH. Serotonin-containing neurons in brain: depression of firing by monoamine oxidase inhibitors. Science. 1970;169(3950):1100-2. Epub 1970/09/11.

[28] Gartside SE, Umbers V, Sharp T. Inhibition of 5-HT cell firing in the DRN by non-selective 5-HT reuptake inhibitors: studies on the role of 5-HT1A autoreceptors and noradrenergic mechanisms. Psychopharmacology. 1997;130(3):261-8. Epub 1997/04/01.

[29] Scuvee-Moreau JJ, Dresse AE. Effect of various antidepressant drugs on the spontaneous firing rate of locus coeruleus and dorsal raphe neurons of the rat. European journal of pharmacology. 1979;57(2-3):219-25. Epub 1979/08/01.

[30] Sharp T, Gartside SE, Umbers V. Effects of co-administration of a monoamine oxidase inhibitor and a 5-HT1A receptor antagonist on 5-hydroxytryptamine cell firing and release. European journal of pharmacology. 1997;320(1):15-9. Epub 1997/02/05.

[31] Blier P, de Montigny C. Effect of chronic tricylic antidepressant treatment on the serotoninergic autoreceptor: a microiontophoretic study in the rat. Naunyn-Schmiedeberg's archives of pharmacology. 1980;314(2):123-8. Epub 1980/11/01.

[32] Blier P, de Montigny C. Serotoninergic but not noradrenergic neurons in rat central nervous system adapt to long-term treatment with monoamine oxidase inhibitors. Neuroscience. 1985;16(4):949-55. Epub 1985/12/01.

[33] Blier P, de Montigny C. Current advances and trends in the treatment of depression. Trends in pharmacological sciences. 1994;15(7):220-6. Epub 1994/07/01.

[34] Sleight AJ, Marsden CA, Palfreyman MG, Mir AK, Lovenberg W. Chronic MAO A and MAO B inhibition decreases the 5-HT1A receptor-mediated inhibition of forskolin-stimulated adenylate cyclase. European journal of pharmacology. 1988;154(3):255-61. Epub 1988/09/23.

[35] Berendsen HH, Broekkamp CL. Attenuation of 5-HT1A and 5-HT2 but not 5-HT1C receptor mediated behaviour in rats following chronic treatment with 5-HT receptor agonists, antagonists or anti-depressants. Psychopharmacology. 1991;105(2):219-24. Epub 1991/01/01.

[36] Shen C, Li H, Meller E. Repeated treatment with antidepressants differentially alters 5-HT1A agonist-stimulated [35S]GTP gamma S binding in rat brain regions. Neuropharmacology. 2002;42(8):1031-8. Epub 2002/07/20.

[37] Celada P, Artigas F. Monoamine oxidase inhibitors increase preferentially extracellular 5-hydroxytryptamine in the midbrain raphe nuclei. A brain microdialysis study in the awake rat. Naunyn-Schmiedeberg's archives of pharmacology. 1993;347(6):583-90. Epub 1993/06/01.

[38] Sleight AJ, Smith RJ, Marsden CA, Palfreyman MG. The effects of chronic treatment with amitriptyline and MDL 72394 on the control of 5-HT release in vivo. Neuropharmacology. 1989;28(5):477-80. Epub 1989/05/01.

[39] Blier P, Chaput Y, de Montigny C. Long-term 5-HT reuptake blockade, but not monoamine oxidase inhibition, decreases the function of terminal 5-HT autoreceptors: an electrophysiological study in the rat brain. Naunyn-Schmiedeberg's archives of pharmacology. 1988;337(3):246-54. Epub 1988/03/01.

[40] Haddjeri N, Blier P, de Montigny C. Long-term antidepressant treatments result in a tonic activation of forebrain 5-HT1A receptors. The Journal of neuroscience : the official journal of the Society for Neuroscience. 1998;18(23):10150-6. Epub 1998/11/21.

[41] Evrard A, Malagie I, Laporte AM, Boni C, Hanoun N, Trillat AC, et al. Altered regulation of the 5-HT system in the brain of MAO-A knock-out mice. The European journal of neuroscience. 2002;15(5):841-51. Epub 2002/03/22.

[42] Lanoir J, Hilaire G, Seif I. Reduced density of functional 5-HT1A receptors in the brain, medulla and spinal cord of monoamine oxidase-A knockout mouse neonates. The Journal of comparative neurology. 2006;495(5):607-23. Epub 2006/02/25.

[43] Fabre V, Beaufour C, Evrard A, Rioux A, Hanoun N, Lesch KP, et al. Altered expression and functions of serotonin 5-HT1A and 5-HT1B receptors in knock-out mice lacking the 5-HT transporter. The European journal of neuroscience. 2000;12(7):2299-310. Epub 2000/08/18.

[44] Hensler JG. Differential regulation of 5-HT1A receptor-G protein interactions in brain following chronic antidepressant administration. Neuropsychopharmacology : official publication of the American College of Neuropsychopharmacology. 2002;26(5):565-73. Epub 2002/04/03.

[45] Rossi DV, Valdez M, Gould GG, Hensler JG. Chronic administration of venlafaxine fails to attenuate 5-HT1A receptor function at the level of receptor-G protein interaction. The international journal of neuropsychopharmacology / official scientific journal of the Collegium Internationale Neuropsychopharmacologicum. 2006;9(4):393-406. Epub 2005/07/23.

[46] Chaput Y, de Montigny C, Blier P. Presynaptic and postsynaptic modifications of the serotonin system by long-term administration of antidepressant treatments. An in vivo electrophysiologic study in the rat. Neuropsychopharmacology : official publication of

the American College of Neuropsychopharmacology. 1991;5(4):219-29. Epub 1991/12/01.

[47] Mandrioli R, Mercolini L, Saracino MA, Raggi MA. Selective serotonin reuptake inhibitors (SSRIs): therapeutic drug monitoring and pharmacological interactions. Current medicinal chemistry. 2012;19(12):1846-63. Epub 2012/03/15.

[48] Reed CR, Kajdasz DK, Whalen H, Athanasiou MC, Gallipoli S, Thase ME. The efficacy profile of vilazodone, a novel antidepressant for the treatment of major depressive disorder. Current medical research and opinion. 2012;28(1):27-39. Epub 2011/11/24.

[49] Pejchal T, Foley MA, Kosofsky BE, Waeber C. Chronic fluoxetine treatment selectively uncouples raphe 5-HT(1A) receptors as measured by [(35)S]-GTP gamma S autoradiography. British journal of pharmacology. 2002;135(5):1115-22. Epub 2002/03/06.

[50] Czachura JF, Rasmussen K. Effects of acute and chronic administration of fluoxetine on the activity of serotonergic neurons in the dorsal raphe nucleus of the rat. Naunyn-Schmiedeberg's archives of pharmacology. 2000;362(3):266-75. Epub 2000/09/21.

[51] El Mansari M, Sanchez C, Chouvet G, Renaud B, Haddjeri N. Effects of acute and long-term administration of escitalopram and citalopram on serotonin neurotransmission: an in vivo electrophysiological study in rat brain. Neuropsychopharmacology : official publication of the American College of Neuropsychopharmacology. 2005;30(7): 1269-77. Epub 2005/02/11.

[52] Invernizzi R, Belli S, Samanin R. Citalopram's ability to increase the extracellular concentrations of serotonin in the dorsal raphe prevents the drug's effect in the frontal cortex. Brain research. 1992;584(1-2):322-4. Epub 1992/07/03.

[53] Mansari ME, Wiborg O, Mnie-Filali O, Benturquia N, Sanchez C, Haddjeri N. Allosteric modulation of the effect of escitalopram, paroxetine and fluoxetine: in-vitro and in-vivo studies. The international journal of neuropsychopharmacology / official scientific journal of the Collegium Internationale Neuropsychopharmacologicum. 2007;10(1): 31-40. Epub 2006/02/02.

[54] Mnie-Filali O, El Mansari M, Espana A, Sanchez C, Haddjeri N. Allosteric modulation of the effects of the 5-HT reuptake inhibitor escitalopram on the rat hippocampal synaptic plasticity. Neuroscience letters. 2006;395(1):23-7. Epub 2005/12/07.

[55] Smith JE, Lakoski JM. Electrophysiological effects of fluoxetine and duloxetine in the dorsal raphe nucleus and hippocampus. European journal of pharmacology. 1997;323(1):69-73. Epub 1997/03/26.

[56] Aznavour N, Rbah L, Riad M, Reilhac A, Costes N, Descarries L, et al. A PET imaging study of 5-HT(1A) receptors in cat brain after acute and chronic fluoxetine treatment. NeuroImage. 2006;33(3):834-42. Epub 2006/09/26.

[57] Riad M, Zimmer L, Rbah L, Watkins KC, Hamon M, Descarries L. Acute treatment with the antidepressant fluoxetine internalizes 5-HT1A autoreceptors and reduces the in

vivo binding of the PET radioligand [18F]MPPF in the nucleus raphe dorsalis of rat. The Journal of neuroscience : the official journal of the Society for Neuroscience. 2004;24(23):5420-6. Epub 2004/06/11.

[58] Descarries L, Riad M. Effects of the antidepressant fluoxetine on the subcellular localization of 5-HT1A receptors and SERT. Philosophical transactions of the Royal Society of London Series B, Biological sciences. 2012;367(1601):2416-25. Epub 2012/07/25.

[59] Rutter JJ, Auerbach SB. Acute uptake inhibition increases extracellular serotonin in the rat forebrain. The Journal of pharmacology and experimental therapeutics. 1993;265(3): 1319-24. Epub 1993/06/01.

[60] Le Poul E, Laaris N, Doucet E, Laporte AM, Hamon M, Lanfumey L. Early desensitization of somato-dendritic 5-HT1A autoreceptors in rats treated with fluoxetine or paroxetine. Naunyn-Schmiedeberg's archives of pharmacology. 1995;352(2):141-8. Epub 1995/08/01.

[61] Mnie-Filali O, Faure C, Mansari ME, Lambas-Senas L, Berod A, Zimmer L, et al. R-citalopram prevents the neuronal adaptive changes induced by escitalopram. Neuroreport. 2007;18(15):1553-6. Epub 2007/09/22.

[62] Riad M, Rbah L, Verdurand M, Aznavour N, Zimmer L, Descarries L. Unchanged density of 5-HT(1A) autoreceptors on the plasma membrane of nucleus raphe dorsalis neurons in rats chronically treated with fluoxetine. Neuroscience. 2008;151(3):692-700. Epub 2008/01/02.

[63] Moulin-Sallanon M, Charnay Y, Ginovart N, Perret P, Lanfumey L, Hamon M, et al. Acute and chronic effects of citalopram on 5-HT1A receptor-labeling by [18F]MPPF and -coupling to receptors-G proteins. Synapse. 2009;63(2):106-16. Epub 2008/11/20.

[64] Castro ME, Diaz A, del Olmo E, Pazos A. Chronic fluoxetine induces opposite changes in G protein coupling at pre and postsynaptic 5-HT1A receptors in rat brain. Neuropharmacology. 2003;44(1):93-101. Epub 2003/02/01.

[65] Hanoun N, Mocaer E, Boyer PA, Hamon M, Lanfumey L. Differential effects of the novel antidepressant agomelatine (S 20098) versus fluoxetine on 5-HT1A receptors in the rat brain. Neuropharmacology. 2004;47(4):515-26. Epub 2004/09/24.

[66] Rossi DV, Burke TF, McCasland M, Hensler JG. Serotonin-1A receptor function in the dorsal raphe nucleus following chronic administration of the selective serotonin reuptake inhibitor sertraline. Journal of neurochemistry. 2008;105(4):1091-9. Epub 2008/01/10.

[67] Mannoury la Cour C, El Mestikawy S, Hanoun N, Hamon M, Lanfumey L. Regional differences in the coupling of 5-hydroxytryptamine-1A receptors to G proteins in the rat brain. Molecular pharmacology. 2006;70(3):1013-21. Epub 2006/06/15.

[68] Castro E, Diaz A, Rodriguez-Gaztelumendi A, Del Olmo E, Pazos A. WAY100635 prevents the changes induced by fluoxetine upon the 5-HT1A receptor functionality. Neuropharmacology. 2008;55(8):1391-6. Epub 2008/09/24.

[69] Blier P, Bouchard C. Modulation of 5-HT release in the guinea-pig brain following long-term administration of antidepressant drugs. British journal of pharmacology. 1994;113(2):485-95. Epub 1994/10/01.

[70] Vidal R, Valdizan EM, Mostany R, Pazos A, Castro E. Long-term treatment with fluoxetine induces desensitization of 5-HT4 receptor-dependent signalling and functionality in rat brain. Journal of neurochemistry. 2009;110(3):1120-7. Epub 2009/06/16.

[71] Mnie-Filali O, Faure C, Lambas-Senas L, El Mansari M, Belblidia H, Gondard E, et al. Pharmacological blockade of 5-HT7 receptors as a putative fast acting antidepressant strategy. Neuropsychopharmacology : official publication of the American College of Neuropsychopharmacology. 2011;36(6):1275-88. Epub 2011/02/18.

[72] Sleight AJ, Carolo C, Petit N, Zwingelstein C, Bourson A. Identification of 5-hydroxytryptamine7 receptor binding sites in rat hypothalamus: sensitivity to chronic antidepressant treatment. Molecular pharmacology. 1995;47(1):99-103. Epub 1995/01/01.

[73] Jing Y, Kalsekar I, Curkendall SM, Carls GS, Bagalman E, Forbes RA, et al. Intent-to-treat analysis of health care expenditures of patients treated with atypical antipsychotics as adjunctive therapy in depression. Clinical therapeutics. 2011;33(9):1246-57. Epub 2011/08/16.

[74] Lin CH, Lin SH, Jang FL. Adjunctive low-dose aripiprazole with standard-dose sertraline in treating fresh major depressive disorder: a randomized, double-blind, controlled study. Journal of clinical psychopharmacology. 2011;31(5):563-8. Epub 2011/08/27.

[75] Trivedi MH, Thase ME, Fava M, Nelson CJ, Yang H, Qi Y, et al. Adjunctive aripiprazole in major depressive disorder: analysis of efficacy and safety in patients with anxious and atypical features. The Journal of clinical psychiatry. 2008;69(12):1928-36. Epub 2009/02/05.

[76] Chernoloz O, El Mansari M, Blier P. Effects of sustained administration of quetiapine alone and in combination with a serotonin reuptake inhibitor on norepinephrine and serotonin transmission. Neuropsychopharmacology : official publication of the American College of Neuropsychopharmacology. 2012;37(7):1717-28. Epub 2012/03/01.

[77] Dremencov E, El Mansari M, Blier P. Distinct electrophysiological effects of paliperidone and risperidone on the firing activity of rat serotonin and norepinephrine neurons. Psychopharmacology. 2007;194(1):63-72. Epub 2007/05/29.

[78] Marcus MM, Jardemark K, Malmerfelt A, Gertow J, Konradsson-Geuken A, Svensson TH. Augmentation by escitalopram, but not citalopram or R-citalopram, of the effects

of low-dose risperidone: behavioral, biochemical, and electrophysiological evidence. Synapse. 2012;66(4):277-90. Epub 2011/11/29.

[79] Lucas G, Rymar VV, Du J, Mnie-Filali O, Bisgaard C, Manta S, et al. Serotonin(4) (5-HT(4)) receptor agonists are putative antidepressants with a rapid onset of action. Neuron. 2007;55(5):712-25. Epub 2007/09/06.

[80] Licht CL, Kirkegaard L, Zueger M, Chourbaji S, Gass P, Aznar S, et al. Changes in 5-HT4 receptor and 5-HT transporter binding in olfactory bulbectomized and glucocorticoid receptor heterozygous mice. Neurochemistry international. 2010;56(4):603-10. Epub 2010/01/12.

[81] Licht CL, Marcussen AB, Wegener G, Overstreet DH, Aznar S, Knudsen GM. The brain 5-HT4 receptor binding is down-regulated in the Flinders Sensitive Line depression model and in response to paroxetine administration. Journal of neurochemistry. 2009;109(5):1363-74. Epub 2009/05/30.

[82] Licht CL, Knudsen GM, Sharp T. Effects of the 5-HT(4) receptor agonist RS67333 and paroxetine on hippocampal extracellular 5-HT levels. Neuroscience letters. 2010b; 476(2):58-61. Epub 2010/04/13.

[83] Lucas G, Du J, Romeas T, Mnie-Filali O, Haddjeri N, Pineyro G, et al. Selective serotonin reuptake inhibitors potentiate the rapid antidepressant-like effects of serotonin4 receptor agonists in the rat. PloS one. 2010;5(2):e9253. Epub 2010/02/20.

[84] Abbas AI, Hedlund PB, Huang XP, Tran TB, Meltzer HY, Roth BL. Amisulpride is a potent 5-HT7 antagonist: relevance for antidepressant actions in vivo. Psychopharmacology. 2009;205(1):119-28. Epub 2009/04/02.

[85] Adell A. Lu-AA21004, a multimodal serotonergic agent, for the potential treatment of depression and anxiety. IDrugs : the investigational drugs journal. 2010;13(12):900-10. Epub 2010/12/15.

[86] Baldwin DS, Hansen T, Florea I. Vortioxetine (Lu AA21004) in the long-term open-label treatment of major depressive disorder. Current medical research and opinion. 2012;28(10):1717-24. Epub 2012/09/18.

[87] Bang-Andersen B, Ruhland T, Jorgensen M, Smith G, Frederiksen K, Jensen KG, et al. Discovery of 1-[2-(2,4-dimethylphenylsulfanyl)phenyl]piperazine (Lu AA21004): a novel multimodal compound for the treatment of major depressive disorder. Journal of medicinal chemistry. 2011;54(9):3206-21. Epub 2011/04/14.

[88] Ishibashi T, Horisawa T, Tokuda K, Ishiyama T, Ogasa M, Tagashira R, et al. Pharmacological profile of lurasidone, a novel antipsychotic agent with potent 5-hydroxytryptamine 7 (5-HT7) and 5-HT1A receptor activity. The Journal of pharmacology and experimental therapeutics. 2010;334(1):171-81. Epub 2010/04/21.

[89] Hedlund PB, Huitron-Resendiz S, Henriksen SJ, Sutcliffe JG. 5-HT7 receptor inhibition and inactivation induce antidepressantlike behavior and sleep pattern. Biological psychiatry. 2005;58(10):831-7. Epub 2005/07/16.

[90] Altman J, Das GD. Autoradiographic and histological evidence of postnatal hippocampal neurogenesis in rats. The Journal of comparative neurology. 1965;124(3):319-35. Epub 1965/06/01.

[91] Eriksson PS, Perfilieva E, Bjork-Eriksson T, Alborn AM, Nordborg C, Peterson DA, et al. Neurogenesis in the adult human hippocampus. Nature medicine. 1998;4(11):1313-7. Epub 1998/11/11.

[92] Murrell W, Bushell GR, Livesey J, McGrath J, MacDonald KP, Bates PR, et al. Neurogenesis in adult human. Neuroreport. 1996;7(6):1189-94. Epub 1996/04/26.

[93] Takahashi T, Nowakowski RS, Caviness VS, Jr. BUdR as an S-phase marker for quantitative studies of cytokinetic behaviour in the murine cerebral ventricular zone. Journal of neurocytology. 1992;21(3):185-97. Epub 1992/03/11.

[94] Hanson ND, Owens MJ, Nemeroff CB. Depression, antidepressants, and neurogenesis: a critical reappraisal. Neuropsychopharmacology : official publication of the American College of Neuropsychopharmacology. 2011;36(13):2589-602. Epub 2011/09/23.

[95] Garcia-Verdugo JM, Doetsch F, Wichterle H, Lim DA, Alvarez-Buylla A. Architecture and cell types of the adult subventricular zone: in search of the stem cells. Journal of neurobiology. 1998;36(2):234-48. Epub 1998/08/26.

[96] Benraiss A, Chmielnicki E, Lerner K, Roh D, Goldman SA. Adenoviral brain-derived neurotrophic factor induces both neostriatal and olfactory neuronal recruitment from endogenous progenitor cells in the adult forebrain. The Journal of neuroscience : the official journal of the Society for Neuroscience. 2001;21(17):6718-31. Epub 2001/08/23.

[97] Magavi SS, Leavitt BR, Macklis JD. Induction of neurogenesis in the neocortex of adult mice. Nature. 2000;405(6789):951-5. Epub 2000/07/06.

[98] Pencea V, Bingaman KD, Wiegand SJ, Luskin MB. Infusion of brain-derived neurotrophic factor into the lateral ventricle of the adult rat leads to new neurons in the parenchyma of the striatum, septum, thalamus, and hypothalamus. The Journal of neuroscience : the official journal of the Society for Neuroscience. 2001;21(17):6706-17. Epub 2001/08/23.

[99] Campbell S, Marriott M, Nahmias C, MacQueen GM. Lower hippocampal volume in patients suffering from depression: a meta-analysis. The American journal of psychiatry. 2004;161(4):598-607. Epub 2004/04/02.

[100] Videbech P, Ravnkilde B. Hippocampal volume and depression: a meta-analysis of MRI studies. The American journal of psychiatry. 2004;161(11):1957-66. Epub 2004/10/30.

[101] MacQueen GM, Yucel K, Taylor VH, Macdonald K, Joffe R. Posterior hippocampal volumes are associated with remission rates in patients with major depressive disorder. Biological psychiatry. 2008;64(10):880-3. Epub 2008/08/30.

[102] Santarelli L, Saxe M, Gross C, Surget A, Battaglia F, Dulawa S, et al. Requirement of hippocampal neurogenesis for the behavioral effects of antidepressants. Science. 2003;301(5634):805-9. Epub 2003/08/09.

[103] Perera TD, Dwork AJ, Keegan KA, Thirumangalakudi L, Lipira CM, Joyce N, et al. Necessity of hippocampal neurogenesis for the therapeutic action of antidepressants in adult nonhuman primates. PloS one. 2011;6(4):e17600. Epub 2011/04/29.

[104] Li YF, Zhang YZ, Liu YQ, Wang HL, Yuan L, Luo ZP. Moclobemide up-regulates proliferation of hippocampal progenitor cells in chronically stressed mice. Acta pharmacologica Sinica. 2004;25(11):1408-12. Epub 2004/11/05.

[105] Malberg JE, Eisch AJ, Nestler EJ, Duman RS. Chronic antidepressant treatment increases neurogenesis in adult rat hippocampus. The Journal of neuroscience : the official journal of the Society for Neuroscience. 2000;20(24):9104-10. Epub 2000/01/11.

[106] Chen F, Madsen TM, Wegener G, Nyengaard JR. Imipramine treatment increases the number of hippocampal synapses and neurons in a genetic animal model of depression. Hippocampus. 2010;20(12):1376-84. Epub 2009/11/19.

[107] Pechnick RN, Zonis S, Wawrowsky K, Cosgayon R, Farrokhi C, Lacayo L, et al. Antidepressants stimulate hippocampal neurogenesis by inhibiting p21 expression in the subgranular zone of the hipppocampus. PloS one. 2011;6(11):e27290. Epub 2011/11/15.

[108] Kodama M, Fujioka T, Duman RS. Chronic olanzapine or fluoxetine administration increases cell proliferation in hippocampus and prefrontal cortex of adult rat. Biological psychiatry. 2004;56(8):570-80. Epub 2004/10/13.

[109] Snyder JS, Kee N, Wojtowicz JM. Effects of adult neurogenesis on synaptic plasticity in the rat dentate gyrus. Journal of neurophysiology. 2001;85(6):2423-31. Epub 2001/06/02.

[110] Ge S, Goh EL, Sailor KA, Kitabatake Y, Ming GL, Song H. GABA regulates synaptic integration of newly generated neurons in the adult brain. Nature. 2006;439(7076): 589-93. Epub 2005/12/13.

[111] Halim ND, Weickert CS, McClintock BW, Weinberger DR, Lipska BK. Effects of chronic haloperidol and clozapine treatment on neurogenesis in the adult rat hippocampus. Neuropsychopharmacology : official publication of the American College of Neuropsychopharmacology. 2004;29(6):1063-9. Epub 2004/03/11.

[112] Hanson ND, Nemeroff CB, Owens MJ. Lithium, but not fluoxetine or the corticotropin-releasing factor receptor 1 receptor antagonist R121919, increases cell proliferation in the adult dentate gyrus. The Journal of pharmacology and experimental therapeutics. 2011;337(1):180-6. Epub 2011/01/12.

[113] Luo C, Xu H, Li XM. Quetiapine reverses the suppression of hippocampal neurogenesis caused by repeated restraint stress. Brain research. 2005;1063(1):32-9. Epub 2005/11/08.

[114] Jaholkowski P, Kiryk A, Jedynak P, Ben Abdallah NM, Knapska E, Kowalczyk A, et al. New hippocampal neurons are not obligatory for memory formation; cyclin D2

knockout mice with no adult brain neurogenesis show learning. Learning & memory. 2009;16(7):439-51. Epub 2009/06/26.

[115] Sahay A, Scobie KN, Hill AS, O'Carroll CM, Kheirbek MA, Burghardt NS, et al. Increasing adult hippocampal neurogenesis is sufficient to improve pattern separation. Nature. 2011;472(7344):466-70. Epub 2011/04/05.

[116] Gorman JM, Docherty JP. A hypothesized role for dendritic remodeling in the etiology of mood and anxiety disorders. The Journal of neuropsychiatry and clinical neurosciences. 2010;22(3):256-64. Epub 2010/08/06.

[117] Duman RS, Li N. A neurotrophic hypothesis of depression: role of synaptogenesis in the actions of NMDA receptor antagonists. Philosophical transactions of the Royal Society of London Series B, Biological sciences. 2012;367(1601):2475-84. Epub 2012/07/25.

[118] Holtmaat A, Svoboda K. Experience-dependent structural synaptic plasticity in the mammalian brain. Nature reviews Neuroscience. 2009;10(9):647-58. Epub 2009/08/21.

[119] Yoshihara Y, De Roo M, Muller D. Dendritic spine formation and stabilization. Current opinion in neurobiology. 2009;19(2):146-53. Epub 2009/06/16.

[120] Bhatt DH, Zhang S, Gan WB. Dendritic spine dynamics. Annual review of physiology. 2009;71:261-82. Epub 2009/07/07.

[121] Bourne JN, Harris KM. Balancing structure and function at hippocampal dendritic spines. Annual review of neuroscience. 2008;31:47-67. Epub 2008/02/21.

[122] Matsuzaki M, Honkura N, Ellis-Davies GC, Kasai H. Structural basis of long-term potentiation in single dendritic spines. Nature. 2004;429(6993):761-6. Epub 2004/06/11.

[123] Zhou Q, Homma KJ, Poo MM. Shrinkage of dendritic spines associated with long-term depression of hippocampal synapses. Neuron. 2004;44(5):749-57. Epub 2004/12/02.

[124] Conrad CD. What is the functional significance of chronic stress-induced CA3 dendritic retraction within the hippocampus? Behavioral and cognitive neuroscience reviews. 2006;5(1):41-60. Epub 2006/07/04.

[125] Michelsen KA, van den Hove DL, Schmitz C, Segers O, Prickaerts J, Steinbusch HW. Prenatal stress and subsequent exposure to chronic mild stress influence dendritic spine density and morphology in the rat medial prefrontal cortex. BMC neuroscience. 2007;8:107. Epub 2007/12/21.

[126] Sousa N, Lukoyanov NV, Madeira MD, Almeida OF, Paula-Barbosa MM. Reorganization of the morphology of hippocampal neurites and synapses after stress-induced damage correlates with behavioral improvement. Neuroscience. 2000;97(2):253-66. Epub 2000/05/09.

[127] Cook SC, Wellman CL. Chronic stress alters dendritic morphology in rat medial prefrontal cortex. Journal of neurobiology. 2004;60(2):236-48. Epub 2004/07/22.

[128] Radley JJ, Sisti HM, Hao J, Rocher AB, McCall T, Hof PR, et al. Chronic behavioral stress induces apical dendritic reorganization in pyramidal neurons of the medial prefrontal cortex. Neuroscience. 2004;125(1):1-6. Epub 2004/03/31.

[129] Arnone D, McIntosh AM, Ebmeier KP, Munafo MR, Anderson IM. Magnetic resonance imaging studies in unipolar depression: systematic review and meta-regression analyses. European neuropsychopharmacology : the journal of the European College of Neuropsychopharmacology. 2012;22(1):1-16. Epub 2011/07/05.

[130] Kang HJ, Voleti B, Hajszan T, Rajkowska G, Stockmeier CA, Licznerski P, et al. Decreased expression of synapse-related genes and loss of synapses in major depressive disorder. Nature medicine. 2012;18(9):1413-7. Epub 2012/08/14.

[131] Holderbach R, Clark K, Moreau JL, Bischofberger J, Normann C. Enhanced long-term synaptic depression in an animal model of depression. Biological psychiatry. 2007;62(1):92-100. Epub 2006/12/05.

[132] Li W, Liu L, Liu YY, Luo J, Lin JY, Li X, et al. Effects of electroconvulsive stimulation on long-term potentiation and synaptophysin in the hippocampus of rats with depressive behavior. The journal of ECT. 2012;28(2):111-7. Epub 2012/04/26.

[133] Xu L, Anwyl R, Rowan MJ. Behavioural stress facilitates the induction of long-term depression in the hippocampus. Nature. 1997;387(6632):497-500. Epub 1997/05/29.

[134] Bhagya V, Srikumar BN, Raju TR, Rao BS. Chronic escitalopram treatment restores spatial learning, monoamine levels, and hippocampal long-term potentiation in an animal model of depression. Psychopharmacology. 2011;214(2):477-94. Epub 2010/11/06.

[135] Matsumoto M, Tachibana K, Togashi H, Tahara K, Kojima T, Yamaguchi T, et al. Chronic treatment with milnacipran reverses the impairment of synaptic plasticity induced by conditioned fear stress. Psychopharmacology. 2005;179(3):606-12. Epub 2004/12/25.

[136] Cooke JD, Grover LM, Spangler PR. Venlafaxine treatment stimulates expression of brain-derived neurotrophic factor protein in frontal cortex and inhibits long-term potentiation in hippocampus. Neuroscience. 2009;162(4):1411-9. Epub 2009/05/26.

[137] O'Connor JJ, Rowan MJ, Anwyl R. Use-dependent effects of acute and chronic treatment with imipramine and buspirone on excitatory synaptic transmission in the rat hippocampus in vivo. Naunyn-Schmiedeberg's archives of pharmacology. 1993;348(2): 158-63. Epub 1993/08/01.

[138] Stewart CA, Reid IC. Repeated ECS and fluoxetine administration have equivalent effects on hippocampal synaptic plasticity. Psychopharmacology. 2000;148(3):217-23. Epub 2001/02/07.

[139] Huang GJ, Ben-David E, Tort Piella A, Edwards A, Flint J, Shifman S. Neurogenomic evidence for a shared mechanism of the antidepressant effects of exercise and chronic fluoxetine in mice. PloS one. 2012;7(4):e35901. Epub 2012/05/05.

[140] Wang JW, David DJ, Monckton JE, Battaglia F, Hen R. Chronic fluoxetine stimulates maturation and synaptic plasticity of adult-born hippocampal granule cells. The Journal of neuroscience : the official journal of the Society for Neuroscience. 2008;28(6): 1374-84. Epub 2008/02/08.

[141] Hajszan T, MacLusky NJ, Leranth C. Short-term treatment with the antidepressant fluoxetine triggers pyramidal dendritic spine synapse formation in rat hippocampus. The European journal of neuroscience. 2005;21(5):1299-303. Epub 2005/04/09.

[142] Bedrosian TA, Weil ZM, Nelson RJ. Chronic citalopram treatment ameliorates depressive behavior associated with light at night. Behavioral neuroscience. 2012;126(5):654-8. Epub 2012/08/15.

[143] Norrholm SD, Ouimet CC. Altered dendritic spine density in animal models of depression and in response to antidepressant treatment. Synapse. 2001;42(3):151-63. Epub 2001/12/18.

[144] Restivo L, Roman F, Dumuis A, Bockaert J, Marchetti E, Ammassari-Teule M. The promnesic effect of G-protein-coupled 5-HT4 receptors activation is mediated by a potentiation of learning-induced spine growth in the mouse hippocampus. Neuropsychopharmacology : official publication of the American College of Neuropsychopharmacology. 2008;33(10):2427-34. Epub 2007/12/14.

[145] Tajiri M, Hayata-Takano A, Seiriki K, Ogata K, Hazama K, Shintani N, et al. Serotonin 5-HT(7) receptor blockade reverses behavioral abnormalities in PACAP-deficient mice and receptor activation promotes neurite extension in primary embryonic hippocampal neurons: therapeutic implications for psychiatric disorders. Journal of molecular neuroscience : MN. 2012;48(3):473-81. Epub 2012/07/31.

[146] Luthl A, Laurent JP, Figurov A, Muller D, Schachner M. Hippocampal long-term potentiation and neural cell adhesion molecules L1 and NCAM. Nature. 1994;372(6508):777-9. Epub 1994/12/22.

[147] Gascon E, Vutskits L, Kiss JZ. Polysialic acid-neural cell adhesion molecule in brain plasticity: from synapses to integration of new neurons. Brain research reviews. 2007;56(1):101-18. Epub 2007/07/31.

[148] Guirado R, Sanchez-Matarredona D, Varea E, Crespo C, Blasco-Ibanez JM, Nacher J. Chronic fluoxetine treatment in middle-aged rats induces changes in the expression of plasticity-related molecules and in neurogenesis. BMC neuroscience. 2012;13:5. Epub 2012/01/10.

[149] Murphy KJ, Foley AG, O'Connell A W, Regan CM. Chronic exposure of rats to cognition enhancing drugs produces a neuroplastic response identical to that obtained by complex environment rearing. Neuropsychopharmacology : official publication of the American College of Neuropsychopharmacology. 2006;31(1):90-100. Epub 2005/07/01.

[150] Sairanen M, O'Leary OF, Knuuttila JE, Castren E. Chronic antidepressant treatment selectively increases expression of plasticity-related proteins in the hippocampus and medial prefrontal cortex of the rat. Neuroscience. 2007;144(1):368-74. Epub 2006/10/20.

[151] Varea E, Blasco-Ibanez JM, Gomez-Climent MA, Castillo-Gomez E, Crespo C, Martinez-Guijarro FJ, et al. Chronic fluoxetine treatment increases the expression of PSA-NCAM in the medial prefrontal cortex. Neuropsychopharmacology : official publication of the American College of Neuropsychopharmacology. 2007;32(4):803-12. Epub 2006/08/11.

[152] Frasca A, Fumagalli F, Ter Horst J, Racagni G, Murphy KJ, Riva MA. Olanzapine, but not haloperidol, enhances PSA-NCAM immunoreactivity in rat prefrontal cortex. The international journal of neuropsychopharmacology / official scientific journal of the Collegium Internationale Neuropsychopharmacologicum. 2008;11(5):591-5. Epub 2008/07/03.

[153] Mackowiak M, Dudys D, Chocyk A, Wedzony K. Repeated risperidone treatment increases the expression of NCAM and PSA-NCAM protein in the rat medial prefrontal cortex. European neuropsychopharmacology : the journal of the European College of Neuropsychopharmacology. 2009;19(2):125-37. Epub 2008/12/02.

[154] Evans GJ, Cousin MA. Tyrosine phosphorylation of synaptophysin in synaptic vesicle recycling. Biochemical Society transactions. 2005;33(Pt 6):1350-3. Epub 2005/10/26.

[155] Drigues N, Poltyrev T, Bejar C, Weinstock M, Youdim MB. cDNA gene expression profile of rat hippocampus after chronic treatment with antidepressant drugs. Journal of neural transmission. 2003;110(12):1413-36. Epub 2003/12/11.

[156] Rapp S, Baader M, Hu M, Jennen-Steinmetz C, Henn FA, Thome J. Differential regulation of synaptic vesicle proteins by antidepressant drugs. The pharmacogenomics journal. 2004;4(2):110-3. Epub 2004/01/07.

[157] Rodriguez JJ, Davies HA, Silva AT, De Souza IE, Peddie CJ, Colyer FM, et al. Long-term potentiation in the rat dentate gyrus is associated with enhanced Arc/Arg3.1 protein expression in spines, dendrites and glia. The European journal of neuroscience. 2005;21(9):2384-96. Epub 2005/06/04.

[158] Chowdhury S, Shepherd JD, Okuno H, Lyford G, Petralia RS, Plath N, et al. Arc/Arg3.1 interacts with the endocytic machinery to regulate AMPA receptor trafficking. Neuron. 2006;52(3):445-59. Epub 2006/11/08.

[159] Peebles CL, Yoo J, Thwin MT, Palop JJ, Noebels JL, Finkbeiner S. Arc regulates spine morphology and maintains network stability in vivo. Proceedings of the National Academy of Sciences of the United States of America. 2010;107(42):18173-8. Epub 2010/10/06.

[160] Rial Verde EM, Lee-Osbourne J, Worley PF, Malinow R, Cline HT. Increased expression of the immediate-early gene arc/arg3.1 reduces AMPA receptor-mediated synaptic transmission. Neuron. 2006;52(3):461-74. Epub 2006/11/08.

[161] Pei Q, Zetterstrom TS, Sprakes M, Tordera R, Sharp T. Antidepressant drug treatment induces Arc gene expression in the rat brain. Neuroscience. 2003;121(4):975-82. Epub 2003/10/29.

[162] Huang EJ, Reichardt LF. Trk receptors: roles in neuronal signal transduction. Annual review of biochemistry. 2003;72:609-42. Epub 2003/04/05.

[163] Berry A, Bellisario V, Capoccia S, Tirassa P, Calza A, Alleva E, et al. Social deprivation stress is a triggering factor for the emergence of anxiety- and depression-like behaviours and leads to reduced brain BDNF levels in C57BL/6J mice. Psychoneuroendocrinology. 2012;37(6):762-72. Epub 2011/10/07.

[164] De Vry J, Prickaerts J, Jetten M, Hulst M, Steinbusch HW, van den Hove DL, et al. Recurrent long-lasting tethering reduces BDNF protein levels in the dorsal hippocampus and frontal cortex in pigs. Hormones and behavior. 2012;62(1):10-7. Epub 2012/05/16.

[165] Hamani C, Machado DC, Hipolide DC, Dubiela FP, Suchecki D, Macedo CE, et al. Deep brain stimulation reverses anhedonic-like behavior in a chronic model of depression: role of serotonin and brain derived neurotrophic factor. Biological psychiatry. 2012;71(1):30-5. Epub 2011/10/18.

[166] Nibuya M, Takahashi M, Russell DS, Duman RS. Repeated stress increases catalytic TrkB mRNA in rat hippocampus. Neuroscience letters. 1999;267(2):81-4. Epub 1999/07/10.

[167] Yazir Y, Utkan T, Aricioglu F. Inhibition of neuronal nitric oxide synthase and soluble guanylate cyclase prevents depression-like behaviour in rats exposed to chronic unpredictable mild stress. Basic & clinical pharmacology & toxicology. 2012;111(3): 154-60. Epub 2012/03/06.

[168] Zhang Y, Gu F, Chen J, Dong W. Chronic antidepressant administration alleviates frontal and hippocampal BDNF deficits in CUMS rat. Brain research. 2010;1366:141-8. Epub 2010/10/06.

[169] Burke TF, Advani T, Adachi M, Monteggia LM, Hensler JG. Sensitivity of hippocampal 5-HT1A receptors to mild stress in BDNF-deficient mice. The international journal of neuropsychopharmacology / official scientific journal of the Collegium Internationale Neuropsychopharmacologicum. 2012:1-15. Epub 2012/05/12.

[170] Taliaz D, Stall N, Dar DE, Zangen A. Knockdown of brain-derived neurotrophic factor in specific brain sites precipitates behaviors associated with depression and reduces neurogenesis. Molecular psychiatry. 2010;15(1):80-92. Epub 2009/07/22.

[171] Gonul AS, Akdeniz F, Taneli F, Donat O, Eker C, Vahip S. Effect of treatment on serum brain-derived neurotrophic factor levels in depressed patients. European archives of psychiatry and clinical neuroscience. 2005;255(6):381-6. Epub 2005/04/06.

[172] Karege F, Perret G, Bondolfi G, Schwald M, Bertschy G, Aubry JM. Decreased serum brain-derived neurotrophic factor levels in major depressed patients. Psychiatry research. 2002;109(2):143-8. Epub 2002/04/03.

[173] Lee BH, Kim H, Park SH, Kim YK. Decreased plasma BDNF level in depressive patients. Journal of affective disorders. 2007;101(1-3):239-44. Epub 2006/12/19.

[174] Shimizu E, Hashimoto K, Okamura N, Koike K, Komatsu N, Kumakiri C, et al. Alterations of serum levels of brain-derived neurotrophic factor (BDNF) in depressed patients with or without antidepressants. Biological psychiatry. 2003;54(1):70-5. Epub 2003/07/05.

[175] Choi MJ, Kang RH, Lim SW, Oh KS, Lee MS. Brain-derived neurotrophic factor gene polymorphism (Val66Met) and citalopram response in major depressive disorder. Brain research. 2006;1118(1):176-82. Epub 2006/09/19.

[176] Kang RH, Chang HS, Wong ML, Choi MJ, Park JY, Lee HY, et al. Brain-derived neurotrophic factor gene polymorphisms and mirtazapine responses in Koreans with major depression. Journal of psychopharmacology. 2010;24(12):1755-63. Epub 2009/06/06.

[177] Laje G, Lally N, Mathews D, Brutsche N, Chemerinski A, Akula N, et al. Brain-Derived Neurotrophic Factor Val66Met Polymorphism and Antidepressant Efficacy of Ketamine in Depressed Patients. Biological psychiatry. 2012;72(11):e27-8. Epub 2012/07/10.

[178] Mamounas LA, Altar CA, Blue ME, Kaplan DR, Tessarollo L, Lyons WE. BDNF promotes the regenerative sprouting, but not survival, of injured serotonergic axons in the adult rat brain. The Journal of neuroscience : the official journal of the Society for Neuroscience. 2000;20(2):771-82. Epub 2000/01/13.

[179] Mamounas LA, Blue ME, Siuciak JA, Altar CA. Brain-derived neurotrophic factor promotes the survival and sprouting of serotonergic axons in rat brain. The Journal of neuroscience : the official journal of the Society for Neuroscience. 1995;15(12):7929-39. Epub 1995/12/01.

[180] Assareh N, ElBatsh MM, Marsden CA, Kendall DA. The effects of chronic administration of tranylcypromine and rimonabant on behaviour and protein expression in brain regions of the rat. Pharmacology, biochemistry, and behavior. 2012;100(3):506-12. Epub 2011/11/01.

[181] Balu DT, Hoshaw BA, Malberg JE, Rosenzweig-Lipson S, Schechter LE, Lucki I. Differential regulation of central BDNF protein levels by antidepressant and non-antidepressant drug treatments. Brain research. 2008;1211:37-43. Epub 2008/04/25.

[182] De Foubert G, Carney SL, Robinson CS, Destexhe EJ, Tomlinson R, Hicks CA, et al. Fluoxetine-induced change in rat brain expression of brain-derived neurotrophic factor varies depending on length of treatment. Neuroscience. 2004;128(3):597-604. Epub 2004/09/24.

[183] Khundakar AA, Zetterstrom TS. Biphasic change in BDNF gene expression following antidepressant drug treatment explained by differential transcript regulation. Brain research. 2006;1106(1):12-20. Epub 2006/07/18.

[184] Zhang F, Zhou H, Wilson BC, Shi JS, Hong JS, Gao HM. Fluoxetine protects neurons against microglial activation-mediated neurotoxicity. Parkinsonism & related disorders. 2012;18 Suppl 1:S213-7. Epub 2011/12/23.

[185] Serra-Millas M, Lopez-Vilchez I, Navarro V, Galan AM, Escolar G, Penades R, et al. Changes in plasma and platelet BDNF levels induced by S-citalopram in major depression. Psychopharmacology. 2011;216(1):1-8. Epub 2011/02/11.

[186] Yoshimura R, Mitoma M, Sugita A, Hori H, Okamoto T, Umene W, et al. Effects of paroxetine or milnacipran on serum brain-derived neurotrophic factor in depressed patients. Progress in neuro-psychopharmacology & biological psychiatry. 2007;31(5): 1034-7. Epub 2007/04/27.

[187] Tamburella A, Micale V, Navarria A, Drago F. Antidepressant properties of the 5-HT4 receptor partial agonist, SL65.0155: behavioral and neurochemical studies in rats. Progress in neuro-psychopharmacology & biological psychiatry. 2009;33(7):1205-10. Epub 2009/07/15.

[188] Agostinho FR, Reus GZ, Stringari RB, Ribeiro KF, Pfaffenseller B, Stertz L, et al. Olanzapine plus fluoxetine treatment increases Nt-3 protein levels in the rat prefrontal cortex. Neuroscience letters. 2011;497(2):99-103. Epub 2011/05/07.

[189] Pae CU, Marks DM, Han C, Patkar AA, Steffens D. Does neurotropin-3 have a therapeutic implication in major depression? The International journal of neuroscience. 2008;118(11):1515-22. Epub 2008/10/15.

[190] Araque A, Navarrete M. Glial cells in neuronal network function. Philosophical transactions of the Royal Society of London Series B, Biological sciences. 2010;365(1551): 2375-81. Epub 2010/07/07.

[191] Butt AM. ATP: a ubiquitous gliotransmitter integrating neuron-glial networks. Seminars in cell & developmental biology. 2011;22(2):205-13. Epub 2011/03/08.

[192] Paradise MB, Naismith SL, Norrie LM, Graeber MB, Hickie IB. The role of glia in late-life depression. International psychogeriatrics / IPA. 2012;24(12):1878-90. Epub 2012/08/10.

[193] Oh DH, Son H, Hwang S, Kim SH. Neuropathological abnormalities of astrocytes, GABAergic neurons, and pyramidal neurons in the dorsolateral prefrontal cortices of patients with major depressive disorder. European neuropsychopharmacology : the journal of the European College of Neuropsychopharmacology. 2012;22(5):330-8. Epub 2011/10/04.

[194] Rajkowska G, Miguel-Hidalgo JJ. Gliogenesis and glial pathology in depression. CNS & neurological disorders drug targets. 2007;6(3):219-33. Epub 2007/05/22.

[195] Connor TJ, Leonard BE. Depression, stress and immunological activation: the role of cytokines in depressive disorders. Life sciences. 1998;62(7):583-606. Epub 1998/02/24.

[196] Khairova RA, Machado-Vieira R, Du J, Manji HK. A potential role for pro-inflammatory cytokines in regulating synaptic plasticity in major depressive disorder. The international journal of neuropsychopharmacology / official scientific journal of the Collegium Internationale Neuropsychopharmacologicum. 2009;12(4):561-78. Epub 2009/02/20.

[197] Sheline YI, Price JL, Yan Z, Mintun MA. Resting-state functional MRI in depression unmasks increased connectivity between networks via the dorsal nexus. Proceedings of the National Academy of Sciences of the United States of America. 2010;107(24): 11020-5. Epub 2010/06/11.

[198] Kavalali ET, Monteggia LM. Synaptic Mechanisms Underlying Rapid Antidepressant Action of Ketamine. The American journal of psychiatry. 2012. Epub 2012/10/05.

[199] Salvadore G, van der Veen JW, Zhang Y, Marenco S, Machado-Vieira R, Baumann J, et al. An investigation of amino-acid neurotransmitters as potential predictors of clinical improvement to ketamine in depression. The international journal of neuropsychopharmacology / official scientific journal of the Collegium Internationale Neuropsychopharmacologicum. 2012;15(8):1063-72. Epub 2011/11/02.

[200] Scheidegger M, Walter M, Lehmann M, Metzger C, Grimm S, Boeker H, et al. Ketamine decreases resting state functional network connectivity in healthy subjects: implications for antidepressant drug action. PloS one. 2012;7(9):e44799. Epub 2012/10/11.

[201] Blier P, de Montigny C. Serotonin and drug-induced therapeutic responses in major depression, obsessive-compulsive and panic disorders. Neuropsychopharmacology : official publication of the American College of Neuropsychopharmacology. 1999;21(2 Suppl):91S-8S. Epub 1999/08/05.

[202] Watanabe Y, Gould E, McEwen BS. Stress induces atrophy of apical dendrites of hippocampal CA3 pyramidal neurons. Brain research. 1992;588(2):341-5. Epub 1992/08/21.

[203] Pavlides C, Nivon LG, McEwen BS. Effects of chronic stress on hippocampal long-term potentiation. Hippocampus. 2002;12(2):245-57. Epub 2002/05/10.

[204] Cieslik K, Sowa-Kucma M, Ossowska G, Legutko B, Wolak M, Opoka W, et al. Chronic unpredictable stress-induced reduction in the hippocampal brain-derived neurotrophic factor (BDNF) gene expression is antagonized by zinc treatment. Pharmacological reports : PR. 2011;63(2):537-43. Epub 2011/05/24.

[205] Liu W, Zhou C. Corticosterone reduces brain mitochondrial function and expression of mitofusin, BDNF in depression-like rodents regardless of exercise preconditioning. Psychoneuroendocrinology. 2012;37(7):1057-70. Epub 2012/01/17.

[206] Wellman CL. Dendritic reorganization in pyramidal neurons in medial prefrontal cortex after chronic corticosterone administration. Journal of neurobiology. 2001;49(3): 245-53. Epub 2001/12/18.

[207] Pavlides C, Watanabe Y, McEwen BS. Effects of glucocorticoids on hippocampal long-term potentiation. Hippocampus. 1993;3(2):183-92. Epub 1993/04/01.

[208] Novati A, Hulshof HJ, Koolhaas JM, Lucassen PJ, Meerlo P. Chronic sleep restriction causes a decrease in hippocampal volume in adolescent rats, which is not explained by changes in glucocorticoid levels or neurogenesis. Neuroscience. 2011;190:145-55. Epub 2011/07/02.

[209] Mirescu C, Peters JD, Noiman L, Gould E. Sleep deprivation inhibits adult neurogenesis in the hippocampus by elevating glucocorticoids. Proceedings of the National Academy of Sciences of the United States of America. 2006;103(50):19170-5. Epub 2006/12/01.

[210] Tartar JL, Ward CP, McKenna JT, Thakkar M, Arrigoni E, McCarley RW, et al. Hippocampal synaptic plasticity and spatial learning are impaired in a rat model of sleep fragmentation. The European journal of neuroscience. 2006;23(10):2739-48. Epub 2006/07/05.

[211] Zobel A, Jessen F, von Widdern O, Schuhmacher A, Hofels S, Metten M, et al. Unipolar depression and hippocampal volume: impact of DNA sequence variants of the glucocorticoid receptor gene. American journal of medical genetics Part B, Neuropsychiatric genetics : the official publication of the International Society of Psychiatric Genetics. 2008;147B(6):836-43. Epub 2008/02/21.

[212] Janssen J, Hulshoff Pol HE, de Leeuw FE, Schnack HG, Lampe IK, Kok RM, et al. Hippocampal volume and subcortical white matter lesions in late life depression: comparison of early and late onset depression. Journal of neurology, neurosurgery, and psychiatry. 2007;78(6):638-40. Epub 2007/01/11.

[213] McKinnon MC, Yucel K, Nazarov A, MacQueen GM. A meta-analysis examining clinical predictors of hippocampal volume in patients with major depressive disorder. Journal of psychiatry & neuroscience : JPN. 2009;34(1):41-54. Epub 2009/01/07.

[214] Li CT, Lin CP, Chou KH, Chen IY, Hsieh JC, Wu CL, et al. Structural and cognitive deficits in remitting and non-remitting recurrent depression: a voxel-based morphometric study. NeuroImage. 2010;50(1):347-56. Epub 2009/11/26.

[215] Cheng YQ, Xu J, Chai P, Li HJ, Luo CR, Yang T, et al. Brain volume alteration and the correlations with the clinical characteristics in drug-naive first-episode MDD patients: a voxel-based morphometry study. Neuroscience letters. 2010;480(1):30-4. Epub 2010/07/03.

[216] Cole J, Costafreda SG, McGuffin P, Fu CH. Hippocampal atrophy in first episode depression: a meta-analysis of magnetic resonance imaging studies. Journal of affective disorders. 2011;134(1-3):483-7. Epub 2011/07/13.

[217] Kronmuller KT, Schroder J, Kohler S, Gotz B, Victor D, Unger J, et al. Hippocampal volume in first episode and recurrent depression. Psychiatry research. 2009;174(1):62-6. Epub 2009/10/06.

[218] Sexton CE, Mackay CE, Ebmeier KP. A Systematic Review and Meta-Analysis of Magnetic Resonance Imaging Studies in Late-Life Depression. The American journal of geriatric psychiatry : official journal of the American Association for Geriatric Psychiatry. 2012. Epub 2012/03/03.

[219] Geerlings MI, Brickman AM, Schupf N, Devanand DP, Luchsinger JA, Mayeux R, et al. Depressive symptoms, antidepressant use, and brain volumes on MRI in a population-based cohort of old persons without dementia. Journal of Alzheimer's disease : JAD. 2012;30(1):75-82. Epub 2012/03/02.

[220] Steffens DC, McQuoid DR, Payne ME, Potter GG. Change in hippocampal volume on magnetic resonance imaging and cognitive decline among older depressed and nondepressed subjects in the neurocognitive outcomes of depression in the elderly study. The American journal of geriatric psychiatry : official journal of the American Association for Geriatric Psychiatry. 2011;19(1):4-12. Epub 2010/09/03.

[221] Chu CL, Liang CK, Chou MY, Lin YT, Pan CC, Lu T, et al. Decreased plasma brain-derived neurotrophic factor levels in institutionalized elderly with depressive disorder. Journal of the American Medical Directors Association. 2012;13(5):434-7. Epub 2011/09/29.

[222] Nifosi F, Toffanin T, Follador H, Zonta F, Padovan G, Pigato G, et al. Reduced right posterior hippocampal volume in women with recurrent familial pure depressive disorder. Psychiatry research. 2010;184(1):23-8. Epub 2010/09/08.

[223] Boccardi M, Almici M, Bresciani L, Caroli A, Bonetti M, Monchieri S, et al. Clinical and medial temporal features in a family with mood disorders. Neuroscience letters. 2010;468(2):93-7. Epub 2009/10/31.

[224] Ansell EB, Rando K, Tuit K, Guarnaccia J, Sinha R. Cumulative adversity and smaller gray matter volume in medial prefrontal, anterior cingulate, and insula regions. Biological psychiatry. 2012;72(1):57-64. Epub 2012/01/06.

Chapter 7

Biological Markers and Genetic Factors of Major Depressive Disorder

Hwa-Young Lee and Yong-Ku Kim

Additional information is available at the end of the chapter

http://dx.doi.org/10.5772/54388

1. Introduction

Major depressive disorder (MDD) is very prevalent and severe psychiatric disorder with prevalence estimates ranging 5% to 20% [1, 2] and has been a growing public health concern due to its recurrent, deliberate, and lethal nature. According to projections, MDD will become the second leading cause of disability worldwide by the year 2020. [3]

MDD is considered to be a clinically heterogeneous disorder which result from multiple genes interacting with environmental factors such as early stressful life events [4] and the diagnosis is based on a patient's symptoms, not on laboratory test.

Although recent decades have witnessed a tremendous revolution in the development of antidepressant drugs, the neurochemical effects that underlie the therapeutic action of these agents remain largely unknown. Antidepressant drugs acutely increase levels of monoamines, but it takes 2–3 weeks to show a clinical response after the administration of an antidepressant drug, [5] and the initial response rate in patients with major depressive disorders is about 70%. [6]

For the further understanding of the pathogenesis or the prediction of treatment response of MDD, biological approach for depression is needed.

The term 'biological marker' means biological change associated with depression that could be used to indicate the presence and severity of the condition and predict drug or other treatments' response as well as the clinical prognosis. So, the research for biological markers of depressive disorders is helpful for finding diagnostic method and useful to distinguish the effectiveness and early improvement after antidepressant administration.

Although work in this area has been inconclusive, many animal, post-mortem, clinical, and genetic studies have produced results implicating at least 3 neurobiological systems in the pathogenesis in major depression: dysfunction in the serotonergic system, hyperactivity of the hypothalamic-pituitary-adrenal axis, and decreased neuroplasticity. Additionally, other neurotransmitters, biochemical factors including inflammatory markers, neurophysiologic markers and neuroimaging markers may be associated with MDD.

In this chapter, we discuss biological markers involved in the pathogenesis of major depressive disorder.

2. Biological marker and genetic factor

2.1. Neurotransmitters

2.1.1. Serotonergic system

It has been hypothesized that a deficit in serotonin may be a crucial determinant in the pathophysiology of major depression. The serotonin system has been widely investigated in studies of major depression. The innervations of the serotonin system project from the dorsal raphe nucleus to all of the regions of the brain, including the cerebral cortex and hippocampus. Decreased function and activity of the serotonergic system in patients with major depression have been also confirmed in postmortem, serotonin transporter and serotonin receptor studies.

In suicide victims with major depression, enhanced radioligand binding of an agonist to inhibitory serotonin-1A autoreceptors in the human dorsal raphe nucleus provides pharmacological evidence to support the hypothesis of diminished activity of serotonin neurons. [7]

A trend of decreased 5-HT1A receptor expression appears to be a robust finding in major depression. A functional genetic variant of the 5-HT1A receptor, the C-1019G promoter polymorphism (rs6295), has been investigated in major depression. The G allele was more frequent in major depression. [8] By contrast, polymorphisms of HTR1A showed no association in Caucasians, while a significant association was observed in several studies of Asians. [9]

Imipramine binds to the serotonin transporter (5-HTT) on platelets, and it has been suggested that decreased platelet imipramine binding may be a putative biological marker of depressive disorder. A meta-analysis has shown that imipramine binding to platelets is indeed a robust biological marker of depression. [10]

Tryptophan hydroxylase (TPH), which has two isoforms (TPH1 and TPH2), is one of the rate limiting factors in serotonin synthesis, Postmortem studies have reported significantly higher numbers and higher densities of TPH immunoreactive neurons in the dorsal raphe nuclei of alcohol dependent, depressed suicide victims [11] when compared to controls. We have found that the TPH2 -703G/T SNP may have an important effect on susceptibility to suicidal behavior in those with major depressive disorder. Additionally, an increased frequency of the G allele of the TPH2 SNP is associated with elevated risk of suicidal behavior itself rather than with the diagnosis of major depression. [12]

Collectively, serotonin receptor, TPH and 5-HTT studies suggest that deficient or impaired serotonin activity is involved in major depression.

2.1.2. *Noradrenergic and dopaminergic systems*

The mechanism of action of tricyclic and monoamine oxidase inhibitor antidepressants involves the monoaminergic neurobiology. Recently, dual-acting antidepressants such as serotonin norepinephrine reuptake inhibitors (SNRIs) are introduced and have presented clinicians with a wider range of antidepressants. The action of the antidepressants is based on alterations in the functions of neurotransmitter systems and changes in the monoamine systems. [13, 14] Catecholamine metabolites, particularly 3-methoxy-4-hydroxy phenylglycol (MHPG), did not sufficiently distinguish depressed from other groups. Work in this area then underwent a subtle but significant shift toward the use of catecholamine metabolites to predict the response to tricyclic antidepressants. [15, 16] Nonetheless, research into the levels of monoamine transmitters and their metabolites have not found convincing evidence of a primary dysfunction into a particular transmitter system in depression, or a critical role in helping predict antidepressant response. [17]

The norepinephrine (NE) system has been studied in depression, particularly the action of NE reuptake inhibitors and SNRIs, which act at the NE transporter. Although polymorphisms the NET gene have not shown consistent association regarding susceptibility to depression, [18-20] but it cannot be denied that it may be an important candidate.

The Antidepressant effect of mirtazapine appears to be related to the dual enhancement of central noradrenergic and serotonergic neurotransmission via the blockade of adrenergic $\alpha 2$ receptors. [21-23] Previous studies have outlined the functional aspects of $\alpha 2$ receptors in depression, reporting reduced $\alpha 2$ inhibition of platelet adenylate cyclase activity [24] and increased adrenergic $\alpha 2$ agonist-induced platelet aggregation in depressed patients. [25] Three genes that encode human adrenergic $\alpha 2$ receptors have been cloned: $\alpha 2a$, $\alpha 2B$, and $\alpha 2C$. [26] The adrenergic $\alpha 2a$ receptor (ADRA2A) subtype is expressed in the central nervous system and peripheral tissues. [27] According to this classification, the classic $\alpha 2$ receptor studied in mood disorders is the $\alpha 2a$ receptor.

Previous study didn't show any association between this polymorphism and mood disorders, including depressive and bipolar disorders. [28] Regarding the prediction of antidepressant treatment, the ADRA2A −1291C/G genotypes did not show consistent results. [29, 30]

The dopamine (DA) system is also highly asssocitated with the symptomatology of depression, with the proposed pathophysiology of melancholic depression involving decreased DA transmission. [31] A VNTR in exon 15 of the DA transporter gene (SLC6A3), which affects the expression levels of the transporter, [32] is associated with a faster onset of antidepressant-treatment response. [33] The DA receptors have also been involved in pharmacogenetic studies of antidepressants in depression. The exon 3 VNTR of the DRD4 gene was also investigated in antidepressant drug response, with some studies finding no association, [34, 35] and one study finding a significant modulation of this polymorphism on various antidepressant drugs. [36]

2.2. Hypothalamic-pituitary- adrenal axis (HPA axis)

Hyperactivity of the hypothalamic-pituitaryadrenal (HPA) axis is one of the most consistent neuroendocrine abnormalities in major depressive disorder. [37] Specifically, patients with MDD show increased concentrations of cortisol in the plasma, urine and cerebrospinal fluid (CSF) and an exaggerated cortisol response to adrenocorticotrophic hormone (ACTH). [38-40] The corticosteroid receptor hypothesis has been proposed for the pathogenesis of MDD, which focuses on impaired corticosteroid receptor signalling, leading to a reduced negative feedback of cortisol, an increased production of corticotropin-releasing hormone (CRH) and hypercortisolism. [38]

Interestingly, cortisol and CRH affect the serotonin (5-HT) system. [39, 41] During the stress response, glucocorticoids (GCs) stimulate all these features of 5-HT transmission. [42] Conversely, 5-HT transmission is impaired and noradrenergic transmission in the hippocampus is suppressed during chronic psychosocial stress and hypercortisolism, which is similar to the series of events evident during depression. [43] It is reported HPA axis dysregulation could be a trait genetically determined which contributes to an increased risk for depression. From the fact that this trait is found both in affected subjects and in healthy relatives with a high familial risk, HPA axis is an interesting candidate endophenotype for affective disorders. [44, 45]

Studies investigating the hypothetical causes of an impaired regulation of HPA axis in depression have mainly focused on two elements: i) glucocorticoid receptor (GR) feedback mechanisms and ii) CRH signaling system.

Reduced GR function has been pointed out as the responsible of diminished sensitivity to cortisol which would lead to an inefficient feedback mechanism. [46] On the other hand, CRH peptide mediates the regulation of HPA axis as well as autonomic and behavioral responses in front of stress. [47] Moreover, dysregulation of HPA axis has also been suggested to play a central role in the mechanisms of action of antidepressants. [38, 48] Normalization of disturbances at HPA axis has been considered a prerequisite of a proper clinical response to antidepressant treatment. [39, 49]

It was reported that Bcl1 polymorphism was associated with the susceptibility to MDD, not the prediction of treatment response. [50] Genetic association studies have yielded preliminary evidence for a role of GR genetic variations in the genetic vulnerability for MDD. Taken together, the evidence for a role of GR and the GR gene in the neurobiology of MDD is building rapidly. [51]

2.3. Neuroplasticity

A time-lag in clinical response after the administration of an antidepressant drug suggests that alterations in monoamine metabolism alone cannot explain the entire antidepressant effect. In this respect, it was suggested that the mechanism of action might be associated with intracellular signal transduction pathways that are linked to the expression of specific genes. [52]

The neural plasticity hypothesis proposes that depression results from an inability to make appropriate adaptive responses to stress. [53] By stimulating intracellular pathways, antidepressants lead to upregulation of cAMP response element-binding (CREB) protein and an increase in the expression of neurotrophic factors, particularly BDNF. Brain-derived neurotrophic factor (BDNF), an important member of the neurotrophin family, affects the survival and function of neurons in the central nervous system and is abundant in the brain and peripheral nervous system. BDNF is the neurotrophic factor in the focus of intense research for the last years. BDNF acts on neurons at both presynaptic and postsynaptic sites by binding to its tyrosine kinase receptor TrkB, and internalization of the BDNF TrkB complex-signalling endosome. [54]

It has many effects on the nervous system, such as neuronal growth, differentiation, and repair. [55] It has been shown that stress decreases the synthesis of hippocampal BDNF in adult animals [33, 56] and induces atrophy of the apical dendrites of CA3 neurons. [57-59] Growing evidence suggests that BDNF may play a crucial role in depression. [60-63] So far, considerable work on the involvement of neurotrophic factors in the pathophysiology of depression has been carried out. Direct infusion of BDNF into the rat midbrain has antidepressant effects in the learned helplessness and forced swim behavioral models of depression in rodents. [62] In addition, long-term antidepressant drug treatment and electroconvulsive therapy can increase BDNF expression. [64]

BDNF and serotonin (5-hydroxytryptamine, 5-HT) are known to regulate synaptic plasticity, neurogenesis and neuronal survival in the adult brain. These two signals co-regulate one another such that 5-HT stimulates the expression of BDNF, and BDNF enhances the growth and survival of 5-HT neurons. [65]

Several lines of research show that the BDNF molecule is probably the "final common pathway" for different antidepressant approaches. These include antidepressants [64], electroconvulsive therapy, [64, 66] exercise [67, 68] and repetitive transcranial magnetic stimulation. [69] A large body of evidence, in humans, shows the similar result with direct measurements of BDNF in the bloodstream. [70-72] Treatment of depressed patients with antidepressants increases the serum BDNF levels close to the levels of normal controls. [73-75] In addition, they support the possibility that the enhancement of BDNF expression may be an important element in the clinical response to antidepressant treatment. [76]

Measurements of BDNF levels in sera or plasma in previous studies have been challenged. Our research group has also examined plasma BDNF levels among patients with major depression who both have and have not attempted suicide. One study found that plasma BDNF levels were significantly lower among depressed patients than among normal controls. [77]

The BDNF gene has several polymorphic markers, including an intronic microsatellite (GT)n dinucleotide repeat [78] and a functional coding region single-nucleotide polymorphism (SNP) at position 196/758, which results in a valine (Val) to methionine (Met) amino acid change at codon 66 (rs6265). Because this codon lies in region of the BDNF precursor protein that is cleaved away, it is not apparent in the mature BDNF protein. On pharmacogenetic study of BDNF, it was suggested that the Val66Met polymorphism of BDNF is associated with citalopram efficacy, with Met allele carriers responding better to citalopram treatment. [79] However, other studies suggested that BDNF polymorphism does not affect the clinical outcome of antidepressant administration. [80, 81]

2.4. Neuroimaging marker

Positron emission tomography (PET) imaging studies have revealed multiple abnormalities of regional cerebral blood flow (CBF) and glucose metabolism in brain regions. In PET imaging of unmedicated subjects with major depression, regional CBF and metabolism are consistently increased in the amygdala, orbital cortex, and medial thalamus, and decreased in the dorsomedial/dorsal anterolateral PFC and anterior cingulate cortex ventral to the genu of the corpus callosum (subgenual PFC) relative to healthy controls. [82, 83] These circuits have also been implicated more generally in emotional behavior.

Recent neuroimaging studies have focused on the neurobiological abnormalities that are associated with MDD, such as dysfunctional or structural differences in cerebral regions, including the prefrontal cortex, amygdala, anterior cingulate cortex (ACC), and hippocampus, in patients with MDD compared with healthy controls. [84-87]

Reductions in hippocampal volume may not antedate illness onset, but volume may decrease at the greatest rate in the early years after illness onset. [87] In the absence of a significant correlation between hippocampal volume and age in either post-depressive or control subjects, a significant correlation with total lifetime duration of depression was found. This suggest that repeated stress during recurrent depressive episodes may result in cumulative hippocampal injury as reflected in volume loss. [88]

Previous structural magnetic resonance imaging (MRI) studies using region-of-interest (ROI) analyses have shown a variety of findings. [89, 90] These inconsistencies can be explained by the variability in the ROI criteria among studies and an inconsistency in ROI validation. [89, 91, 92] Consequently, voxel-based morphometry (VBM) [93] is being increasingly used as a viable alternative methodology for detecting structural abnormalities in patients with neuropsychiatric disorders, including MDD. [94-97] Previous MDD VBM studies have also shown reduced gray matter density in the hippocampus. [95, 96, 98] Recently, it is reported that gray matter density of several regions associated with emotion regulation, particularly dorsal raphe nucleus, was lower in MDD patients. [99]

Findings to directly compare unipolar depressed and bipolar depressed individuals, [100] more widespread abnormalities in white matter connectivity and white matter hyperintensities in bipolar depression than unipolar depression, habenula volume reductions in bipolar but not unipolar depression, and differential patterns of functional abnormalities in emotion regulation and attentional control neural circuitry in the two depression types.

Neuroimaging technology has provided unprecedented opportunities for elucidating the anatomical correlates of major depression. [82] Nowadays, researches that combine brain imaging and genetics have been emerging. The first imaging genetics research reported that carriers of the short allele of the serotonin transporter promoter polymorphism exhibit greater amygdala neuronal activity, as assessed by functional magnetic resonance imaging, in response to fearful stimuli compared with individuals homozygous for the long allele. [101] Since then, however, it has been reported that homozygosity for the l or s allele is associated with decreased hippocampal volumes in patients with major depression. [102, 103] Even though these results inconsistent, future direction for imaging genetics is promising.

3. Conclusions

Major depressive disorder is considered to be a clinically heterogeneous disorder and the diagnosis is based on a patient's symptoms, not on laboratory test. So, the pathogenesis of major depressive disorder is not clear. MDD results from multiple genes interacting with environmental factors such as early stressful life events. Although recent decades have witnessed a tremendous revolution in the development of antidepressant drugs, the neurochemical effects that underlie the therapeutic action of these agents remain largely unknown. Antidepressants alter the levels of neurotransmitters such as serotonin in the synaptic cleft several minutes after their administration, and this alters the activity of the neurotransmission system. Nevertheless, an improvement in the symptoms of depression takes 2–6 weeks of treatment, during which time the neuronal response and morphology of cells change.

The research results for the monoamine system, hyperactivity of the hypothalamic-pituitary-adrenal axis, decreased neuroplasticity, and neuroimaging will be helpful to understand the pathogenesis of major depressvie disorder. To find biological markers for diagnosing MDD and predicting the individual responses to antidepressants, genetic case-control association studies are used widely because they are relatively easy to conduct and can discover genetic variants with small influences on phenotype.

Researchers have searched for biological markers of diagnosis and treatment response, and will try to understand the pathogenesis of depression and the mechanisms underlying the delayed response to antidepressant treatment.

Author details

Hwa-Young Lee[1] and Yong-Ku Kim[2*]

*Address all correspondence to: yonkgu@korea.ac.kr

1 Department of Psychiatry, College of Medicine, Soonchunhyang University, Republic of Korea

2 Department of Psychiatry, College of Medicine, Korea University, Republic of Korea

References

[1] Bierut, L.J., et al., Major depressive disorder in a community-based twin sample: are there different genetic and environmental contributions for men and women? Arch Gen Psychiatry, 1999. 56(6): p. 557-63.

[2] Hamet, P. and J. Tremblay, Genetics and genomics of depression. Metabolism, 2005. 54(5 Suppl 1): p. 10-5.

[3] Murray, C.J. and A.D. Lopez, Global mortality, disability, and the contribution of risk factors: Global Burden of Disease Study. Lancet, 1997. 349(9063): p. 1436-42.

[4] Caspi, A., et al., Influence of life stress on depression: moderation by a polymorphism in the 5-HTT gene. Science, 2003. 301(5631): p. 386-9.

[5] Hindmarch, I., Expanding the horizons of depression: beyond the monoamine hypothesis. Hum Psychopharmacol, 2001. 16(3): p. 203-218.

[6] Nemeroff, C.B., Psychopharmacology of affective disorders in the 21st century. Biol Psychiatry, 1998. 44(7): p. 517-25.

[7] Stockmeier, C.A., et al., Increase in serotonin-1A autoreceptors in the midbrain of suicide victims with major depression-postmortem evidence for decreased serotonin activity. J Neurosci, 1998. 18(18): p. 7394-401.

[8] Lemonde, S., et al., Impaired repression at a 5-hydroxytryptamine 1A receptor gene polymorphism associated with major depression and suicide. J Neurosci, 2003. 23(25): p. 8788-99.

[9] Horstmann, S. and E.B. Binder, Pharmacogenomics of antidepressant drugs. Pharmacol Ther, 2009. 124(1): p. 57-73.

[10] Ellis, P.M. and C. Salmond, Is platelet imipramine binding reduced in depression? A meta-analysis. Biol Psychiatry, 1994. 36(5): p. 292-9.

[11] Bonkale, W.L., G. Turecki, and M.C. Austin, Increased tryptophan hydroxylase immunoreactivity in the dorsal raphe nucleus of alcohol-dependent, depressed suicide subjects is restricted to the dorsal subnucleus. Synapse, 2006. 60(1): p. 81-5.

[12] Yoon, H.K. and Y.K. Kim, TPH2 -703G/T SNP may have important effect on susceptibility to suicidal behavior in major depression. Prog Neuropsychopharmacol Biol Psychiatry, 2009. 33(3): p. 403-9.

[13] Blier, P. and C. de Montigny, Current advances and trends in the treatment of depression. Trends Pharmacol Sci, 1994. 15(7): p. 220-6.

[14] Delgado, P.L., et al., Monoamines and the mechanism of antidepressant action: effects of catecholamine depletion on mood of patients treated with antidepressants. Psychopharmacol Bull, 1993. 29(3): p. 389-96.

[15] Schildkraut, J.J., The catecholamine hypothesis of affective disorders: a review of supporting evidence. 1965. J Neuropsychiatry Clin Neurosci, 1995. 7(4): p. 524-33; discussion 523-4.

[16] Mooney, J.J., et al., Urinary 3-methoxy-4-hydroxyphenylglycol and the depression-type score as predictors of differential responses to antidepressants. J Clin Psychopharmacol, 1991. 11(6): p. 339-43.

[17] Delgado, P.L., Depression: the case for a monoamine deficiency. J Clin Psychiatry, 2000. 61 Suppl 6: p. 7-11.

[18] Ryu, S.H., et al., Association between norepinephrine transporter gene polymorphism and major depression. Neuropsychobiology, 2004. 49(4): p. 174-7.

[19] Chang, C.C., et al., Lack of association between the norepinephrine transporter gene and major depression in a Han Chinese population. J Psychiatry Neurosci, 2007. 32(2): p. 121-8.

[20] Zill, P., et al., Identification of a naturally occurring polymorphism in the promoter region of the norepinephrine transporter and analysis in major depression. Neuropsychopharmacology, 2002. 26(4): p. 489-93.

[21] Herman, G.M., Pharmacology of Antidepressant: Selectivity or Multiplicity? J Clin Psychiatry 1999. 60 suppl 17: p. 4-8.

[22] Kasper, S., Efficacy of antidepressants in the treatment of severe depression: the place of mirtazapine. J Clin Psychopharmacol, 1997. 17 Suppl 1: p. 19S-28S.

[23] Preskorn, S.H., Selection of an antidepressant: mirtazapine. J Clin Psychiatry, 1997. 58 Suppl 6: p. 3-8.

[24] Siever, L.J., et al., Platelet alpha-adrenergic binding and biochemical responsiveness in depressed patients and controls. Psychiatry Res, 1984. 11(4): p. 287-302.

[25] Garcia-Sevilla, J.A., et al., Alpha 2-adrenoceptor-mediated inhibition of platelet adenylate cyclase and induction of aggregation in major depression. Effect of long-term cyclic antidepressant drug treatment. Arch Gen Psychiatry, 1990. 47(2): p. 125-32.

[26] Bylund, D.B., et al., International Union of Pharmacology nomenclature of adrenoceptors. Pharmacol Rev, 1994. 46(2): p. 121-36.

[27] Lorenz, W., et al., Expression of three alpha 2-adrenergic receptor subtypes in rat tissues: implications for alpha 2 receptor classification. Mol Pharmacol, 1990. 38(5): p. 599-603.

[28] Ohara, K., et al., Polymorphism in the promoter region of the alpha 2A adrenergic receptor gene and mood disorders. Neuroreport, 1998. 9(7): p. 1291-4.

[29] Lee, H.Y., et al., Association of the adrenergic alpha 2a receptor--1291C/G polymorphism with weight change and treatment response to mirtazapine in patients with major depressive disorder. Brain Res, 2009. 1262: p. 1-6.

[30] Wakeno, M., et al., The alpha 2A-adrenergic receptor gene polymorphism modifies antidepressant responses to milnacipran. J Clin Psychopharmacol, 2008. 28(5): p. 518-24.

[31] Geracitano, R., et al., On the effects of psychostimulants, antidepressants, and the antiparkinsonian drug levodopa on dopamine neurons. Ann N Y Acad Sci, 2006. 1074: p. 320-9.

[32] Fuke, S., et al., The VNTR polymorphism of the human dopamine transporter (DAT1) gene affects gene expression. Pharmacogenomics J, 2001. 1(2): p. 152-6.

[33] Smith, M.A., et al., Stress and glucocorticoids affect the expression of brain-derived neurotrophic factor and neurotrophin-3 mRNAs in the hippocampus. J Neurosci, 1995. 15(3 Pt 1): p. 1768-77.

[34] Serretti, A., et al., No association between dopamine D(2) and D(4) receptor gene variants and antidepressant activity of two selective serotonin reuptake inhibitors. Psychiatry Res, 2001. 104(3): p. 195-203.

[35] Serretti, A., et al., Dopamine receptor D4 is not associated with antidepressant activity of sleep deprivation. Psychiatry Res, 1999. 89(2): p. 107-14.

[36] Garriock, H.A., et al., Number of risk genotypes is a risk factor for major depressive disorder: a case control study. Behav Brain Funct, 2006. 2: p. 24.

[37] Holsboer, F., The rationale for corticotropin-releasing hormone receptor (CRH-R) antagonists to treat depression and anxiety. J Psychiatr Res, 1999. 33(3): p. 181-214.

[38] Holsboer, F., The corticosteroid receptor hypothesis of depression. Neuropsychopharmacology, 2000. 23(5): p. 477-501.

[39] Holsboer, F. and N. Barden, Antidepressants and hypothalamic-pituitary-adrenocortical regulation. Endocr Rev, 1996. 17(2): p. 187-205.

[40] Nemeroff, C.B., The corticotropin-releasing factor (CRF) hypothesis of depression: new findings and new directions. Mol Psychiatry, 1996. 1(4): p. 336-42.

[41] De Kloet, E.R., et al., Brain corticosteroid receptor balance in health and disease. Endocr Rev, 1998. 19(3): p. 269-301.

[42] Meijer, O.C. and E.R. de Kloet, Corticosterone and serotonergic neurotransmission in the hippocampus: functional implications of central corticosteroid receptor diversity. Crit Rev Neurobiol, 1998. 12(1-2): p. 1-20.

[43] Wolkowitz, O.M., et al., Ketoconazole administration in hypercortisolemic depression. Am J Psychiatry, 1993. 150(5): p. 810-2.

[44] Holsboer, F., et al., Altered hypothalamic-pituitary-adrenocortical regulation in healthy subjects at high familial risk for affective disorders. Neuroendocrinology, 1995. 62(4): p. 340-7.

[45] Modell, S., et al., Hormonal response pattern in the combined DEX-CRH test is stable over time in subjects at high familial risk for affective disorders. Neuropsychopharmacology, 1998. 18(4): p. 253-62.

[46] Pariante, C.M. and A.H. Miller, Glucocorticoid receptors in major depression: relevance to pathophysiology and treatment. Biol Psychiatry, 2001. 49(5): p. 391-404.

[47] Arborelius, L., et al., The role of corticotropin-releasing factor in depression and anxiety disorders. J Endocrinol, 1999. 160(1): p. 1-12.

[48] Nemeroff, C.B. and M.J. Owens, Treatment of mood disorders. Nat Neurosci, 2002. 5 Suppl: p. 1068-70.

[49] Nemeroff, C.B., The role of corticotropin-releasing factor in the pathogenesis of major depression. Pharmacopsychiatry, 1988. 21(2): p. 76-82.

[50] Lee, H., et al., Association of glucocorticoid receptor polymorphisms with the susceptibility to major depressive disorder and treatment responses in Korean depressive patients. Acta Neuropsychiatrica, 2009. 21(1): p. 11-17.

[51] Claes, S., Glucocorticoid receptor polymorphisms in major depression. Ann N Y Acad Sci, 2009. 1179: p. 216-28.

[52] Duman, R.S., et al., Neuronal plasticity and survival in mood disorders. Biol Psychiatry, 2000. 48(8): p. 732-9.

[53] Popoli, M., M. Gennarelli, and G. Racagni, Modulation of synaptic plasticity by stress and antidepressants. Bipolar Disord, 2002. 4(3): p. 166-82.

[54] Lu, B., BDNF and activity-dependent synaptic modulation. Learn Mem, 2003. 10(2): p. 86-98.

[55] Lewin, G.R. and Y.A. Barde, Physiology of the neurotrophins. Annu Rev Neurosci, 1996. 19: p. 289-317.

[56] Nibuya, M., et al., Repeated stress increases catalytic TrkB mRNA in rat hippocampus. Neurosci Lett, 1999. 267(2): p. 81-4.

[57] Gould, E., et al., Neurogenesis in the dentate gyrus of the adult tree shrew is regulated by psychosocial stress and NMDA receptor activation. J Neurosci, 1997. 17(7): p. 2492-8.

[58] Gould, E., et al., Proliferation of granule cell precursors in the dentate gyrus of adult monkeys is diminished by stress. Proc Natl Acad Sci U S A, 1998. 95(6): p. 3168-71.

[59] Magarinos, A.M. and B.S. McEwen, Stress-induced atrophy of apical dendrites of hippocampal CA3c neurons: involvement of glucocorticoid secretion and excitatory amino acid receptors. Neuroscience, 1995. 69(1): p. 89-98.

[60] Duman, R.S., G.R. Heninger, and E.J. Nestler, A molecular and cellular theory of depression. Arch Gen Psychiatry, 1997. 54(7): p. 597-606.

[61] Altar, C.A., Neurotrophins and depression. Trends Pharmacol Sci, 1999. 20(2): p. 59-61.

[62] Siuciak, J.A., et al., Antidepressant-like effect of brain-derived neurotrophic factor (BDNF). Pharmacol Biochem Behav, 1997. 56(1): p. 131-7.

[63] Chen, B., et al., Increased hippocampal BDNF immunoreactivity in subjects treated with antidepressant medication. Biol Psychiatry, 2001. 50(4): p. 260-5.

[64] Nibuya, M., S. Morinobu, and R.S. Duman, Regulation of BDNF and trkB mRNA in rat brain by chronic electroconvulsive seizure and antidepressant drug treatments. J Neurosci, 1995. 15(11): p. 7539-47.

[65] Mattson, M.P., S. Maudsley, and B. Martin, BDNF and 5-HT: a dynamic duo in age-related neuronal plasticity and neurodegenerative disorders. Trends Neurosci, 2004. 27(10): p. 589-94.

[66] Altar, C.A., et al., Effects of electroconvulsive seizures and antidepressant drugs on brain-derived neurotrophic factor protein in rat brain. Biol Psychiatry, 2003. 54(7): p. 703-9.

[67] Oliff, H.S., et al., Exercise-induced regulation of brain-derived neurotrophic factor (BDNF) transcripts in the rat hippocampus. Brain Res Mol Brain Res, 1998. 61(1-2): p. 147-53.

[68] Garcia, C., et al., The influence of specific noradrenergic and serotonergic lesions on the expression of hippocampal brain-derived neurotrophic factor transcripts following voluntary physical activity. Neuroscience, 2003. 119(3): p. 721-32.

[69] Muller, M.B., et al., Long-term repetitive transcranial magnetic stimulation increases the expression of brain-derived neurotrophic factor and cholecystokinin mRNA, but not neuropeptide tyrosine mRNA in specific areas of rat brain. Neuropsychopharmacology, 2000. 23(2): p. 205-15.

[70] Karege, F., et al., Decreased serum brain-derived neurotrophic factor levels in major depressed patients. Psychiatry Res, 2002. 109(2): p. 143-8.

[71] Karege, F., et al., Low brain-derived neurotrophic factor (BDNF) levels in serum of depressed patients probably results from lowered platelet BDNF release unrelated to platelet reactivity. Biol Psychiatry, 2005. 57(9): p. 1068-72.

[72] Shimizu, E., et al., Alterations of serum levels of brain-derived neurotrophic factor (BDNF) in depressed patients with or without antidepressants. Biol Psychiatry, 2003. 54(1): p. 70-5.

[73] Aydemir, O., A. Deveci, and F. Taneli, The effect of chronic antidepressant treatment on serum brain-derived neurotrophic factor levels in depressed patients: a preliminary study. Prog Neuropsychopharmacol Biol Psychiatry, 2005. 29(2): p. 261-5.

[74] Gervasoni, N., et al., Partial normalization of serum brain-derived neurotrophic factor in remitted patients after a major depressive episode. Neuropsychobiology, 2005. 51(4): p. 234-8.

[75] Gonul, A.S., et al., Effect of treatment on serum brain-derived neurotrophic factor levels in depressed patients. Eur Arch Psychiatry Clin Neurosci, 2005. 255(6): p. 381-6.

[76] Russo-Neustadt, A., et al., Physical activity-antidepressant treatment combination: impact on brain-derived neurotrophic factor and behavior in an animal model. Behav Brain Res, 2001. 120(1): p. 87-95.

[77] Lee, B.H., et al., Decreased plasma BDNF level in depressive patients. J Affect Disord, 2007. 101(1-3): p. 239-44.

[78] Proschel, M., et al., Dinucleotide repeat polymorphism at the human gene for the brain-derived neurotrophic factor (BDNF). Hum Mol Genet, 1992. 1(5): p. 353.

[79] Choi, M.J., et al., Brain-derived neurotrophic factor gene polymorphism (Val66Met) and citalopram response in major depressive disorder. Brain Res, 2006. 1118(1): p. 176-82.

[80] Kang, R.H., et al., Brain-derived neurotrophic factor gene polymorphisms and mirtazapine responses in Koreans with major depression. J Psychopharmacol, 2010. 24(12): p. 1755-63.

[81] Tsai, S.J., et al., Association study of a brain-derived neurotrophic-factor genetic polymorphism and major depressive disorders, symptomatology, and antidepressant response. Am J Med Genet B Neuropsychiatr Genet, 2003. 123B(1): p. 19-22.

[82] Drevets, W.C., Neuroimaging and neuropathological studies of depression: implications for the cognitive-emotional features of mood disorders. Curr Opin Neurobiol, 2001. 11(2): p. 240-9.

[83] Manji, H.K., W.C. Drevets, and D.S. Charney, The cellular neurobiology of depression. Nat Med, 2001. 7(5): p. 541-7.

[84] Canli, T., et al., Brain activation to emotional words in depressed vs healthy subjects. Neuroreport, 2004. 15(17): p. 2585-8.

[85] Frodl, T., et al., Hippocampal and amygdala changes in patients with major depressive disorder and healthy controls during a 1-year follow-up. J Clin Psychiatry, 2004. 65(4): p. 492-9.

[86] Henriques, J.B., Davidson, R.J., Decreased responsiveness to reward in depression. COGNITION AND EMOTION, 2000. 15(5): p. 711-724.

[87] MacQueen, G.M., et al., Course of illness, hippocampal function, and hippocampal volume in major depression. Proc Natl Acad Sci U S A, 2003. 100(3): p. 1387-92.

[88] Sheline, Y.I., et al., Depression duration but not age predicts hippocampal volume loss in medically healthy women with recurrent major depression. J Neurosci, 1999. 19(12): p. 5034-43.

[89] Konarski, J.Z., et al., Volumetric neuroimaging investigations in mood disorders: bipolar disorder versus major depressive disorder. Bipolar Disord, 2008. 10(1): p. 1-37.

[90] Lorenzetti, V., et al., Structural brain abnormalities in major depressive disorder: a selective review of recent MRI studies. J Affect Disord, 2009. 117(1-2): p. 1-17.

[91] Goldstein, J.M., et al., Cortical abnormalities in schizophrenia identified by structural magnetic resonance imaging. Arch Gen Psychiatry, 1999. 56(6): p. 537-47.

[92] Wolkin, A., et al., Structural magnetic resonance image averaging in schizophrenia. Am J Psychiatry, 1998. 155(8): p. 1064-73.

[93] Ashburner, J. and K.J. Friston, Voxel-based morphometry--the methods. Neuroimage, 2000. 11(6 Pt 1): p. 805-21.

[94] Leung, K.K., et al., Neural correlates of attention biases of people with major depressive disorder: a voxel-based morphometric study. Psychol Med, 2009. 39(7): p. 1097-106.

[95] Shah, P.J., et al., Cortical grey matter reductions associated with treatment-resistant chronic unipolar depression. Controlled magnetic resonance imaging study. Br J Psychiatry, 1998. 172: p. 527-32.

[96] Vasic, N., et al., Gray matter reduction associated with psychopathology and cognitive dysfunction in unipolar depression: a voxel-based morphometry study. J Affect Disord, 2008. 109(1-2): p. 107-16.

[97] Cheng, Y.Q., et al., Brain volume alteration and the correlations with the clinical characteristics in drug-naive first-episode MDD patients: a voxel-based morphometry study. Neurosci Lett, 2010. 480(1): p. 30-4.

[98] Bergouignan, L., et al., Can voxel based morphometry, manual segmentation and automated segmentation equally detect hippocampal volume differences in acute depression? Neuroimage, 2009. 45(1): p. 29-37.

[99] Lee, H.Y., et al., Demonstration of decreased gray matter concentration in the midbrain encompassing the dorsal raphe nucleus and the limbic subcortical regions in major depressive disorder: an optimized voxel-based morphometry study. J Affect Disord, 2011. 133(1-2): p. 128-36.

[100] Almeida, J.R. and M.L. Phillips, Distinguishing between Unipolar Depression and Bipolar Depression: Current and Future Clinical and Neuroimaging Perspectives. Biol Psychiatry, 2012.

[101] Hariri, A.R., et al., Serotonin transporter genetic variation and the response of the human amygdala. Science, 2002. 297(5580): p. 400-3.

[102] Frodl, T., et al., Reduced hippocampal volumes associated with the long variant of the tri- and diallelic serotonin transporter polymorphism in major depression. Am J Med Genet B Neuropsychiatr Genet, 2008. 147B(7): p. 1003-7.

[103] Eker, M.C., et al., Smaller hippocampus volume is associated with short variant of 5-HTTLPR polymorphism in medication-free major depressive disorder patients. Neuropsychobiology, 2011. 63(1): p. 22-8.

Chapter 8

Mood Disorders and Mother-Infant Relationship – The Supportive Role of a Midwife

Ana Polona Mivšek and Tita Stanek Zidarič

Additional information is available at the end of the chapter

http://dx.doi.org/10.5772/53253

1. Introduction

It was Freud in 1940 [1] who referred to the mother's bond with a child as "unique, without parallel", and who has asserted that the mother is "established unalterably for a whole lifetime as our first and strongest love object… the prototype of all later love relations". It is the trust created in the mother-baby bond that sets the stage for the adult's later relationships. At core, this trust comes from the most basic level of relating, including with touch that can be felt both literally and symbolically. Successful relating comes from the mother's ability to connect with her baby from one mind to another as associated to empathic identification with baby's state of mind; the Winnicott's primarily preoccupation. It is also important that mother connects with her infant from one body to another, defining boundary between internal and external space, forever impacting psychological development. These early sensorial encounters than become the basis for our experiences of self and identity.

The psychological well-being of a mother during the pregnancy and after the birth can have a profound effect on the care she provides for the baby. The baby needs eye contact, affectionate handling and sound stimulation for successful development. Postnatal depression (PND) can impair mother's ability to provide a baby with these stimulations [2]. Parental psychological influences and adverse lifestyle choices have consistently demonstrated an impact upon the outcome for newborn infants and have impact on them also in their adulthood. One of such situations is also maternal depression. Therefore the aim of intervention strategies for this condition is to break this cycle [3].

Improving maternal depression does not, in itself, necessarily improve mother–infant interaction [4]. Different interventions that enhance creation of mother-infant relationship can be therefore considered as crucial for the benefits of parent-infant dyad when mother is depressed. Already in 1977 Field [5] has recommended teaching mothers both - about infants' cues and also about the baby massage.

Based upon these recommendations, the following chapter aims to present arguments of benefits to improve PND for two interventions (Newborn Behavioural Observation – NBO and infant massage).

2. Background

Postnatal period can be very demanding for a new mother; acceptance of new role, changes of a lifestyle and continuous care for the baby can be tiring. In the postnatal period family with a baby receives postnatal care at home. Ideally by the midwife who cared for the woman during the pregnancy and birth. Beside the check-up for the woman's physical changes and care of the newborn, midwives should offer support and advice on adaptation to parenthood and be aware of signs of poor emotional well-being [6]. Postpartum mood disorders represent the most frequent form of maternal morbidity following delivery [7]. Midwife can include certain practices in the routine postnatal care that can help women raise her self-esteem in transition to motherhood and consequently alleviate depressive mood.

2.1. Postnatal period and postnatal depression

There is no specific definition of PND [8]; the debate, whether this is a general depression, incidentally occurring after the birth of a child or whether it is an entity on its own, still lasts. PND is categorized as major depressive disorder. Symptoms are similar to a general major depressive episode [9]. Three of the symptoms from the seven listed in the ICD 10 classification or four from the eight symptoms listed by DSM IV [10] must be present in order for woman to be diagnosed with PND. However symptoms may be masked by the common changes of postnatal period (fatigue, weight loss, tiredness ect.) [11].

As the definition of PND, also the duration and the onset of PND are not clearly defined. The crucial time for onset is around third [9] to sixth week postpartum [8,11], but some women can develop PND from pre-existing depressive states prenatally [3,12]. If untreated, PND can last up to the end of first postpartum year [11] or even longer.

Longitudinal and epidemiological studies have estimated different prevalence rates of PND, ranging from 3% to more than 28% of women [7]. Beck and Gable [13] report 12% prevalence of severe depression and 19% of minor.

It is still not known exactly what triggers the outbreak of mental disturbances in the postnatal period [14]. The literature regarding the aetiology of PND is inconclusive and many researchers support the theory of a synergistic effect of several factors [15,16.] The quantity of the risk factors identified in the literature calls into question their usefulness at predicting PND [17]. According to experts [18] the presentation of PND varies individually. Since women are individuals, a healthcare professional would be required to have in-depth knowledge about their personality, life situation and expectations regarding the motherhood in order to successfully interpret their behaviour postnatally.

Women with PND rarely seek help on their own (sometimes because they are not aware of the reason for their bad mood or might be afraid of stigma associated with mental illnesses), it is estimated that approximately 50% of cases of PND go undetected by health workers [13]. It is therefore recommended that screening should be performed as a part of routine postnatal care [19].

In depression with mild to moderate symptoms, non-pharmacological treatment is proposed [20]. Because many women decline pharmacological treatments, these interventions are often the first line treatment [21]. Despite the fact that some experts believe that these therapies are unhelpful in the long term, they admit that there is an improvement in maternal mood right after their application [4,22]. Antidepressants may be considered for use in women with mild, moderate or severe PND, only when they are unresponsive or reluctant to participate in non-drug management programmes [23], if the woman is at risk of suicide or infanticide, or has severe depression that does not respond to non-pharmacological treatment [20]. A lot of new methods of complementary treatment are currently being evaluated in order to help women with PND, for example acupuncture [24], massage therapy [25], bright light therapy [26,27], kangaroo (skin to skin) therapy [28] or regular physical activity [29,30] ect.

There is an on-going debate whether PND is an illness or normal and understandable response to difficulties of motherhood [31]. However it was never denied that women need help to cope with these feelings. It is a general tendency that woman should be treated at home in a known environment with the support of partner and other family members. PND can affect all family members, therefore all interventions should be family centred [32].

2.1.1. *Impact of maternal depression on infant*

It has been suggested that the child may be a factor in the development of PND, particularly in the case of multiple pregnancies, when the child is immature or has special needs [33]. Others have suggested that demanding childcare on its own could be a trigger for PND [34]. McIntosh [35] interviewed mothers to identify the main cause of PND. Women perceived motherhood as such to be the strongest risk factor, because it entails cyclic, demanding and responsible work that isolates them and robs them of their freedom. Additional burdens were lack of support and lack of time for themselves. Depressed mothers report significantly higher perceived stress, related to the child care and lower self-esteem in connection to motherhood abilities [36]. They often perceive their infants to be demanding [37,38] although there is no evidence as to whether PND is a condition which is provoked by the demanding temperament of the child or whether the mothers' perception of the child's behaviour is distorted or made more sensitive to the child's demands by the presence of PND [39-41].

Ambivalent feelings towards pregnancy and child or other stress related situations prenatally may provoke antenatal depression [11]. The maternal depression during the pregnancy may takes its toll on the well-being of the foetus. Depressed pregnant woman may eat and sleep less well [42] and are more likely to live unhealthy [43]. Prolonged anxiety and depression can change ability of mother's body to absorb nourishment; therefore newborn babies can be of low weight [44]. Prenatal depression has been clearly associated with the risk of prematurity and/or low birth weight [45]. Besides that, some researchers [46] found that physiological markers of individual differences in infant temperament are identifiable in the foetal period, and possibly shaped by the prenatal environment; that is in this case affected with prenatal depression and therefore exposed to stress hormones [47-49] and effects of biochemical imbalance [50]. Neonates of antenataly depressed mothers, tested with Brazelton Neonatal Behavior Assessment Scale (NBAS) showed inferior performance on orientation, reflex, excitability and withdrawal clusters [51]. Because they were exposed to the high level of stress hormones during the pregnancy, babies of antenatally depressed mothers usually cry more and for longer periods [44] and can be therefore perceived as more demanding by mothers.

Postnatally depression continues to have negative impact on child development [52]; especially from the aspect of the emotional, behavioural, and cognitive functioning [53,54]. PND occurs at a time when the foundation of the mother-child relationship is being laid. It has an effect on the mother's parenting abilities, which can have an adverse impact on the child [4], as the infant's need for love may be unsatisfied [55] and later the communication between them is impaired [4]. Hagen [56] claims women with PND exhibit fewer positive emotions towards their children, are less responsive and less sensitive to infant cues, have a less successful maternal role attainment, and have consequently infants, who are less securely attached. Their parenting style is more punitive; with less positive engagement [4]. Depression could act to weaken parents' ability to regulate child's emotions, potentially affecting temperament development [57]. A depressed mother is less positive, less contingent, and shows less vocal and play interactions to her child. Maternal responsiveness has been viewed as important element of child development that gives infant social, emotional and cognitive competencies [58] and promotes development of communication [59,60]. Therefore some researchers claim that mother's sensitivity is crucial [61], however it is impaired when mother is depressed [62]. Resulting from the mother's depressive symptoms, the infant shows less positive affection, less contingent behaviour [63- 67], sleep and eat less [64] and can have problems in regulating emotions at 7 months; therefore is perceived as child with difficult temperament by mothers [68,69]. A wealth of empirical evidence demonstrates that maternal and parental depression has been strongly associated with an increased incidence of attachment maladaptation, behavioural and emotional problems, altered cognitive and motor development and reduced social interaction abilities in infants [70-76]. Studies showed also poor physical status of infants of depressed mothers [77]; they are at the relative risk to be underweighted, maternal depression predicts poorer growth and frequent illnesses later in childhood [78]. Depressed mothers relate to their infants less and therefore infants of depressed mothers show fewer positive facial expressions [79,80]. Children of depressed mothers might be less active, irritable, can suffer from palpitations and have lower muscle tone [81]. Babies can suffer from micro-depression as they mirror their mother's feelings in order to stay connected to her [82,83]. Mother-infant dyad is often treated as inseparable in the first 3 months after the birth; some [84] naming it the fourth trimester of the pregnancy. Therefore child must be included in the treatment of maternal depression.

Beck [34] writes that depressive mood disorder not only have adverse effects on maternal-infant interaction during the first year of age, but may also have long-term effects on child over the age of one year. There is a more strong connection between maternal depressive mood and infants [85]; long-term paternal depression has affected only male children [40,76]. The mother's on-going depression can cause harmful effects also for siblings and can contribute to emotional, behavioural, cognitive, interpersonal [4,81,86] and psychomotor problems [87] of children later in life. Evidence show that they can be at risk for learning deficit [88]. Besides, children whose mothers develop PND are themselves proned to anxiety, depression and other mental illnesses later in life [45,89,90,91].

2.1.2. Impact of maternal depression on mother – infant interaction

The passing on of life from parent to child is one of the greatest privileges that come to women and man. But with the privilege there comes the responsibility. Most mothers find gratification in the maternal role despite the challenges, however depressed mothers experience less gratification [92].

At the beginning of the newborn's life his survival is completely dependent on another person who feeds, protects and nurtures him. There is evidence emphasising the importance of a quality of early infant – mother, or other caregiver's interaction and the quality of attachment to child's development [93]. One of the unique properties of humankind is the capacity to form and maintain relationships. The importance of effective human relationships lies in the fact that in many ways they determine the quality of our lives [94].

Human development occurs within relationship from the beginning of life. Newborn baby experiences and internalizes what mother experiences and feels. All relationships and encounters with mother, baby, and father during this primary period affect the quality of life and baby's foundation, therefore supportive, loving, and healthy relationships are integral to optimizing primary foundations for baby [95].

There is a clear difference between bonding and attachment. Nevertheless, many healthcare professionals and non-professionals continue to use the terms interchangeably [96]. Bonding is the initial emotional connection mothers make with their newborns [97], whereas attachment which is more complex than bonding [98] is the relationship that develops between mother–baby couple during the first year of the child's life [97] and includes an emotional component that requires time to process [98]. The importance of distinction between bonding and attachment lies in the fact that bonding has not been shown to predict any aspect of child outcome, whereas attachment is a powerful predictor of a child's later social and emotional outcome [96]. Nevertheless, if bonding is disturbed, then maternal-infant attachment can also be interrupted [99].The maternal–infant attachment begins to develop as early as in pregnancy [100]. The nine month period of pregnancy is not solely concerned with the physical development of the fetus. It is suggested that the development of women into a mother is equally dynamic and integral to the woman's own identity, her role identity, the identity of the developing fetus and the relationship between them [97]. After birth the production of oxytocin during lactation increases parasympathetic activity which reduces anxiety and foster mother to infant emotional evolvement. Maternal oxytocin circulation can therefore predispose women to form bonds and show bonding behaviour [100]. This is also one of the reasons why the first minutes after birth are so important. It is believed that birth and bonding are critical developmental process for mother, baby, and father that form core patterns with life-long implications. The best outcomes for the baby and mother occur when mother feels empowered and supported. The natural process of birth is to be allowed; to unfold with minimal intervention and no interruption in mother-baby connection and physical contact [95]. Sensitive nurturing care is supposed to be the basis of secure attachment [97] which forms the most important basis for the child's psychological growth and development [101].

It is well known, that the postpartum period is the most sensitive period of life for development of mother-child interaction. Childbirth experience and transition to motherhood are very special experiences that make a mother incomparably capable of caring for her child [102]. The first few months of an infant's life have been shown to affect later infant attachment [103]. Because after birth mother's physical and emotional state can be adversely affected by exsostion, pain, anaesthesia, ect. a delay or block in attachment can occur [104].

The first few months after birth could be regarded as a highly sensitive period for the development of the mother–infant relationship [105]. Unfortunately, some mothers find it hard to relate to their new baby, and such failure may have long-term effects on the infant [106]. Nevertheless, bonding is a complex, personal experience that takes time and luckily the baby whose basic needs are usually being met won't suffer if the bond is delayed for some time at first [107].

Even though many researchers have investigated the emotional tie between a mother and her infant [108] studies on attachment are largely focused on attachment from a child's perspective, while studies on attachment of the mother to her child are limited [97]. The research showed that women with more or stronger depressive or anxiety symptoms show less feelings of bonding with their infants. Feelings of hostility, rejection, anxiety and dissatisfaction in the relationship with their newborn infants were noticed [108]. Depressed mothers are often unable to meet their children social and emotional needs and even a mild maternal depression has a significant impact on maternal bonding [105]. This may lead to so called insecure attachment, which is associated with unresponsive, rejecting and insensitive parenting [109].

As shown in Table 1 There are four types of infant-parent attachment; three organized types - secure, avoidant and resistant, and one disorganized type [96].

Quality of caregiving	**Strategies to deal with distress**				**Type of attachment**
Sensitive	Loving	→	Organized	→	Secure
Insensitive	Rejecting	→	Organized	→	Insecure - avoidant
Insensitive	Inconsistent	→	Organized	→	Insecure - resistant
Atypical	Atypical	→	Disorganized	→	Insecure - disorganized

Table 1. Types of attachment and antecedents [96]

Links between maternal depression and maternal attachment disorganization were made, but as described by George and Solomon [110] the researchers aren't in agreement since the results are inconsistent; some of them found positive while others found negative associations. Nevertheless, children that have disorganized attachment are usually exposed to specific forms of distorted parenting and unusual caregiver's behaviour that are atypical [96]. Because depression can alter behaviour [111] we can say that depressed mothers show atypical behaviour towards their children.

The consequences of disorganized attachment relationships have been the focus of considerable developmental and clinical research in the past two decades [112]. Mostly because there are many consequences of parent–infant disorganized attachment. Disorganized attachment in infancy and early childhood was recognized as a powerful predictor for serious deficits in the child's social, emotional, behavioural functioning [112] and psychopathology and maladjustment in children [113]. Therefore, caregiving behaviours are clearly influential in providing children with the appropriate support to manage and regulate their own emotions and behaviour [114].

Disturbances in maternal–infant interaction may occur even before a baby is born, therefore depressive symptoms during the latter part of pregnancy were found to be an important risk factor for lower maternal attachment [115]. It is clear that mothers with current depressive symptoms and those with histories of severe depressive disorders displayed less positive behaviour toward their children [116], have less balanced attachment style [117] which leads to a mother's inability to interact in a responsive and sensitive manner with her baby and might consequently disrupt the development of secure attachment.

Depressed mothers are more likely to have attachment issues with their infants and their insecurity regarding motherhood further creates an unsteady attachment process [118]. As a consequence the lack of maternal-newborn attachment can cause distress in the newborn, making the newborn fussier and irritable, which in turn causes the new mother more stress and can deeper her own depression and anxiety [118].

2.2. Midwifery skills that enhance mother-infant relationship

By early screening and intervention programmes for PND, it may be possible to avoid the adverse effects of parental depression on child temperament. The nature of the optimum intervention strategy remains to be determined. Although treatments aimed at parental depression undoubtedly have benefits for the parents involved, two well-designed studies [118,119] cast doubt on the idea that treatment of postnatal depression alone is sufficient to prevent adverse child outcomes [40]. The direct relationship between mother and infant is one vital consideration, which can intercept cyclical downward spiral [121]. Much is known about detection and treatment of PND, but less is known about interventions to facilitate re-attachment [122]. Therapies of PND should therefore target also the mother–infant relationship [123] to improve their interaction [50].

2.2.1. Touch and infant massage

Touch is the most social sense; it typically implies an interaction with another person. Therefore is an extremely important part of non-verbal communication [124]. Skin is the largest and the most sensitive organ. The skin and the nervous system arise from the same embryonic cell layer (ectoderm). We could consider skin an exposed portion of the nervous system. Therefore some write of the psychological function of the skin [125] and a skin ego [1]. As sir Richard Bowlby said [1] words are not necessary to communicate feelings and develop relationship. Touch has strong effect on our bodies, since stimulation is quickly transmitted to the sensory cortex [126]. Touch can be considered a type of food, necessary for the infant's well-being; on the most basic instinctual level, physical contact is essential to sustain human life [44,127].

The sense of touch is the most developed sense after the birth. It is the first sense developed in utero. The sensory cortex, where touch is consciously perceived, is the most developed area of the brain at birth [128,129]. Early contact stimulation of the baby can begin already from the beginning of pregnancy. Foetus gets continuous massage for the entire nine months by the amniotic fluid and with mother's stroking the abdomen. Despite the fact that the effects of maternal massage in pregnancy are not sufficiently proved [130], researchers [131] claim that women who are being massaged during pregnancy and birth are using more touch stimulation for their newborn infants. Massaging mother during the pregnancy and birth can be therefore beneficial also for the child. Uterine contractions in pregnancy that can be also caused with massaging the belly are perceived by child as touch stimulation. Touch alters oxytocin level and therefore baby is more relaxed [124]. That can be of major importance for the babies whose mothers are suffering for prenatal depression and are therefore exposed to higher levels of stress hormones.

Caring touch plays a critical role in the development of relationship with the child during pregnancy and [132] after the birth. It affects baby's physical and emotional development [129]. It was shown that babies who are touched frequently after the birth develop better; for example score higher on IQ and language tests [133], sleep, eat better and cry less [81]. Massage, as a systematic touch has several positive effects on physical, mental and emotional state of the baby. In infants, massage reduces colic, pain associated with teething, enhance growth, ect. Massage stimulates and promotes growth and development, but at the same time relaxes; lowers levels of hormones that cause tension [124,134]. Infant massage may improve newborn's sleep organization, lowers level of kortizol, helps baby gain weight [129,135-138] and deep touch helps them in organizing [139]. Sensory stimulation like massage speeds myelination of the nervous system, thus enhancing rapid brain-body communication. This has long lasting effects; massage can affect the ability to handle stress in adulthood – baby, who in a womb experienced fear-producing biochemical environment, can unconsciously perceive world as a place of anxiety and fear (his/her structure of cells has been intrauterine programmed as such) and massage can help him/her to reshape this interpretations [44].

Furthermore, massage is likely to nurture the parent as much or more than does the infant, who receives it. Infant massage could be a tool for building mother-infant bond by deeply communicative means of touch [140]. Massage gives parents an opportunity to realize baby's behavioural cues; signs that child uses for communicating his/her needs [127]. With this they become more sensitive for baby's expressions, which helps them to understand infant [128]. Result is raised self-confidence for acquisiting the parenting role, enhanced development of role related skills and perception of lower parental stress [141,142].

Depressed mothers touch their infants less than non-depressed mothers. As a result infants of depressed mothers spend longer periods of time in touching self rather than toys or mother, compensating the lack of positive tactile stimulation [143]. Touch deprivation can have several negative effects on a child, such as sleep disturbance, growth restriction and immune system decompensation [124]. Baby massage can improve the mood of depressed mothers [144] and promotes mother-infant relationship [137]. While other benefits of infant massage are not clearly defined, the evidence for improvements of mother-infant relationship in connection with maternal depression is compelling [145].

2.2.2. *Mother-infant relationship and newborn behavioural observation*

Newborn Behavioral Observation System (NBO) is a relationship-building, a structured set of observations, designed to help the clinician and parent together, to observe the infant's behavioural capacities and identify the kind of support the infant needs for successful growth and development. The goal of the NBO is to strengthen the relationship between parents and their infant and also to promote a positive relationship between clinician and family. Although the NBO attempts to reveal the full reaches of the newborn behavioural repertoire, the clinical focus is on the infant's individuality and includes observations of the infant's; capacity to habituate to external light and sound stimuli, the quality of motor tone and activity level, capacity for self-regulation, response to stress, and visual, auditory and social interactive capacities [128].

The NBO is based on the assumption that newborns come into the world as competent persons [128] and the sooner the communication between parents and infant is established the greater attachment and less frustration parents may experience.

NBO should become a part of routine family cantered midwifery postpartum care [147]. Midwives after birth have the opportunity to enlighten parents about their infants' unique capabilities [146]. The more the parent knows; the better can respond appropriately to the infant without abuse or neglect [146]. NBO promotes active role of parents and can therefore help to establish early attachment between the parents and the newborn which is a foundation for development of a healthy and competent child and later an adult [147].

Healthcare professionals should use the knowledge of newborn behaviour to facilitate connections that parents will use throughout their parenting lives. Using the infant's behaviour as his language, they can sensitize parents to what their infant is "saying" and help parents to accurately interpret baby's cues and respond appropriately.

Interventions such as the NBO that help mothers learn to recognize, understand, and respond to the behavioural cues of their infants could be used with those mothers identified as being at risk for ineffective maternal role transition [148]. NBO can therefore, similar as found by Jung et al. [121] help the depressed mothers and their families to develop effective ways of managing and comforting the infant when distressed, and to understand the 'meaning' of infant's behaviours and how contingent responses to infant cues increase positive interactions. As a consequence, it is expected that an infant who begins to more frequently show interest in the mother, smile and sustain eye contact, is also likely to evoke more enjoyable and arousing experiences for the mother [121]. Positive responsiveness and involvement between depressed mothers and their infants is very likely to be demonstrated by an increase in the infant's positive emotion expressions while engaged with the mother. Infant's responses to the mother's vocalizations and attempts at engagement encourage the mother to continue [92].

Throughout an NBO session the midwife can encourage depressed mother to explore the knowledge she already posses about their infant and make predictions and observations. This shared exploration of the infant's responses guides the midwife in providing anticipatory guidance for caregiving and to enhance mother infant relationship. NBO is a family-centered tool [128] and should also include extended family or friends which are in case of a mother's depression more than invited to help embrace, hold, and interact with the infant so that the infant is not deprived of warmth, love, and affection [99].

2.3. Evaluation of the proposed midwifery interventions

Mother needs to be, despite the depression, active participant in the baby's care, not only for the well-being of an infant but also for her own [124]. Therefore midwives should include in the management of postnatally depressed mothers activities that help them building relationship with there babies. Infant massage and NBO seemed appropriate interventions, therefore authors gathered more data on their effectiveness.

2.3.1. Methodology

Since the benefits of infant massage and maternal depression has been clearly shown in past reviews [144,151], the search for the new evidence was performed only for the period from 2008 to 2012. We searched the following databases: Cochrane Library, CINAHL, EIFL direct, MEDLINE, ScienceDirect, ProQuest, Springer Link, BMJ Journals, IngentaConnect, Oxford Journals, Embase, Eric and Midirs. For the search, we used key words: postnatal/postpartum/maternal depression AND Infant/baby massage in the title. Exclusion criteria were: non-academic papers. Inclusion criteria were: appropriateness of the content, English language. The search gave 3 results that are discussed below.

The following databases: Cochrane Library, CINAHL, EIFL direct, MEDLINE, ScienceDirect, ProQuest, Springer Link, BMJ Journals, IngentaConnect, Oxford Journals, Embase, Eric and Midirs were also searched for evidence of research on NBO and maternal depression. For the search, we used key words: postnatal/postpartum/maternal depression AND newborn behavioural observation in the title but the search didn't give us any results.

2.3.2. *Effect of baby massage on maternal depressive symptoms*

The results of the recent studies confirm the findings of the past research. O'Higins et al. [149] performed randomized controlled trial among 62 postnatal women, who scored above 12 on Edinburgh Postnatal Depression Scale (EPDS) at four weeks postpartum. In the control group were 34 women, who scored 9 on EPDS. They were randomly assigned to infant massage course (International Associaltion of Infant Massage – IAIM scheme) or in a group for support intervention. Women in experimental group were tested again with EPDS after six sessions of intervention and after one year. EPDS showed statistically significant improvement in the mood of depressed mothers after the intervention in both groups, but slightly more in the infant massage group. At one year, massage-group mothers had non-depressed levels of sensitivity of interaction with their babies. It can be concluded that infant massage improves mother-infant interaction, consequently preventing possible side effects of maternal depression on child emotional and psychological development, as described in the literature review.

Similar conclusions were made also by Gürol and Polat [150], who performed randomized controlled trial among 117 mother-infant couples, observing attachment before and after 38-days long infant massage intervention, using Maternal Attachment Inventory (MAI). 57 mothers in the experimental group showed statistically significantly higher post-test mean values of the MAI.

Underdown and Barlow [151] performed a research among socioeconomically deprivileged mothers, who are said to be at higher risk for postnatal depression, due to their life situation. Their sample consisted of 39 mother-infant couples, assigned to eight infant massage classes (using the structure and philosophy of IAIM programme). They collected data with observation, in-depth interviews and quantitatively with several measurement scales, also EPDS. Besides the evaluation of the effect of baby massage course on the mental state of the mother, their aim was also to define crucial elements of good infant massage programme. It became obvious that the important elements of the course are, beside the actual massage, also the topics, discussed during the sessions, especially information on baby's cry and baby's cues that facilitates parents interaction.

3. Discussion and conclusions

Today modern science is rediscovering age-old treatments and the medical sciences are incorporating these interventions into scientific protocols [152]. Touching and understanding baby's behaviour are one of them. As obvious it can be particularly beneficial for women suffering PND.

Teaching depressed mothers and their family member's infant massage and/or go through NBO with them can help them understand the fact that their child is a competent person. Doing infant massage on their own while understanding their child's cues can help depressed mothers to reduce the display of atypical behaviour and therefore ovoid or minimize the risk of insecure - disorganized attachment. This is so important because of the negative long-term consequences associated with this condition.

Interventions that focus on what mothers do with their infants instead of focusing only on how they feel can be effective in increasing infants' positive responsiveness and improving infant outcomes. Such interventions can be an essential component of treatment when mothers suffer from PND [121]. Similar conclusions were made by Ewell Foster et al. [116] whose findings highlight the importance of providing parenting interventions for depressed mothers.

Studies of touch and discussion with parents about infant behaviour and temperament showed beneficial effect on postnatally depressed mothers and their infants. There were no side effects mentioned in any study. On the basis of this review, we can conclude that infant massage and NBO could be included into the routine postnatal midwifery care. Infant massage and NBO should therefore become an intervention tool for midwives to support mothers with postnatal depression in order to develop a positive relationship with their newborn children.

More studies relating NBO with postpartum depression are needed, since there is no study directly testing improvements of maternal depressed mood after a session(s) of NBO.

Author details

Ana Polona Mivšek and Tita Stanek Zidarič

*Address all correspondence to: polona.mivsek@zf.uni-lj.si

Faculty of health Ljubljana, Midwifery department, Slovenia

References

[1] Lucier P. The skin as a psychic organ: the use of infant massage as a psychotherapeutic tool in infant-parent psychotherapy. Journal of prenatal and perinatal psychology and health 2007; 22(2) 113-127.

[2] Johnston PGB, Flood K, Spinks K. The newborn child. 9th ed. Edinburgh: Churchill Livingstone; 2003.

[3] Evans C. History taking and the newborn examination: an evolving perspective. In: Lomax A, ed. Examination of the newbor: an evidence-based guide, Chester: Willey-Blackwell ltd; 2011. 13-47.

[4] Cooper P, Murray L. The impact of psychological treatments of postpartum depression on maternal mood and development. In: Murray L, Cooper PJ, eds. Postpartum Depression and Child Development. London: The Guilford Press; 1997. 201–220.

[5] Field T. Effect of early separation, interactive deficits, and experimental manipulations on infant–mother interaction. Child Development 1977; 48 763–771.

[6] Baston H, Hall J. Midwifery essentials: Postnatal. 4th vol. Edinburgh: Churchill Livingstone; 2009.

[7] Letourneau NL, Fedick CB, Willms JD, Dennis CL, Hegadoren K, Stewart MJ. Longitudinal study of postpartum depression, maternal-child relationships and children's behaviour to 8 years of age. In: Devore D, editor. Parent-child relations: New research. New York: Nova Science; 2006. 45–63.

[8] Wisner KL, Parry BL, Piontek CM. Clinical practice – postpartum depression. New England Journal of Medicine 2002; 347(3) 194-9.

[9] APA. Diagnostic and statistical manual of mental disorders IV 4th ed. Washington: APA; 1994.

[10] Clement S, Elliott S. Psychological health before, during and after chilbirth. In: Marsh G, Renfrew M, eds. Community based maternity care. Oxford: Oxford university press; 1999.

[11] Yonkers KA, Ramin SM, Rush AJ, Navarrete CA, Carmody T, March D, Hartwell SF, Leveno KJ. Onset and persistence of postpartum depression in an inner-city maternal health clinic system. American Journal of Psychiatry 2001; 158(11) 1856-63.

[12] Josefsson A, Berg G, Nordin C, Sydsjo G. Prevalence of depressivesymptoms in late pregnancy and postpartum. Acta Obstetricia et Gynecologica Scandinavica 2001; 80(3) 251-255.

[13] Beck CT, Gable RK. Further validation of the postpartum depression screening scale, Nursing Research 2001; 50(3) 155-64.

[14] Dietch KV, Bunney B. The silent disease: diagnosing and treating depression in women. Lifeliness 2002; 6(2) 140-5.

[15] LoCicero AK, Weiss DM, Issokson D. Postpartum depression: a proposal for prevention through an integrated care and support network. Applied and preventive psychology 1997; 6(4) 169-78.

[16] Clarke-Akalanue E, Myles P. Supporting new mothers with PND: an evaluation, Journal of Community Nursing 2002; 16(12) 18-20.

[17] Wylie L, Hollins Martin CJ, Martin CR, Rankin J. The enigma of PND: an update. Journal of Psychiatric Mental Health Nursing 2011; 18 48-58.

[18] Sit DK, Wisner KL. Identification of postpartum depression. Clinical Obstetrics and Gynecology 2009; 52 456–468.

[19] Bowe S, Watson A. Perinatal depression: a randomised controlled trial of an antenatal education intervention for primiparas. Obstetrical and gynaecological survey 2001; 56(10): 597-9.

[20] Misri S, Kostaras X. Benefits and risks to mother and infant of drug treatment for postnatal depression. Drug Safety 2002; 25 (13) 903-911.

[21] Austin MP, Lumley J. Antenatal screening for postnatal depression: a systematic review. Acta Psychiatrica Scandinavica 2003; 107(1): 10-7.

[22] Dennis CL, Hodnett E. (2007). Psychosocial and psychological interventions for treating postpartum depression DOI: 10.1002/14651858.CD006116.pub2, Cochrane Database of Systematic Reviews 4(CD006116).

[23] NICE. Intrapartm care: care of healthy women and their babies during childbirth: clinical guideline. London: RCOG Press; 2007.

[24] Schnyer RN, Manber R, Fitzcharles AJ. Acupuncture treatment for depression during pregnancy: conceptual framework and two case reports. Alternative health practitioner 2003; 8(1) 40-53.

[25] Boath E, Henshaw C. The treatment of PND: a comprehensive literature review. Journal of reproductive and infant psychology 2001; 19(3) 215-48.

[26] Corral M, Kuan A, Kostaras D. Bright light therapy's effect on postpartum depression. American journal of psychiatry 2000; 157(2): 303-4.

[27] Oren DA, Wisner KL, Spinelli M, Epperson CN, Peindl KS, Terman SUJ, Terman M. An open trial of morning light therapy for treatment of antepartum depression. The American journal of psychiatry 2002; 159(4) 666-9.

[28] Dombrowski MAS, Anderson GC, Santori C, Burkhammer M. Kangaroo (skin to skin) care with a postpartum women who felt depressed. American journal of maternal child nursing 2001; 26(4) 214-6.

[29] Powell-Kennedy H, Beck CT, Driscoll JW. A light in the fog: caring for women with postpartum depression. Journal of Midwifery and Women Health 2002; 47(5) 318-30.

[30] Armstrong K, Edwards H. The effect of exercise and social support on mothers reporting depressive symptoms: a pilot randomised controlled trial. International journal of mental health nursing 2003; 12(2): 130-8.

[31] Ussher J. Depression in the postnatal period: a normal response to motherhood. In: Stewart, M., ed. Pregnancy, birth and maternity care: feminist perspectives. Edinburgh: Books for midwives; 2004.

[32] Mivšek AP, Zakšek T. Mood Disorders in the Puerperium and the Role of the Midwife: Study on Improvement of Midwives' Knowledge About Post-Natal Depression After an Educational Intervention. In: Juruena MFP, ed. Clinical, Research and Treatment Approaches to Affective Disorders. Rijeka: Intech; 2011.

[33] Leonard LG. Depression and anxiety disorders during multiple pregnancy and parenthood. JOGNN 1998; 27(3) 329-37.

[34] Beck CT. Theoretical perspectives of postpartum depression and their treatment implications. MCN 2002; 27(5) 282-7.

[35] McIntosh J. Postpartum depression: women's help-seeking behaviour and perceptions of cause. JAN 1993; 18(2) 178-84.

[36] Wang S, Chen C, Chin C, Lee S. Impact of postpartum depression on the mother-infant couple. Birth 2005; 32(1) 39-44.

[37] Littlewood J, McHugh N. Maternal distress and PND: the mith of Madonna. Houndsmills: MacMillan, 1997.

[38] Bruder-Costello B, Warner V, Talati A, Nomura Y, Bruder G, Weissman M. Temperament among offspring at high and low risk for depression. Psychiatry Research 2007; 153 145–151.

[39] Stein A, Arteche A, Lehtonen A, Craske M, Harvey A, Counsell N, Murray L. Interpretation of infant facial expression in the context of maternal postnatal depression. Infant Behaviour and development 2010; 33 273-8.

[40] Hanington L, Ramchandani P, Stein A. Parental depression and child temperament: assessing child to parent effect in a longitudional population study. Infant behaviour and development 2010; 33 88-95.

[41] McGrath JM, Records K, Rice M. Maternal depression and infant tempeament characteristics. Infant behavior and development 2008; 31(1) 71-80.

[42] Davies L. Influences on the health of the newborn, before and during pregnancy. In: Davies L, McDonald S, eds. Examination of the newborn and neonatal health: a multidimensional approach. Edinburgh: Churchill Livingstone, Elsevier; 2008. 79-95.

[43] Zuckerman AH, Bauchner H, Cabral H. Depressive symptoms during pregnancy: relationships to poor health Behaviors. American journal of obstetrics and gynaecology 1989; 160 110-111.

[44] McClure V. Infant massage: a handbook forloving parents. Rev ed. London: Souvenir press; 2001.

[45] Field T. Prenatal depression effect on early development: a review. Infant behavior and development 2011; 34(1) 1-14.

[46] Werner EA, Myers MM, Fifer WP, Cheng B, Fang Y, Allen R, Monk C. Prenatal predictors of infant temperament. Developmental Psychobiology 2007; 49 474-84.

[47] Waxler E, Thelen K, Muzik M. Maternal perinatal depression – impact on infant and child development. European Psychiatric review 2011; 4(1) 41-7.

[48] Poggi Davis E, Glynn LM, Dunkel Schetter C, Hobel C, Chicz-Demet A, Sandman CA. Prenatal exposure to maternal depression and cortisol influences infant temperament. Journal of the American academy of child and adolescent psychiatry 2007; 46(6) 737-46.

[49] Melley M, Crozier K. Maternal and family health and the impact on the fetus and neonate. In: Williamson A, Crozier K, eds. Neonatal care. Devon: Reflect press; 2008. 11-33.

[50] Field T. Maternal depression effects on infants and early interventions. Preventive medicine 1998; 27(2) 200-203.

[51] Lundy BL, Jones NA, Field T, Nearing G, Davalos M, Pietro PA, Schanberg S, Kuhn C. Prenatal depression effects on neonates. Infant behavior and development 1999; 22(1) 119-129.

[52] Davis E. Heart and hands: a midwife's guide to pregnancy and birth. Berkeley: Celestial arts; 2004.

[53] Sobey SW. Barriers to postpartum depression prevention and treatment: a policy analysis. Journal of Midwifery and Women Health 2002; 47(5) 331-6.

[54] Martins C, Gaffan EA. Effects of early maternal depression on patterns of infant–mother attachment: A meta-analytic investigation. Journal of Child Psychology and Psychiatry 2000; 41(6) 737–746.

[55] Beck CT. A check list to identify women at risk for developing postpartum depression, JOGNN 1998; 27(1) 39-45.

[56] Hagen EH. The functions of postpartum depression. Evolution and Human Behavior 1999; 20 325-359.

[57] Lovejoy MC, Graczyk PA, O'Hare E, Neuman G. Maternal depression and parenting behavior: A meta-analytic review. Clinical Psychology Review 2000; 20(5) 561–592.

[58] Stern DN. The interpersonal world of the infant. New York: Basic books; 1985.

[59] Sohr-Preston SL, Scaramella LV. Implications of timing of maternal depressive symptoms for early cognitive and language development. Clinical Child Family Psychological Review 2006; 9 65-83.

[60] Stein A, Malmberg LE, Sylva K, Barnes J, Leach P. The influence of maternal depression, caregiving, and socioeconomic status in the post-natal year on children's language development. Child Care Health Development 2008; 34 603-12.

[61] Kaplan LA, Evans L, Monk C. Effects of mothers' prenatal psychiatric status and postnatal caregiving on infant biobehavioral regulation: Can prenatal programming be modified? Early Human Development 2008; 84: 249-56.

[62] Milgrom J, Westley DT, Gemmill AW. The mediating role of maternal responsiveness in some longer term effects of postnatal depression on infant development. Infant behavior and development 2004; 27(4) 443-454.

[63] Murray L, Fiori-Cowley A, Hooper R. The impact of postnatal depression and associated adversity on early motherinfant interactions and later infant outcome. Child Development 1996; 67 2512–26.

[64] Righetti-Veltema M, Conne-Perreard E, Bousquet A, Manzano J. Postpartum depression and mother-infant relationship at 3-months old. Journal of affective disorders 2002; 70(3) 291-306.

[65] Campbell SB, Cohn JF, Meyers T. Depression in first-time mothers: mother–infant interaction and depression chronicity. Developmental Psychology 1995; 31 349–357.

[66] Field TF. Early interactions between infants and their postpartum depressed mothers. Infant Behavioral Development 2002; 7 517–522.

[67] Bagner DM, Pettit JW, Lewinsohn PM, Seeley JR. Effect of maternal depression on child behavior: a sensitive period? Journal of the American academy of child and adolescent psychiatry 2010; 49(7) 699-707.

[68] Muzik M. Maternal perinatal depression: impact on infant emotional regulation and later toddler behavior problems. In: 4th world congress on women's mental health. Madrid: Springer Wien; 2011. 107-108.

[69] Donovan WL, Leavitt LA, Walsh RO. Conflict and depression predict maternal sensitivity to infant cries. Infant behavior and development 1998; 21(3) 505-517.

[70] Field T, Lang C, Martinez A, Yando R, Pickens J, Bendell D. Preschool follow-up of infants of dysphoric mothers. Journal of Clinical Child Psychology 1996; 25 272-279.

[71] Dawson G, Frey K, Self J, Panagiotides H, Hessl D, Yamada E, Rinaldi J. Frontal brain electrical activity in infants of depressed and nondepressed mothers: relation to variations in infant behavior. Development and psychopathology 1999; 11(3) 589-605.

[72] Sato T, Uehara T, Narita T, Sakado K, Yoichiro F. Parental bonding and personality in relation to lifetime history of depression. Psychiatry and clinical neurosciences 2000; 54 121-130.

[73] O'Connor TG, Heron J, Golding J, Beveridge M, Glover V. Maternal antenatal anxiety and children's behavioural problems at four years'. British Journal of psychiatry 2002; 180 502-508.

[74] Casey P, Goolsby S, Berkowitz C, Frank D, Cook J, Cutts D, Black MM, Zaldivar N, Levenson S, Heeren T, Meyers A. Maternal depression, changing public assistance, food security and child health issues. Pediatrics 2004; 113 298-304.

[75] Toth SL, Rogosch FA, Sturge-Apple M. Maternal depression, children's attachment security and representational development : an organizational perspective: Child development 2009; 80(1) 192-208.

[76] Ramchandani P, Stein A, Evans J, O'Connor TG. Paternal depression in the postnatal period and child development: A prospective population study. The Lancet 2005; 365 2201–2205.

[77] O'Brien LM, Heycock EG, Hanna M, Jones PW, Cox JL. Postnatal depression and faltering growth: A community study. Pediatrics 2004; 113(5) 1242–1247.

[78] Rahman A, Iqbal Z, Bunn J, Lovel H, Harrington R. Impact of maternal depression on infant nutritional status and Illness: cohort study. Archives of Gen Psychiatry 2004; 61 946-52.

[79] Lamberg L. Safety of antidepressants use in pregnant and nursing women. Journal of the american medical association 1999; 282 222-223.

[80] Gress-Smith JL, Luecken LJ, Lemery-Chalfant K, Howe R. Postpartum depression prevalence and impact on infant health, weight and sleep in low-income and ethnic minority women and infants. Maternal and Child Health Journal 2012; 16(4) 887-893.

[81] Field T. Massage therapy for infants and children. Developmental and behavioral pediatrics 1995; 16(2) 106.

[82] Agnew T. Mother's ruin: mothers with severe mental health problems. Nursing times 1999; 95(44) 16.

[83] van Os J, Jones P, Lewis G, Wadsworth M, Murray R. Developmental precursors of affective illness in a general population birth cohort. Archives of General Psychiatry 1997; 54 625–631

[84] Kitzinger S. Me, matere. Ljubljana: Ganeš; 1994.

[85] Durbin CE, Klein DN, Hayden EP, Buckley ME, Moerk KC. Temperamental emotionality in preschoolers and parental mood disorders. Journal of Abnormal Psychology 2005; 114(1) 28–37.

[86] Miller LJ. Postpartum depression. Journal of the American Medical Association 2002; 287 762-765.

[87] Cornish A M, McMahon CA, Ungerer JA, Barnett B, Kowalenko N, Tennant C. Postnatal depression and infant cognitive and motor development in the second postnatal year: impact of depression chronicity andinfant gender. Infant behavior and development 2005; 28(4) 407-417.

[88] Kaplan PS, Danko CM, Diaz A, Kalinka CJ. An associative learning deficit in 1-year-old infants of depressed mothers: role of depression duration. Infant behavior and development 2011; 34(1) 35-44.

[89] DeAngelis T. There's a new hope for women with postpartum blues. American psychological association monitor; 1997 22.

[90] Halligan SL, Murray L, Martins C, Cooper PJ. Maternal depression and psychiatric outcomes in adolescent offspring: a 13-year longitudional study. Journal of affective disorders 2007; 97(1-3) 145-154.

[91] Murray L, Arteche A, Fearon P, Halligan S, Goodyer I, Cooper P. Maternal postnatal depression and the development of depression in offspring up to 16 years of age. Journal of the American academy of child and adolescent psychiatry 2011; 50(5) 460-470.

[92] Logsdon CM, Wisner KL, Pinto-Foltz MD. The Impact of Postpartum Depression on Mothering. Journal of Obstetric, Gynecologic, and Neonatal Nursing 2006; 35 652-658.

[93] Murray L, Woolgar M, Cooper P, Hipwell A. Cognitive vulnerability to depression in 5-year-old children of depressed mothers. J Child Psychol Psychiatry 2001; 42(7) 891 – 899.

[94] Reece BL, Brandt R, Howie KF. Effective Human Relations: Interpersonal and Organizational Applications. 11th ed. Mason: South-Western College Pub; 2010.

[95] McCarty WA, Glenn M. Investing in Human Potential from the Beginning of Life; Key to Maximizing Human Capital. Position Paper; 2008. http://www.naturalfamilylivingsb.org/pdf/PositionPaper_1-09_web.pdf (accessed 23 Avgust 2012).

[96] Benoit D. Infant-parent attachment: Definition, types, antecedents, measurement and outcome. Paediatr Child Health 2004; 9(8): 541-545.

[97] McPhail M, Martin CR, Redshaw M. Maternal – fetal attachment. In: Martin CR. (ed) Perinatal Mental Health; A clinical guide. Cumbria: M&K Update Ltd; 2012. p 431 – 458.

[98] Karl DJ, Beal JA, O'Hare CM, Rissmiller PN. Reconceptualizing the nurse's role in the newborn period as an "attacher." MCN The American Journal of Maternal/Child Nursing 2006; 31 257-262.

[99] Zauderer CR. A Case Study of Postpartum Depression and Altered Maternal – Newborn Attachment. MCN The American Journal of Maternal/Child Nursing 2008; 33(3) 173 – 178.

[100] Thims L. Human Chemistry. Morrisville, North Carolina: LuLu Enterprises; 2007.

[101] Yan-hua D, Xiu X, Zheng-yan W, Hui-rong L, Wei-ping W. Study of mother–infant attachment patterns and influence factors in Shanghai. Early Human Development 2012; 88 295–300.

[102] Nystedt A, Hogberg U, Lundman B. Women's experiences of becoming a mother after prolonged labour. Journal of Advanced Nursing 2008; 63(3) 250 – 258.

[103] Klier CM. Mother-infant bonding disorders in patients with postnatal depression: The Postpartum Bonding Questionnaire in clinical practice. Archives of Women's Mental Health 2006; 9(5) 289–291.

[104] Littleton LY, Engebretson JC. Maternal, Neonatal and Women Health Nursing. New York: Delamar Cengage Learning; 2001.

[105] Moehler E, Brunner R, Wiebel A, Reck C, Resch F. Maternal depressive symptoms in the postnatal period are associated with long – term impairment of mother child bonding. Archives of Women Mental Health 2006; 9(5) 273 – 278.

[106] Taylor A, Atkins R, Kumar R, Adams D, Glover V. A New Mother – to - Infant Bonding Scale: Links with early maternal mood. Archives of Women Mental Health 2005; 8(1) 45 – 51.

[107] Giustardi A, Stablum M, De Martino A. Mother infant relationship and bonding myths and facts. The Journal of Maternal-Fetal and Neonatal Medicine 2011; 24(1) 59-60.

[108] van Bussel J.C.H, Spitz B, Demyttenaere K. Archives of Women Mental Health 2010; 13 373 – 384.

[109] Kompan Erzar K, Poljanec S. Rahločutnost do otrok; Stik z otrokom v prvem letu življenja. Ljubljana : Založba Brat Frančišek in Frančiškanski družinski inštitiut; 2009.

[110] George C, Solomon J. Caregiving Helplessness: The Development of a Screening Measure for Disorganized Maternal Caregiving. In: Solomon J, George C. (ed.) Disorganized Attachment and Caregiving. New York: The Guilford Press; 2011. p133 – 166.

[111] Lindgren K. Relationships Among Maternal-Fetal Attachment, Prenatal Depression, and Health Practices in Pregnancy. Research in Nursing and Health 2001; 24 203-217.

[112] Fearon P, Bakermans-Kranenburg M, Van IJzendoorn, Lapsley AM, Roisman G. The significance of insecure attachment and disorganization in the development of children's externalizing behavior: A meta-analytic study. Child Development 2010; 81 435–456.

[113] Green J, Goldwyn R. Annotation: attachment disorganisation and psychopathology: new findings in attachment research and their potential implications for developmental psychopathology in childhood. J Child Psychol Psychiatry 2002;43 835-46.

[114] Madigan S, Voci S, Benoit D. Stability of atypical caregiver behaviors over six years and associations with disorganized infant–caregiver attachment. Attachment nad Human Development 2011; 13(3) 237-252.

[115] Perry DF, Ettinger AK, Mendelson T, Le, H-N. Prenatal depression predicts postpartum maternal attachment in low-income Latina mothers with infants. Infant Behavior and Development 2011; 34 339–350.

[116] Ewell Foster CJ, Garber J, Durlak JA. Current and past maternal depression, maternal interaction behaviors, and children's externalizing and internalizing symptoms. Journal of Abnormal Child Psychology 2008; 36(4) 527-537.

[117] Korja R, Savonlahti E, Haataja L, Lapinleimu H, Manninen H, Piha J, Lehtonen L, PIPARI Study Group. Attachment representations in mothers of preterm infants. Infant Behavior & Development 2009;32 305–311.

[118] McMahon CA, Barnett B, Kowalenko NM, Tennant CC. Maternal attachment state of mind moderates the impact of postnatal depression on infant attachment. Journal of Child Psychology and Psychiatry2006; 47 660-669.

[119] Cooper P, Murray L. Intergenerational transmission of affective and cognitive processes associated with depression: Infancy and the preschool years. In: Goodyer I, ed. Unipolar depression: A lifespan perspective. Oxford: Oxford University Press; 2003.

[120] Murray L, Cooper PJ, Wilson A, Romaniuk H. Controlled trial of the short- and long-term effect of psychological treatment of post-partum depression. British Journal of Psychiatry. 2003; 182 420–427.

[121] Jung V, Short R, Letourneau N, Andrews D. Interventions with depressed mothers and their infants: Modifying interactive behaviours. Journal of Affective Disorders 2007; 98 199 –205.

[122] McMahon CA, Barnett B, Kowalenko NM, Tennant CC. Maternal attachment state of mind moderates the impact of postnatal depression on infant attachment. Journal of Child Psychology and Psychiatry2006; 47 660-669.

[123] Forman DR, O'Hara MW, Stuart S, Gorman LL, Larsen KE, Coy KC. Effective treatment for postpartum depression is not sufficient to improve the developing mother–child relationship. Development and Psychopathology 2007; 19 585–602.

[124] Field T. Touch. Cambridge: MIT Press; 2003.

[125] Feldman B. A skin for the imaginal. Journal of the analytic psychology 2004; 49 285-311.

[126] Montagu A. Animadversions on the development of a theory of touch. In: In Field TM, ed. Touch in Early Development. Mahwah: Lawrence Erlbaum; 1995. 3-20.

[127] Caplan M. To touch is to live: the need for genuine affection in an impersonal world. 2nd ed. Prescot: Hohm press; 2002.

[128] Nugent K, Keefer CH, Minear S, Johnson LC, Blanchard Y. Understanding newborn behavior and early relationships: The Newborn Behavioral Observations (NBO) system handbook. Baltimore: Paul H. Brookes publishing Co; 2007.

[129] Nugent K, Morell A. Your baby is speaking to you: a visual guide to the amazing behaviors of your newborn and growing baby. Boston: Houghton Mifflin Harcourt; 2011.

[130] Dennis CL, Allen K. (2010) Interventions (other than pharmacological, psychosocial or psychological) for treating antenatal depression. Cochrane Database of Systematic Reviews DOI: 10.1002/14651858.CD006795.pub2 Cochrane Database of Systematic Reviews, Issue 4.

[131] Klaus M. Touching during and after childbirth. In: Field T, ed. Touch in early development. New Jersey: Lawrence Erlbaum Associates, Publishers Inc.; 1995. 19-33.

[132] Leboyer F. Loving hands. New York: Alfred A. Knopf; 1976.

[133] Klaus M, Kennell J. Parent-infant bonding. 2nd ed. St. Louis: Mosby; 1982.

[134] Esquivel-Sibaja AG. Effects of massage on quantitative and qualitative stress parameters in full-term infants. MSc thesis. Costa Rica: Universidad de Costa Rica; 2007.

[135] Ferber SG, Kuint J, Weller A, Feldman R, Dollberg S, Arbel E, Kohelet D. Massage therapy by mothers and trained professionals enhances weight gain in preterm infants. Early human development 2002a; 67(1/2) 37-45.

[136] Ferber SG, Laudon M, Kuint J, Weller A, Zisapel N. Massage therapy by mothers enhances the adjustment of circadian rhytms to the nocturnal period in full-term infants. Journal of developmental and behavioural pediatrics 2002b; 23(6) 410-415.

[137] Onozawa K, Glover V, Adams D, Modi N, Kumar RC. Infant massage improves mother-infant interaction for mothers with postnatal depression. Journal of affective disorders 2001; 63 201-207.

[138] Dieter JNI, Field T, Hernandez-Reif M, Emory EK, Redzepi M. Stable preterm infants gain more waight and sleep less after five days of massage therapy. Journal of pediatric psychology 2003; 28(6) 403-411.

[139] Browne JV. Considerations for touch and massage in the NICU. Neonatal network 2000; 19. 61-64.

[140] Lappin G, Kretschmer RE. Applying infant massage practices: a qualitative study. Journal of visual impairment and blindness 2005; June 355-367.

[141] Beyer K, Strauss L. Infant massage programs may assist in decreasing parental perceived stress levels in new parents. Occupational Therapy in Health Care 2002; 16(4) 53-68.

[142] Fujita M, Endoh Y, Saimon N, Yamaguchi S. Effect of massaging babies on mothers: pilot study on the changes in mood states and salivary cortisol level. Complementary Therapies in Clinical Practice 2006; 12(3) 181-5.

[143] Herrera E, Reissland N, Shepherd J. Maternal touch and maternal child-directed speech: effects of depressed mood in the postnatal period. Journal of affective disorders 2004; 81(1) 29-39.

[144] Dennis CL, Creedy DK. (2008). Psychosocial and psychological interventions for treating postpartum depression. DOI: 10.1002/14651858.CD001134.pub2, Cochrane Database of Systematic Reviews.

[145] Zealey C. The benefits of infant massage: a critical review. Community Practitioner 2005; 78(3) 98-102.

[146] Hotelling BA. Newborn Capabilities: Parent Teaching Is a Necessity. The Journal of Perinatal Education 2004; 13(4) 43 – 49.

[147] Skubic M, Stanek Zidarič T., Mivšek P. Opazovanje vedenja novorojenčkov kot del v družino usmerjene babiške poporodne obravnave/ Newborn behaviour observation as a part of routine familiy centered midwifery postpartum care. In: International Sci-

entific Conference on Nursing and Health Care Research, Evidence-based health care - opportunities for linking health care professions, patient needs and knowledge/Na dokazih podprta zdravstvena obravnava - priložnosti za povezovanje zdravstvenih strok, potreb pacientov in znanj, 9 – 10 June, Jesenice: College of Nursing/Visoka šola za zdravstveno nego; 2011.

[148] Wesley Sanders L, Buckner EB. The Newborn Behavioral Observations System as a Nursing Intervention to Enhance Engagement in First-Time Mothers: Feasibility and Desirability.Pediatric Nursing 2006; 32(5) 455 – 459.

[149] O'Higgins M, St. James Roberts I, Glover V. Postnatal depression and mother and infant outcomes after infant massage Journal of Affective Disorders 2008; 109 (2008) 189–192.

[150] Gürol A, Polat S. The Effects of Baby Massage on Attachment between Mother and their Infants. Asian Nursing Research 2012; 6(1) 35-41.

[151] Underdown A, Barlow J, Chung V, Brown SS. (2009). Massage intervention for promoting mental and physical health in infants aged under six months. DOI: 10.1002/14651858.CD005038.pub2, Cochrane Database of Systematic Reviews http://onlinelibrary.wiley.com/doi/10.1002/14651858.CD005038.pub2/ (22.8.2012).

[152] Muscarella E. Infant massage provides invaluable benefits. PT Bulletin 1996; 3(May) 11-18.

Chapter 9

Cognitive Functions in Euthymic Bipolar Patients and Lithium

Aleksandra Suwalska and Dorota Łojko

Additional information is available at the end of the chapter

http://dx.doi.org/10.5772/55126

1. Introduction

Based on Kraepelin's works we had for many years been distinguishing between manic-depressive illness (bipolar disorder) and dementia praecox (schizophrenia) based on the assumption that bipolar patients tended to experience full remission, whereas the schizophrenic did not. Since the late 1990s, the evidence has been accumulated that the recovery in bipolar disorder is not complete [1]. Persistent psychosocial difficulties and cognitive deficits are common in patients with the bipolar disorder even in euthymic or asymptomatic states [2, 3]. After two decades of scientific work the nature of the cognitive impairments is still the focus of research and debate. The extent and pattern of cognitive impairment in euthymic patients remain uncertain [4]. A meta-analysis of the studies revealed widespread cognitive deficits in patients with schizophrenia and affective disorders in cognitive functioning, speed of information processing, encoding and retrieval, rule discovery, as well as response generation and response inhibition [5]. There is a growing need for clarification regarding the extent and clinical relevance of cognitive impairment in bipolar patients [6].

2. Subjects and methods

2.1. Subjects

Sixty euthymic bipolar patients (25 male, 35 female), aged 26–75 yr (mean±S.D.: 53±10 yr) attending the Outpatient Lithium Clinic at the Department of Psychiatry at the Poznan University of Medical Science were studied. Consensus diagnosis by two psychiatrists was made for each patient, according to DSM-IV criteria (Structured Clinical Interview for DSM-IV Axis I – SCID) [7]. The patients had been treated with lithium carbonate for at least 5 yr. On the day of the study, all patients were euthymic, as defined by a score of <7 on the 17-item Hamilton Depression Rating Scale (HAMD17) [8] and a score of <7 on the Young Mania Rating Scale (YMRS) [9]. Among the patients, 13 were excellent lithium responders, defined as having had no affective episodes on lithium monotherapy for the entire period of lithium administration [10]. Eighty-four healthy controls recruited from the local community were matched by age, gender and education level. The study was approved by the Ethics Committee at the Poznan University of Medical Science. Patients and volunteers gave their written informed consent after hearing a complete description of the study.

2.2. Cognitive assessment- methods

Patients and controls underwent an extensive neuropsychological assessment that included an evaluation of attention, working memory, verbal and visual episodic memory, verbal fluency and executive functions. Neuropsychological testing lasted approximately 2 h. Subjects completed the tests in a fixed order with a break half-way through. The Trail Making Test (TMT) [11], Stroop Colour-Word Interference test [12, 13], verbal fluency tests, as well as selected tests from the Cambridge Automated Neuropsychological Test Battery (CANTAB; CeNeS Ltd, Cambridge, UK) [14-17], were employed.

2.2.1. *Cognitive tests: Paper-and-pencil tests*

The Trail Making Test (TMT) consists of two parts. TMT requires subjects to connect 25 consecutively numbered circles, (part A) and 25 numbered and lettered circles by shifting between the two sets (part B) as quickly as possible, and is very sensitive to cerebral dysfunction. Part A of the test measures psychomotor speed. The results of part B reflect the ability to shift strategy and assess executive function and visuospatial working memory [18]. Time is recorded in seconds.

*The Colour-Word Stroop Interference test (CWST).*The first part of the test (part A)- Reading Colour Names in black (RNCb), measures verbal abilities and attention. The subject is asked to read as quickly as possible words (colour names) printed with black ink on a white card. The second part (part B): Naming the Colour of Word – different (NCWd) – measures verbal working memory and executive functions. The subject is asked to name the colour of each printed word. The colour of the printed word is different from the colour described by the word [12]. Scoring is based on time (seconds).

Verbal fluency tests. Phonologic verbal fluency was studied by asking subjects to generate as many words as possible that begin with each of the letters F, A and S, in consecutive 1-min time periods (FAS Test, from the Controlled Oral Word Association Test) [19]. Semantic verbal fluency was measured with the Category Instant Generation Test, by naming as many items as possible in a given category (animals, vegetables and fruits) within the same time limit. Scores were the sum of all acceptable words produced in the three trials. The Polish version of the FAS test was used. This test was used for the assessment of verbal fluency, which is also a sensitive measure of executive functions, as it requires the subject to generate his/her own strategy.

2.2.2. *Cognitive tests: Selected tests from the Cambridge automated neuropsychological test battery*

Rapid Visual Information Processing (RVP) - a test of visual sustained attention, which is sensitive to dysfunction in the parietal and frontal lobe areas of the brain and is also a sensitive measure of general performance. RVP A' is the signal detection measure of target sensitivity regardless of error tendency (range 0.00 to 1.00; bad to good). This metric is a measure of how good the subject is at detecting target sequences. RVP Mean latency measures the mean time taken to respond and is reported in milliseconds. Response latency in the RVP task is a good indicator of sustained attention function [20].

Stockings of Cambridge (SOC) is a visuospatial planning test based on the Tower of London task [21]. This is a spatial planning test which gives a measure of frontal lobe function. The subject is shown two displays containing three coloured balls. The displays are presented in such a way that they can easily be perceived as stacks of coloured balls held in stockings or socks suspended from a beam. This arrangement makes the 3-D concepts involved apparent to the subject, and fits with the verbal instructions. The subject must use the balls in the lower display to copy the pattern shown in the upper display. The balls may be moved one at a time by touching the required ball, then touching the position to which it should be moved. The time taken to complete the pattern and the number of moves required are taken as measures of the subject's planning ability.

Spatial Span (SSP) - a visuospatial analogue of the Digit Span test assessing working memory capacity. White squares are shown, some of which briefly change colour in a variable sequence. The subject must then touch the boxes which changed colours in the same order that they were displayed by the computer (for clinical mode) or in the reverse order (for reverse mode). The number of boxes increases from 2 at the start of the test to 9 at the end, and the sequence and colour are varied through the test. After an incorrect attempt at choosing the boxes in sequence, the next trial remains at the same difficulty level. The Spatial Span is calculated at the highest level at which the subject successfully remembers at least one sequence of boxes.

Spatial Working Memory (SWM) - is a test of the subject's ability to retain spatial information and to manipulate remembered items in the working memory, which measures the working memory for spatial stimuli and requires the subject to use mnemonic information to work towards a goal. Subjects are required to search through boxes that appear on the screen with the aim of finding the 'blue tokens' hidden inside. The key instruction is that once a token had been taken out of a box, that box would not be used again to hide a token. After two practice trials with two boxes, there were four test trials with each of two, three, four, six and eight boxes. Returning to an 'empty' box already opened and a token removed on a previous search constituted a 'forgetting' or 'Between Search' error (BSE). A Strategy score was calculated from subject's performance on the six and eight box levels, to reflect how often a searching sequence was initiated from the same box during a given trial. Higher Strategy scores represent lower use of strategy (i.e. many sequences beginning with a different box in a given trial), and lower scores represent efficient use of strategy (i.e. many sequences starting with the same box in a given trial).

2.2.2.1. Statistical analyses

Statistical analyses were carried out with Statistica version 10.0 for Windows. To evaluate normality of distribution of the variables, the Shapiro–Wilk test was applied. As most of the investigated variables were not normally distributed, non-parametric tests were employed. Between-group differences in the demographic characteristics and neuropsychological tests were assessed by the Mann–Whitney test (two-groups comparisons) and Kruskal-Wallis ANOVA (multiple comparisons). All the results were expressed as the mean and standard deviation (S.D.). Statistical significance was set at $p<0.05$ for all analyses.

3. Results

Demographic characteristics are presented in table 1.

	Bipolar patients n=60	**ER n=13**	**nonER n=47**	**Controls n=84**
Age (years)	52.6 (10.2)	51.3 (12.1)	52.9 (9.8)	50.6 (14.7)
Gender - Male: Female*	25: 35	7:6	18:29	25:59
Education (years)	13.7 (3.5)	15.1 (2.4)	13.3 (3.7)	13.2 (2.4)
Duration of illness	22.2 (10.8)	21.0 (11.2)	22.6 (10.9)	-
Duration of prophylactic lithium treatment	12.7 (8.9)	12.1 (8.4)	12.9 (9.2)	-
No. of recurrences	13.3 (8.1)	7.2 (5.4)	15.3 (7.9)	-
Intensity of depressive symptoms (HDRS)	2.6 (1.8)	2.3 (0.8)	2.6 (2.0)	0.8 (1.5) [1,2,3]
Intensity of manic symptoms (YMRS)	0.6 (0.9)	0.1 (0.4)	0.7 (1.0)	0.3 (0.7)

* chi-square test

[1] – $p<0.01$ Mann-Whitney test, difference between bipolar patients and controls

[2] – $p<0.05$ ANOVA difference between ER and controls

[3] – $p<0.01$ ANOVA difference between nonER and controls

Table 1. Demographic and clinical characteristic of euthymic bipolar patients and healthy controls. ER - Excellent lithium responders; nonER- non – excellent responders; HAMD - Hamilton Depression Rating Scale; YMRS - Young Mania Rating Scale (values are expressed as mean, standard deviation is shown in brackets).

No differences in age, gender distribution as well as education level between bipolar patients and healthy controls were detected. No difference between excellent responders (ER) and non-excellent responders (nonER) were detected either. Bipolar patients were euthymic but scored significantly worse on Hamilton's depression scale. Both ER and nonER had higher depression sores than the controls. In the bipolar group, 35 patients were treated with lithium as mono-therapy, 13 – lithium in combination with carbamazepine, 4 – lithium+valproate, 8 – lithium+ atypical neuroleptic.

3.1. Assessment of attention, working memory and executive functions

To evaluate working memory planning and executive functions SSP, SWM, SOC from CANTAB Battery and the so-called "paper and pencil test": fluency tests (semantic and phonemic), CWST part B, TMT A and B, were used. To asses sustained attention RVP (CAN-TAB), and part A from CWST were employed. In table 2 the results of the neuropsychological evaluation of bipolar patients treated with lithium and healthy controls are presented. The bipolar group consists of two subgroups: excellent lithium responders and the remaining patients (non- excellent lithium responders).

Subjects with bipolar disorder scored significantly worse than controls on the tests assessing working memory, executive functioning and planning. The longest sequence successfully recalled (SSP Span length) was significantly shorter in the patients group than the controls. SSP total error number was higher in the BD group than in the controls, but the difference was not statistically significant. On the Spatial Working Memory (SWM) test results are presented in two measures: strategy and between errors. Patient scored worse on both of them. On the SOC results were displayed as three dimensions: SOC Mean initial thinking time (5 moves) giving an indication of the time taken to plan the problem solution, SOC Mean subsequent thinking time (5 moves) as well as SOC Problems solved in a minimum number of moves recording the number of occasions upon which the subject has successfully completed a test problem in the minimum possible number of moves. Bipolar patients had significantly worse results in both initial and subsequent thinking times. The controls performed better on fluency tests (verbal and phonemic), and TMT both parts. On the CWST B measuring verbal working memory and executive functions, bipolar patients had significantly worse results than the control subjects. On the sustained attention tests patients also scored significantly worse. Results of RVP A' - the signal detection (a measure of how good the subject is at detecting target sequences) as well RVP Mean latency (a measure of the mean time taken to respond) were significant worse in the patients groups. After dividing lithium-treated patients into ELRs and non-ELRs the differences in cognitive functions between subgroups were observed. The results of excellent lithium responders were similar to those of healthy controls, whereas non-ELRs scored significantly worse on SSP Span length, SWM between errors and strategy, SOC initial thinking time, as well as sustained attention test. The only measure in which ELR scored worse than the controls was RVP mean latency. The results of ELRs were better than the scores of the controls on SSP span length and SOC problems solved in a minimum number of moves, but the difference did not reach statistical significance.

	Bipolar patients	ER	nonER	Controls
Working memory and planning, executive functions				
SSP Span length	5.0 (1.1)	5.8 (1.1)	4.7 (0.9)[3]	5.4 (1.2)[1,4]
SWM Between errors	46.8 (19.7)	40.4 (14.9)	48.6 (20.6)	36.5 (18.7)[2,4]
SWM Strategy	37.3 (4.3)	36.5 (3.7)	37.6 (4.5)	35.2 (4.8)[1,4]
SOC Mean initial thinking time (5 moves)	11376.6 (11785.4)	9580.5 (8738.2)	11873.43 (12532.6)	6853.5 (5823.2)[2,4]
SOC Mean subsequent thinking time (5 moves)	3649.0 (2453.2)	3484.4 (3128.5)	3694.51 (2270.7)	3057.4 (2955.0)[2]
SOC Problems solved in a minimum number of moves	7.6 (1.6)	8.1 (1.7)	7.5 (1.6)	7.4 (1.6)
Semantic fluency (No of words)	40,8(9.0)	44,6(8.9)	39,7(10.0)	47,6(10,0)[2]
Phonemic fluency (No of words)	28,5(8.8)	33,3(9.3)	27,2(12.9)	35,6(12.9)[2]
CWST B (time [sec])	78,7(26.3)	38,2(17.5)	46.0(10.9)	62,9(20,3)[2]
TMT A (time [sec])	44,3(17.3)	89,2(39.0)	119,7(42.7)	36,1(10,9)[2]
TMT B (time [sec])	113,2(46.80	65,5(19.4)	82,9(20.3)	81,3(42,7)[2]
Sustained attention				
RVP A'	0.83 (0.05)	0.86 (0.05)	0.83 (0.05)	0.88 (0.05)[2,4]
RVP Mean latency	604.7 (139.6)	577.6 (164.5)	612.2 (132.9)	482.9 (124.8)[2,3,4]
RVP B''	0.89 (0.21)	0.88 (0.16)	0.89 (0.23)	0.88 (0.28)
CWST A (time [sec])	28,2(5.8)	26,8(5.1)	28,6(9.4)	28,4(9.4)

[1] –difference between BD and controls p< 0.05 Mann-Whitney test

[2] - difference between BD and controls p<0.01 Mann-Whitney test

[3] - difference between ER and controls (p<0.05) ANOVA

[4] – difference between non-ER and controls (p<0.05) ANOVA

Table 2. Neuropsychological evaluation of bipolar patients and healthy controls treated with lithium and healthy controls (values are expressed as mean and standard deviation in brackets). Table presents results of CANTAB tests and paper-and-pencil tests results.

4. Discussion

4.1. Cognitive functions in bipolar patients

Not so long ago it was claimed that bipolar disorder is episodic, and the patient fully recovers between episodes, with no signs of affective, cognitive or psychosocial symptoms [2]. But patients in remission seem to be both affectively disturbed and cognitively impaired which may be a contributory factor to poor psychosocial outcome [2, 22-25]. During the last decade the results of numerous neurocognitive and neuroimaging studies in BD have been reported. They have revealed various dysfunctions in bipolar disorder present during affective episodes and have demonstrated that many neurocognitive deficits persist into periods of clinical remission or euthymia [16, 26]. Patients during affective episodes show significantly lower performance on several measures (tests) of attention, executive function, learning and verbal memory, and psychomotor speed [27-29].

Disturbances of executive functions, verbal and visual memory dysfunctions have been observed in depressive bipolar patients [23, 29-31]. Results of studies in manic patients are less consistent - although impairments in executive functions have been reported [23, 30-35]. Sweeney et al. [30] reported worse results of manic compared to depressive bipolar patients. Manic, but not depressed, patients made suboptimal decisions in Murphy's [35] computerized decision-making task.

Results of neuroimaging scans show structural and functional brain abnormalities in mood disorders in such regions as: basal ganglia frontal lobes, the locus caeruleus, subcortical white matters, hipoccampus, amygdala, temporal lobes, as well as subtle structural deficits in the dorsal raphe [28, 36]. Cognitive dysfunctions were observed in affective acute bipolar patients (attention deficits, flexibility deficits, verbal fluency impairment, memory disturbances) [13, 31, 32, 35] have been reported also during periods of remission [37, 38], independently from residual affective symptoms [1, 16]. Sustained cognitive deficits could be a marker of disease or bipolar traits, it could be a prognostic factor as well [37]. Still, there is ambiguity about those issues [23, 39]. Research results are inconsistent [39], in small groups, diagnosis of bipolar is not precise, and information about treatment is not provided [23].

Recent reports have suggested the presence of persistent cognitive impairments in patients diagnosed with BD even after prolonged euthymic phases [16, 26, 40-48]. Review by Torres et al. [4] revealed widespread cognitive deficits in tests assessing attention, speed of information processing, memory and executive dysfunctions in remitted bipolars versus controls. There was no difference in premorbid intelligence and vocabulary. Some dysfunctions in remitted patients [49] are similar to those observed in patients in acute phase. Cognitive deficits are regarded by several authors as trait-markers or their background (genetic, developmental or associated with illness progression) remains to be evaluated [4]. The studies in euthymic patients are to answer questions concerning the state-dependent (reflecting mood changes) and stable character of cognitive deficits [2, 26, 40, 41, 50, 51].

Disturbances of executive functions, working memory and planning. The results of our study confirmed the reports on disturbances of executive functions in remitted bipolar patients [42-48; 52-54]. Several authors do not show executive dysfunctions [55, 56] or show mild degree dysfunctions [4]. These discrepancies probably result from various definitions of executive function, which lead to the use of different tests and methods as well as problems with clear explanation of the nature of cognitive dysfunction(s). Disturbances of cognitive flexibility and inhibitory control were the most important findings, auditory memory and verbal fluency were more impaired. Intellectual functioning was intact. A recent review of the literature [57] shows deficits in working memory and some aspects of executive functions (inhibitory control).

Larson [58] et al. evaluated two specific aspects of executive functioning: inhibitory control, and spatial delayed working memory. Manic and euthymic patient groups performed similarly in the spatial delayed working memory test. On the inhibitory test manic and euthymic patients committed significantly more perseverative errors than healthy participants. These results indicated that patients had relatively normal working memory abilities, but had a deficit in behavioral self-regulation, which was evident across mood states. In our bipolar remitted group spatial working memory (SWM) was disturbed compared to the control group, and subjects performed worse when it came to updating the working memory continually but strategy planning was less disturbed.

Goswami et al. [59] have measured neurocognitive functions in bipolar disorder and tried to find links to residual mood symptoms, soft neurological signs and psychosocial impairment. They tested attention, memory and executive function in euthymic patients with bipolar disorder and controls. Psychosocial functioning, soft neurological signs and residual mood symptoms were assessed. Tests results on executive function and verbal memory (but not attention) were significantly poorer in bipolar patients. Residual (sub-syndromal) mood symptoms were connected with small cognitive effects, predominantly on verbal memory. Some patients showed a marked social disability which correlated strongly with soft neurological signs but weakly with executive dysfunction, which was linked to the number of episodes. Cognitive dysfunction, social dysfunction and soft signs may represent trait deficits of bipolar illness. Both in the present study and in other authors' results remitted bipolar patients have verbal and nonverbal memory disturbances [4] compared to healthy controls. Those results are consistent through various data [49], a wide spectrum of executive dysfunctions, memory and attention was detected in remitted bipolars [25]. The results of our study are consistent with those of Sole et al. [60] who reported that bipolar patients showed a significantly lower performance on several measures of attention, learning and verbal memory, and executive function compared with healthy controls. Worse performance on TMT is especially important in light of the finding of Sole et al. [60] that the one measure related to executive function (Trail Making Test, part B) was the variable that best predicted psychosocial functioning of bipolar patients. In a two year follow up study in euthymic bipolar patients on lithium executive function and processing speed were affected, and such deficits were maintained over time. Those results show that executive dysfunction is the main long-term neuropsychological deficit of bipolar disorder [61]. After controlling for the effect of subsyndromal depressive symptoms [62] impairment of verbal memory and executive dysfunctions were noticed and this cognitive impairment seems to be related to a worse clinical course and poor functional outcome. Executive dysfunctions are described as a central bipolar trait deficit and due to them bipolars' psychosocial problems are observed [63].

Attention deficits. The results of our study point to the deficits in attention tests. Patients scored worse on sustained attention measurement WCST part B and on RVP test from CANTAB battery. Euthymic bipolar patients have been reported to show persistent deficits in sustained attention tests [53]. Most research shows sustained attention deficits [41, 46], some tests did not show such disturbances [4]. Burdick [64] has not detected a direct relationship between attention deficits and depressive symptoms. Sustained attention deficits apparent during the euthymic period of bipolar disorder cannot be explained in terms of working memory impairment and represent a reduced inherent capacity rather than a changed response bias [16, 42, 44, 45, 53, 65, 66]. Sustained attention deficits are claimed to be a core deficit for bipolar disorder, but those deficits are not dependent on executive dysfunctions, including working memory. Attention deficits and information-processing speed are related to memory processing or other cognitive processes [2, 39, 47, 48]. Furthermore, the data support the view that deficits in verbal memory may be related to genetic factors. [65].

Memory deficits as result of hipoccampal and medial temporal lobe dysfunctions could be a key cognitive problem in bipolar patients [67]. Malhi et al. [68] conducted a review of the literature to compare and contrast the neuropsychological profile of the 3 phases of bipolar disorder to identify potential state and trait deficits. They initially identified more than 100 articles and then excluded reviews and papers in which neuropsychological tests were not administered directly. This left 27 papers, which they further examined and the findings of which they tabulated and discussed. Cognitive and executive functioning deficits were found, including set-shifting, verbal fluency, planning, attention, and memory. In their opinion, those neuropsychological deficits found in bipolar depression, mania or hypomania, and euthymia provide important insights into the pathophysiology of bipolar disorder and may, in future studies, form the basis of clinically meaningful subtypes of bipolar disorder [68]. Deficits in sustaining attention may also help explain the difficulties in psychological and occupational functioning in bipolar disorder patients during remission.

4.2. Factors associated with cognitive deficits

Cognitive impairments result not only from affective disturbances (manic, depression phases) - they are also detectable during the phase free of affective symptoms (remission) Factors associated with cognitive dysfunction in bipolars might be the number of episodes [1, 38, 54], mainly the number of manic episodes [16, 41, 52, 54, 69, 70], chronicity [53, 54], residual affective symptoms, especially depressive ones [27, 38]. Clinical factors associated with cognitive impairment in bipolar patients are medicines such as mood stabilizers, antidepressants and neuroleptics. Drugs used in the treatment for somatic diseases might also influence the cognitive functioning of bipolar patients.The secondary cognitive deficits caused by treatment of bipolar disorder (lithium, antiepileptics, antidepressants, antipsychotics) are similar to the cognitive deficits associated with the disease [71]. Differentiation between cognitive dysfunctions related to the illness and those related to its treatment is difficult. Four studies showed that lithium had a negative effect on memory and speed of information processing, often without subjective complaints or awareness of mental slowness [72, 73], lithium did not cause memory impairment or a change in self-assessment of memory functions [74]. In Engelsmann et al. observation survey mean memory test scores remained remarkably stable over the entire 6-year lithium therapy [75]. A comparison between two groups on lithium therapy: a long- and shorter term group (with means of 12.9 and 5.2 years, respectively) showed no significant differences between these groups on any of the memory tests [31]. Younger bipolars (below 55 yrs) had received lithium therapy for 1-5 years and showed no abnormalities on the Halstead-Reitan Neuropsychological Battery, so lithium therapy was not connected with cognitive impairment [76].

Cognitive function in log-term lithium-treated outpatients were investigated by Lund et al. [77] who tested memory, attention, speed, loss of effort, level of processing, productivity [77]. Results were within normal limits. But further analyses revealed that the performance of the lithium-treated patients indicated a relative lowering of the level of memory and perceptual processing when compared to the level of attention and productivity. Those results support opinion about lithium –influenced worsening in information processing. The effects of blind lithium discontinuation and resumption on measures of cognition, creativity, and fine motor performance in 46 lithium-maintained euthymic out-patients were investigated [72]. Scores on memory measures, tests of tapping speed, and associative productivity all improved significantly during the time off of lithium. The authors analyzed influence of six possible intervening variables: age, sex, lithium concentration in plasma, thyroid function, duration of lithium maintenance, and depressive symptoms. Further analysis suggested that lithium has a greater neuropsychological effect in younger, less-depressed patients having higher plasma lithium concentrations in plasma [72].

In our study lithium-treated patients as a group had poorer results on several tests measures compared to healthy controls, namely SSP span length, SWM between errors, SWM strategy, RVP A, RVP mean latency, and SOC mean initial thinking time as well as on TMT and Stroop test part B. The results of excellent lithium responders did not differ from those of healthy controls (except for one measure in RVP). These might support statement that lithium treatment is associated with a preservation of cognitive functions in ER group. According to literature review [78] neurostructural changes in BD would be hypothetically influenced by the neuroprotective/neurotrophic properties of lithium. These findings are interesting because the pathophysiology of BD involves structural and functional changes in cortical and limbic networks implicated in the regulation of mood and cognition. Reports on the impact of anticonvulsants on cognitive functions in bipolar patients are scarce. Some authors reported that plasma levels of anticonvulsants influence cognitive tests results and carbamazepine or valproinians may be responsible for attention deficits [79, 80]. Neuroleptics have been found to worsen psychomotor function and sustained attention, but higher cognitive functions are relatively unaffected [81]. Zubieta et al. [41] have found negative correlations between Wisconsin Card Sorting Test (WCST) performance and duration of neuroleptics exposition. The use of neuroleptics [82] as well as illness duration and family history were predictive factors for intelligence and memory in bipolar patients. Numerous authors believe that neuroleptics do not influence cognitive functions in bipolars. Cognitive deficits are related

http://dx.doi.org/10.5772/55126

probably to anticholinergics effects of drugs [31]. New neuroleptics (atypical) have positive impact on cognitive functions of schizophrenic patients [83], and probably new neuroleptics improve cognitive function especially in longtime treatment for manic patients [31].

Data on antidepressants are also inconsistent. Literature review shows that antidepresants do not cause cognitive dysfunctions [84]. According to literature review by Knegtering et al. [85] amitriptyline, mianserin and trazodone impair attention and ability to concentrate in elderly, antidepressants with anticholinergic properties (nortriptyline, maprotiline, amitriptyline) might impair working memory. Higher plasma concentrations of nortriptyline correlate with greater cognitive impairment. Tests results about selective serotonin (5-hydroxytryptamine) reuptake inhibitors on cognitive performance in the elderly indicate no detrimental effect. Martinez et al. pointed out that mood stabilizers with antidepressant properties might influence cognitive function and social functioning [31]. Optimal treatment preferring second generation antipsychotics and avoiding drugs with anticholinergic effect, is essential. In Mencier and colleagues opinion prevention of iatrogenic effects of drugs should be now the main therapeutic intervention [71]. Treatment with atypical antipsychotics has been associated with improvement in cognitive tests in patients with schizophrenia, and the little data available in patients with bipolar disorder suggest the potential for similar benefits. MacQueen and Young [86] pointed to the need of further studies to determine if current treatments for bipolar disorder can prevent, delay, or even improve cognitive dysfunctions [86]. Bipolar patient have been treated for years with combination of mood stabilizers, antidepressants and antipsychotics and it is difficult to assess impact of such a combination on various cognitive functions. [28, 34]. Impaired executive functions in bipolars shown in tests might be the feature of bipolar disorder regardless the effects of medication [87]. The contributions of bipolar disorder trait – state cognitive impairment and medications is very complicated to distinguish as well as control [78]. Clinicians treating BD patients should take it into account in prescribing medications for long-term prophylaxis. Medication-related adverse cognitive effects should be taken into consideration. In order to reduce cognitive dysfunction, or at least avoid cognitive deterioration clinicians should use drugs with a favourable or neutral cognitive profile [78]. Cognitive outcome in patients with affective disorders appears to be associated with the number of affective episodes. In the study designed as a controlled cohort study [38] 118 unipolar patients, 28 bipolar patients and 58 controls were included and the analysis results was adjusted to the level of education and subclinical depressive and anxiety symptoms. Patients with recurrent episodes were significantly more impaired than patients with a single episode and more impaired than controls. Some research on bipolar showed negative correlations between number of depressive episodes and executive functions [16, 41, 42]. Verbal learning was correlated with number of depressive episodes [63] or not [42, 52]. Number of manic episodes was connected with worse results in verbal tests and worsening in executive functions tests [16, 41, 52, 54, 62, 63] and visual memory [88]. Systematic literature review by Robinson and Ferrier [25] showed relationship between cognitive dysfunction in bipolar disorder and worse prior course of illness, particularly the number of manic episodes, hospitalizations and length of illness. In their opinion cognitive impairment may be a trait vulnerability factor for bipolar disorder that is present before illness onset and worsens as the illness progresses. Residual affective symptoms might influence cognitive tests results [2, 16,

56, 89]. It is worth to underline that in previous studies usually euthymic patients meant patients free of affective symptoms who did not fulfilled criteria for affective episode. On the other hand 30% of Scott's [90] group of remitted bipolar had patients Beck's score was more than 10 points. In cognitive functions assessment in BD we should consider such factors as pharmacological treatment, course of illness, residual symptoms [2, 16], structural lesions of a neurodegenerative origin [91, 92], functional changes that are most likely genetic in origin [91-93]. There is a close relationship between cognitive impairment and poor treatment adherence, but the causal inferences of these findings are uncertain [94]. Poor treatment adherence may worsen the course of bipolar disorder and so indirectly worsen cognitive performance, or cognitive impairment may contribute to poor treatment adherence and reflect more severe illness.

5. Conclusion and future research

Data concerning cognitive functions in BD are still limited and inconsistent so that further research is necessary. It is worth to underline the growing evidence suggests that the presence of cognitive dysfunction in bipolar affective disorder is a core and enduring deficit of the illness. Impairment in the attention or executive control of action represents an important target for future research. Many clinicians have strongly indicated worse psychosocial functioning of bipolar patients [41, 95], which may be caused by cognitive impairment as neurocognitive deficits could result in psychological and social deficits. Evidence from neuroimaging, molecular genetic, pharmacological and animal studies related to the pathophysiology of bipolar disorder may provide clinicians with new treatment strategies. Neurocognitive impairment in bipolar disorder should be considered a potential therapeutic target, which means that research should focus on new drugs and psychological interventions, including neurocognitive rehabilitation to improve cognitive functions and the functional outcome of bipolar patients [96]. The Cognitive Remediation is defined as a behavioural training based intervention aimed at the improvement of cognitive processes (attention, memory, executive function, social cognition or metacognition) with the goal of durability and generalization [97]. Several cognitive remediation programmes (CR) for patients with schizophrenia have already been developed. The potential benefits of CR in affective disorders may even exceed those of schizophrenia and such approaches hold significant promise for individuals with bipolar disorder [98].

Author details

Aleksandra Suwalska and Dorota Łojko

Department of Adult Psychiatry, Poznan University of Medical Sciences, Poznan, Poland

References

[1] Ferrier, I. N, & Thompson, J. M. Cognitive impairment in bipolar affective disorder: implications for the bipolar diathesis. Br J Psychiatry, (2002). , 293-295.

[2] Ferrier, I. N, et al. Neuropsychological function in euthymic patients with bipolar disorder, in British Journal of Psychiatry. (1999). , 246-251.

[3] Scott, J. Psychotherapy for bipolar disorder. Br J Psychiatry, (1995). , 581-588.

[4] Torres, I. J, Boudreau, V. G, & Yatham, L. N. Neuropsychological functioning in euthymic bipolar disorder: a meta-analysis. Acta Psychiatr Scand Suppl, (2007). , 17-26.

[5] Stefanopoulou, E, et al. Cognitive functioning in patients with affective disorders and schizophrenia: a meta-analysis. Int Rev Psychiatry, (2009). , 336-356.

[6] Latalova, K, et al. Cognitive impairment in bipolar disorder. Biomed Pap Med Fac Univ Palacky Olomouc Czech Repub, (2011). , 19-26.

[7] First, M, et al. Structured Clinical Interview for DSM-IV Axis I Disorders, Research Version. (1997). New York: Biometrics Research.

[8] Hamilton, M. A rating scale for depression. J Neurol Neurosurg Psychiatry, (1960). , 56-62.

[9] Young, R, et al. A rating scale for mania: Reliability, validity, and sensitivity, in British Journal of Psychiatry. (1978). , 429-435.

[10] Grof, P. Excellent lithium responders: people whose lives have been changed by lithium prophylaxis, in Lithium: 50 Years of Psychopharmacology, New Perspectives in Biomedical and Clinical Research, N.J. Birch, V.S. Gallicchio, and R.W. Becker, Editors. (1999). Weidner Publishing Group: Cheshire, Connecticut , 36-51.

[11] Reitan, R. M. The relation of the trail making test to organic brain damage. J Consult Psychol, (1955). , 393-394.

[12] Stroop, J. R. Studies of interference in serial verbal reaction. J Exp Psychol, (1935). , 643-662.

[13] Borkowska, A, & Rybakowski, J. K. Neuropsychological frontal lobe tests indicate that bipolar depressed patients are more impaired than unipolar. Bipolar Disord, (2001). , 88-94.

[14] Elliott, R, et al. Neuropsychological impairments in unipolar depression: the influence of perceived failure on subsequent performance. Psychol Med, (1996). , 975-989.

[15] Purcell, R, et al. Neuropsychological function in young patients with unipolar major depression. Psychol Med, (1997). , 1277-1285.

[16] Clark, L, Iversen, S. D, & Goodwin, G. M. Sustained attention deficit in bipolar disorder. Br J Psychiatry, (2002). , 313-319.

[17] Owen, A. M, et al. Planning and spatial working memory: a positron emission tomography study in humans. Eur J Neurosci, (1996). , 353-364.

[18] Reitan, R. M. Validity of theTrail MakingTest as an indicator of organic brain damage. Percept Mot Skills, (1958).

[19] Borkowski, J, & Benton, A. Word fluency and brain damage. Neuropsychologia, (1967). , 135-140.

[20] Sahakian, B, et al. The effects of nicotine on attention, information processing, and short-term memory in patients with dementia of the Alzheimer type. Br J Psychiatry, (1989). , 797-800.

[21] Shallice, T. Specific impairments of planning. Philos Trans R Soc Lond B Biol Sci, (1982). , 199-209.

[22] Goodwin, F. K, & Jamison, K. R. Manic Depressive Illness (1990). Oxford University Press: Oxford.

[23] Malhi, G. S, et al. Neuropsychological deficits and functional impairment in bipolar depression, hypomania and euthymia. Bipolar Disord, (2007). , 114-125.

[24] Blumberg, H. P, et al. A functional magnetic resonance imaging study of bipolar disorder: state- and trait-related dysfunction in ventral prefrontal cortices. Arch Gen Psychiatry, (2003). , 601-609.

[25] Robinson, L. J, & Ferrier, I. N. Evolution of cognitive impairment in bipolar disorder: a systematic review of cross-sectional evidence. Bipolar Disord, (2006). , 103-116.

[26] Martinez-aran, A, et al. Cognitive impairment in euthymic bipolar patients: implications for clinical and functional outcome. Bipolar Disord, (2004a). , 224-232.

[27] Martinez-aran, A, et al. Cognitive dysfunctions in bipolar disorder: evidence of neuropsychological disturbances. Psychother Psychosom, (2000). , 2-18.

[28] Bearden, C. E, Hoffman, K. M, & Cannon, T. D. The neuropsychology and neuroanatomy of bipolar affective disorder: a critical review. Bipolar Disord, (2001). discussion 151-3., 106-150.

[29] Quraishi, S, & Frangou, S. Neuropsychology of bipolar disorder: a review. J Affect Disord, (2002). , 209-226.

[30] Sweeney, J. A, Kmiec, J. A, & Kupfer, D. J. Neuropsychologic impairments in bipolar and unipolar mood disorders on the CANTAB neurocognitive battery. Biol Psychiatry, (2000). , 674-684.

[31] Martinez-aran, A, et al. Cognitive function across manic or hypomanic, depressed, and euthymic states in bipolar disorder. Am J Psychiatry, (2004). , 262-270.

[32] Clark, L, Iversen, S. D, & Goodwin, G. M. A neuropsychological investigation of prefrontal cortex involvement in acute mania. Am J Psychiatry, (2001). , 1605-1611.

[33] Goldberg, T. E, et al. Contrasts between patients with affective disorders and patients with schizophrenia on a neuropsychological test battery. Am J Psychiatry, (1993). , 1355-1362.

[34] Murphy, F. C, & Sahakian, B. J. Neuropsychology of bipolar disorder. Br J Psychiatry Suppl, (2001). , s120-s127.

[35] Murphy, F. C, et al. Decision-making cognition in mania and depression. Psychol Med, (2001). , 679-693.

[36] Baumann, B, & Bogerts, B. Neuroanatomical studies on bipolar disorder. Br J Psychiatry Suppl, (2001). , s142-s147.

[37] Mckay, A. P, et al. Neuropsychological function in manic-depressive psychosis. Evidence for persistent deficits in patients with chronic, severe illness. Br J Psychiatry, (1995). , 51-57.

[38] Kessing, L. V. Cognitive impairment in the euthymic phase of affective disorder. Psychol Med, (1998). , 1027-1038.

[39] Olley, A, et al. When euthymia is just not good enough: the neuropsychology of bipolar disorder. J Nerv Ment Dis, (2005a). , 323-330.

[40] El-Badri, S. M, et al. Electrophysiological and cognitive function in young euthymic patients with bipolar affective disorder. Bipolar Disord, (2001). , 79-87.

[41] Zubieta, J. K, et al. Cognitive function in euthymic bipolar I disorder. Psychiatry Res, (2001). , 9-20.

[42] Thompson, J. M, et al. Neurocognitive impairment in euthymic patients with bipolar affective disorder. Br J Psychiatry, (2005). , 32-40.

[43] Fleck, D. E, Shear, P. K, & Strakowski, S. M. Processing efficiency and directed forgetting in bipolar disorder. J Int Neuropsychol Soc, (2005). , 871-880.

[44] Clark, L, et al. Sustained attention-deficit confirmed in euthymic bipolar disorder but not in first-degree relatives of bipolar patients or euthymic unipolar depression. Biol Psychiatry, (2005a). , 183-187.

[45] Wilder-willis, K. E, et al. Persistent attentional dysfunction in remitted bipolar disorder. Bipolar Disord, (2001). , 58-62.

[46] Swann, A. C, et al. Impulsivity and phase of illness in bipolar disorder. J Affect Disord, (2003). , 105-111.

[47] Gruber, S. A, Rogowska, J, & Yurgelun-todd, D. A. Decreased activation of the anterior cingulate in bipolar patients: an fMRI study. J Affect Disord, (2004). , 191-201.

[48] Monks, P. J, et al. A functional MRI study of working memory task in euthymic bipolar disorder: evidence for task-specific dysfunction. Bipolar Disord, (2004). , 550-564.

[49] Placais, B, et al. Continuum electrodynamics of type-II superconductors in the mixed state: The dc and ac response. Phys Rev B Condens Matter, (1996). , 13083-13096.

[50] Dixon, T, et al. Effect of symptoms on executive function in bipolar illness. Psychol Med, (2004). , 811-821.

[51] Krabbendam, L, et al. Cognitive dysfunctions and white matter lesions in patients with bipolar disorder in remission. Acta Psychiatr Scand, (2000). , 274-280.

[52] Cavanagh, J. T, et al. Case-control study of neurocognitive function in euthymic patients with bipolar disorder: an association with mania. Br J Psychiatry, (2002). , 320-326.

[53] Harmer, C. J, et al. Sustained attention deficit in bipolar disorder is not a working memory impairment in disguise. Neuropsychologia, (2002). , 1586-1590.

[54] Van Gorp, W. G, et al. Cognitive impairment in euthymic bipolar patients with and without prior alcohol dependence. A preliminary study. Arch Gen Psychiatry, (1998). , 41-46.

[55] Rossi, A, et al. Cognitive function in euthymic bipolar patients, stabilized schizophrenic patients, and healthy controls. J Psychiatr Res, (2000). , 333-339.

[56] Rubinsztein, J. S, et al. Cognitive impairment in remission in bipolar affective disorder. Psychol Med, (2000). , 1025-1036.

[57] Sole, B, et al. Are bipolar II patients cognitively impaired? A systematic review. Psychol Med, (2011). , 1791-1803.

[58] Larson, E. R, et al. Working memory and inhibitory control among manic and euthymic patients with bipolar disorder. J Int Neuropsychol Soc, (2005). , 163-172.

[59] Goswami, U, et al. Neuropsychological dysfunction, soft neurological signs and social disability in euthymic patients with bipolar disorder. Br J Psychiatry, (2006). , 366-373.

[60] Sole, B, et al. Neurocognitive impairment and psychosocial functioning in bipolar II disorder. Acta Psychiatr Scand, (2012). , 309-317.

[61] Mur, M, et al. Long-term stability of cognitive impairment in bipolar disorder: a 2-year follow-up study of lithium-treated euthymic bipolar patients. J Clin Psychiatry, (2008). , 712-719.

[62] Martinez-aran, A, et al. Cognitive impairment in euthymic bipolar patients: implications for clinical and functional outcome. Bipolar Disord, (2004). , 224-232.

[63] Deckersbach, T, et al. Episodic memory impairment in bipolar disorder and obsessive-compulsive disorder: the role of memory strategies. Bipolar Disord, (2004). , 233-244.

[64] Burdick, K. E, et al. Attention and psychomotor functioning in bipolar depression. Psychiatry Res, (2009). , 192-200.

[65] Kieseppa, T, et al. Memory and verbal learning functions in twins with bipolar-I disorder, and the role of information-processing speed. Psychol Med, (2005). , 205-215.

[66] Fleck, D. E, Shear, P. K, & Strakowski, S. M. Processing efficiency and sustained attention in bipolar disorder. J Int Neuropsychol Soc, (2005). , 49-57.

[67] Savitz, J, Solms, M, & Ramesar, R. Neuropsychological dysfunction in bipolar affective disorder: a critical opinion. Bipolar Disord, (2005). , 216-235.

[68] Malhi, G. S, et al. Bipolar disorder: it's all in your mind? The neuropsychological profile of a biological disorder. Can J Psychiatry, (2004). , 813-819.

[69] Altshuler, L. L. Bipolar disorder: are repeated episodes associated with neuroanatomic and cognitive changes? Biol Psychiatry, (1993). , 563-565.

[70] Christensen, M. V, Kyvik, K. O, & Kessing, L. V. Cognitive function in unaffected twins discordant for affective disorder. Psychol Med, (2006). , 1119-1129.

[71] Menecier, P, et al. Bipolar disorders and dementia: fortuitous association or filiation? A case-report and review of the literature.]. Psychol Neuropsychiatr Vieil, (2007). , 23-34.

[72] Kocsis, J. H, et al. Neuropsychologic effects of lithium discontinuation. J Clin Psychopharmacol, (1993). , 268-275.

[73] Honig, A, et al. Lithium induced cognitive side-effects in bipolar disorder: a qualitative analysis and implications for daily practice. Int Clin Psychopharmacol, (1999). , 167-171.

[74] Squire, L. R, et al. Effects of lithium carbonate on memory and other cognitive functions. Am J Psychiatry, (1980). , 1042-1046.

[75] Engelsmann, F, et al. Lithium and memory: a long-term follow-up study. J Clin Psychopharmacol, (1988). , 207-212.

[76] Friedman, M. J, Culver, C. M, & Ferrell, R. B. On the safety of long-term treatment with lithium. Am J Psychiatry, (1977). , 1123-1126.

[77] Lund, Y, Nissen, M, & Rafaelsen, O. J. Long-term lithium treatment and psychological functions. Acta Psychiatr Scand, (1982). , 233-244.

[78] Balanza-martinez, V, et al. Neurocognition in bipolar disorders--a closer look at comorbidities and medications. Eur J Pharmacol, (2010). , 87-96.

[79] Devinsky, O. Cognitive and behavioral effects of antiepileptic drugs. Epilepsia, (1995). Suppl 2: , S46-S65.

[80] Thompson, P. J, & Trimble, M. R. Anticonvulsant drugs and cognitive functions. Epilepsia, (1982). , 531-544.

[81] King, D. J. Psychomotor impairment and cognitive disturbances induced by neuroleptics. Acta Psychiatr Scand Suppl, (1994). , 53-58.

[82] Donaldson, S, et al. The Maudsley Bipolar Disorder Project: the effect of medication, family history, and duration of illness on IQ and memory in bipolar I disorder. J Clin Psychiatry, (2003). , 86-93.

[83] Borkowska, A, et al. Risperidone treatment of schizophrenia: improvement in psychopathology and neuropsychological tests. Neuropsychobiology, (2002). , 85-89.

[84] Thompson, P. J. Antidepressants and memory: a review. Hum Psychopharmacol (1991). , 79-90.

[85] Knegtering, H, Eijck, M, & Huijsman, A. Effects of antidepressants on cognitive functioning of elderly patients. A review. Drugs Aging, (1994). , 192-199.

[86] Macqueen, G, & Young, T. Cognitive effects of atypical antipsychotics: focus on bipolar spectrum disorders. Bipolar Disord, (2003). Suppl 2: , 53-61.

[87] Mur, M, et al. Persistent neuropsychological deficit in euthymic bipolar patients: executive function as a core deficit. J Clin Psychiatry, (2007). , 1078-1086.

[88] Deckersbach, T, et al. Characteristics of non-verbal memory impairment in bipolar disorder: the role of encoding strategies. Psychol Med, (2004). , 823-832.

[89] Clark, L, & Goodwin, G. M. State- and trait-related deficits in sustained attention in bipolar disorder. Eur Arch Psychiatry Clin Neurosci, (2004). , 61-68.

[90] Scott, J, et al. Cognitive vulnerability in patients with bipolar disorder. Psychol Med, (2000). , 467-472.

[91] Ali, S. O, et al. Relationship between prior course of illness and neuroanatomic structures in bipolar disorder: a preliminary study. Neuropsychiatry Neuropsychol Behav Neurol, (2001). , 227-232.

[92] Denicoff, K. D, et al. Relationship between prior course of illness and neuropsychological functioning in patients with bipolar disorder. J Affect Disord, (1999). , 67-73.

[93] Glahn, D. C, et al. The feasibility of neuropsychological endophenotypes in the search for genes associated with bipolar affective disorder. Bipolar Disord, (2004). , 171-182.

[94] Martinez-aran, A, et al. Treatment nonadherence and neurocognitive impairment in bipolar disorder. J Clin Psychiatry, (2009).

[95] Martinez-aran, A, et al. Executive function in patients with remitted bipolar disorder and schizophrenia and its relationship with functional outcome. Psychother Psychosom, (2002)., 39-46.

[96] Goodwin, G. M, et al. Cognitive impairment in bipolar disorder: neurodevelopment or neurodegeneration? An ECNP expert meeting report. Eur Neuropsychopharmacol, (2008)., 787-793.

[97] Wykes, T. Cognitive remediation therapy needs funding. Nature, (2010)., 165-166.

[98] Anaya, C, et al. A systematic review of cognitive remediation for schizo-affective and affective disorders. J Affect Disord, (2012).

Chapter 10

Omega-3 Docosahexaenoic Acid (DHA) and Mood Disorders: Why and How to Provide Supplementation?

Alfonso Valenzuela and Rodrigo Valenzuela

Additional information is available at the end of the chapter

http://dx.doi.org/10.5772/53322

1. Introduction

The cost of brain disorders and mental ill-health has been rising sharply in the last years and in developed and some developing countries now exceeds the cost of other diseases, such as cardiovascular or metabolic diseases (diabetes) [1]. Cognitive decline, particularly in the forms of Alzheimer's disease, has emerged in the last 20 years as a major challenge to health systems affecting the quality of life of the ancient population and of the social and economic environment of the patients and family. Diseases, such as depression, schizophrenia, Huntington's disease and other mood disorders are also rapidly increasing as the life expectancy of the population increases. To reduce the risk of mood disorders and cognitive decline in the elderly it is necessary to consider the possible impact of life style and other non-genetic, but modifiable, risk factors. Diet is one of these modifiable factors that may contribute to the prevention or amelioration of chronic neurodegenerative diseases. Among the dietary nutrients most closely associated with the optimal development and function of the brain and nervous system, docosahexaenoic acid (22:6, DHA) an omega-3 fatty acid, exclusively of marine origin, is at present particularly relevant [2].

In this chapter various functions of DHA in the nervous system, its metabolism into phospholipids, and its involvement in different neurological and mood disorders, such as Alzheimer's diseases, depression and bipolar disorders, cognitive decline, aggression, hostility and antisocial behavior, schizophrenia, among others are revised. It is also discussed the different alternatives now available to provide DHA supplementation to prevent or ameliorate mood disorders. There is now different dietary and supplementary form to provide DHA, such as ethyl esters, triglycerides, partial glycerides, phospholipids, etc. [3]. The importance of nutraceuticals of new development based on DHA and other components is also included in our discussion. Figure 1 shows the molecular structure of DHA.

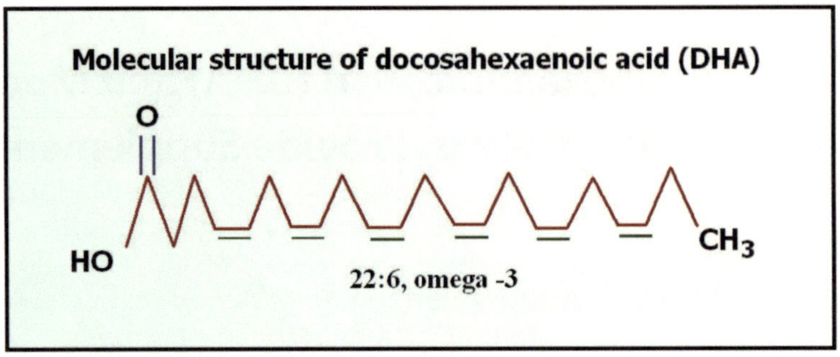

Figure 1.

2. Fatty acids in the brain and nervous system

The brain and the nervous system are the tissues with high content of two polyunsaturated fatty acids: arachidonic acid (20:4, omega-6, AA) and DHA, this last fatty acid being the most important omega-3 long-chain fatty acid in the brain phospholipids, comprising 25% of the total fatty acids of the gray matter. DHA has been the only omega-3 fatty acid used as a major structural and functional component of photoreceptors of the visual system and neurons, and their signaling synaptic structures throughout million years of human evolution [4]. Despite their abundance in these tissues AA and DHA cannot be re-synthesized in mammals. However, the concentration of these fatty acids can be modulated by dietary intake. AA and DHA must be provided by the diet as such (preformed) or through the respective omega-6 and omega-3 precursors from vegetable origin. Linoleic acid (18:2, omega-6, AL) the precursor of AA, is very abundant in the western diet and therefore the formation of AA from AL is not restrictive for humans. On the other hand, alpha linolenic acid, (18:3, omega-3, ALA) the precursor of DHA is less available in our diet and preformed DHA, which is only provided from food of marine origin, is highly restrictive in some populations [5]. The majority of DHA present in the human brain is incorporated during the brain growth spurt which starts at week 26 of gestation and imposes a high demand for the fatty acid until about 2 years of age. DHA is required when neuronal and glial differentiation and migration, and active myelination and synaptogenesis took place in the brain morphogenesis. There is now convincing evidence that neural developmental milestones, determine long-term brain functional capacity in adults [6]. It is supposed that when brain milestones has passed it may be too late to intervene with omega-3 long-chain fatty acids in neurological/neuropsychological disorders such as, depression, and bipolar disorder, mood and cognition, schizophrenia, Alzheimer's disease and Huntington's disease, among others neurological diseases. It has been demonstrate that as the individual ages, a constant reduction of the DHA content of the brain occurs, and in some neurological diseases, such as Alzheimer's disease, a more pronounced reduction of the fatty acid occurs. Epidemiological evidence now suggest that a decrease in brain DHA levels, which normally occurs during aging, and that is exacerbated by reduced dietary intake of DHA, may increase the preva-

http://dx.doi.org/10.5772/53322

lence of neurological diseases. The identification of several DHA-derived metabolites (such as resolvins and neuroprotectins, among others), probably involved in cell signaling suggest that free DHA, liberated from membrane phospholipids, is utilized to perform many other functions beyond a structural role in membrane phospholipids of neuronal cells. The first DHA-derived metabolite is neuroprotectin D1 which can be synthesized from free DHA through a lipoxygenase enzyme [7]. Neuroprotectin D1 is generated during stroke and counteracts pro-inflammatory gene expression that normally results from ischemic damage. Neuroprotectin D1 has anti-inflammatory, antiapoptotic and even neuroregenerative effects, which would help to preserve in general, both the neuronal functioning and the nervous system [8]. This molecule also counteracts potential oxidative damage to DNA in the retinal pigment ephitelium cells [9]. Research about food and/or additives that preferentially provide DHA and molecules that promote its internalization, transport and metabolism will be of basic importance to fully understand the importance in the development, normal function, senescence, and pathology of the nervous system. Basic, clinical and epidemiologic research supports a protective effect of DHA in mood disorders.

3. DHA in the brain cells

Within neurons DHA is almost specifically concentrated in membrane phospholipids, mainly at phosphatidylethanolamine and phosphatidylserine, the latter being the major acidic phospholipid present in brain cell membranes [10]. Phospholipids which make up about one quarter of the solid matter in the brain are also an integral part of the vascular system from which brain cells function and nutrition depend. DHA constitutes 15-20% of the total fatty acid composition of the brain cortex, and when incorporated into phospholipids may improve the efficiency of synaptic membrane vesicles in fusion events (i.e., synaptic vesicles with terminal axonal membrane) which are fundamental for neurotransmission [11]. DHA may also function in synaptic signaling, either as a free fatty acid, as a metabolite (such as, neuroprotectins) or incorporated into phospholipids structure. DHA is also highly concentrated in growth cones during neurite outgrowth were it may be important for maximal neurite growth during brain development, which occurs mainly during the perinatal period [12]. In the adult, DHA is found in neuronal dendrites, where it may be involved in the extension and establishment of the dendritic arborization which occurs during memory formation and acquisition of learning capabilities, modifications which originate the so-called brain plasticity. Additionally, DHA may be important for the efficient regeneration of axons and dendrites in some brain regions, such as cerebellum and hippocampus, after brain injury. Supplementing cultured neuronal cell types with AA and DHA at low concentrations significantly increases neurite outgrowth in several neuronal cell types, principally those from hippocampus [13]. However, there is a limit to the amount of AA to be added because at higher concentrations this fatty acid may be cytotoxic. DHA, however, shows stimulant effects and no cytotoxicity in a wide range of concentrations [14].

3.1. The role of DHA in neuronal phospholipid synthesis

DHA appears to enhance neurite outgrowth be several mechanisms which include an increase in the synthesis of specific phospholipids [13]. In differentiating and mature neurons DHA is preferentially incorporated into phospholipids than into triglycerides. During the synthesis of neuronal phospholipids, DHA is acylated to the sn-2 position of phospholipids to generate phosphatidic acid, which is the precursor of phosphatidylinositol, which in turns is the precursor of inositoltriphosphate (IP3) an important second messenger signal. However, most of the phosphatidic acid is subsequently dephosphorylated to generate diacylglycerol, which is further metabolized into phosphatidylcholine, phosphatidylethanolamine and phosphatidylserine, all of these molecules containing DHA at the sn-2 position [13]. Therefore, it appears that diacylglycerols containing DHA at the sn-2 position are preferentially transformed into phospholipids. This specific transformation occurs through the action of specific enzymes. For example, diacylglycerol molecules that contain DHA at the sn-2 position are the preferred substrate of enzyme ethanolamine phosphotransferase which convert diacylglycerol to phosphatidylethanolamine through the covalent linking of ethanolamine to the sn-3 position of diacylglycerol [15]. Phosphatidylethanolamine may also be converted to phosphatidylserine through the exchange of its nitrogen base with free serine [16].

3.2. The role of DHA in membrane neuronal function

The quantity of double bonds in a fatty acid is directly related to the flexibility of the molecule. Saturated fatty acids, such as palmitic acid (16:0) or stearic acid (18:0) are rigid. This rigidity allows saturated fatty acids to pack together tightly and form a solid structure at lower temperatures. Phospholipids formed by these fatty acids are also rigid structures. The introduction of double bonds into a fatty acid introduces a "kink" in its structure which modifies its spatial conformation. DHA, which has six double bonds, may adopt many countless conformation because the molecule can rotate around C-C bonds but not around the rigid C=C bonds that conform its high polyunsaturation [17]. The highly flexible structure of DHA will not allow phospholipids containing DHA to pack tightly together, resulting in a significant increase in membrane fluidity relative to phospholipids formed only by saturated fatty acids. Membranes having high content of DHA may also increase the efficiency of membrane fusion events which are important in neurotransmission [18]. Additionally, an increased fluidity of membrane appears to be important for increasing the rate at which membrane protein-protein interaction occurs within the phospholipid membrane bilayer. Fluidity is especially relevant in the outer segments of retinal photoreceptors where the activation of G type protein transducin by the rhodopsin-metarhodopsin interaction events occurs within the phospholipids of photoreceptors cells. This process does not occur efficiently when the level of DHA in the phospholipids of vision cells is reduced either during normal aging or by pathological causes [19]. Mitochondrial phospholipids are also enriched in DHA. High DHA in mitochondrial membranes may increase the efficiency of the electron transport chain and the ADP-phosphorilation process by increasing the lateral movement of protein within the membrane bilayer, thus facilitating protein-protein interactions [20]. Additionally, there is a direct correlation between the DHA content of mitochondrial phospholipids and the permeability of the inner membrane to protons [21], thus improving the efficiency of energy production through oxidative phosphorylation. It is generally concluded that DHA positively influences mitochondrial energy production, which is crucial in a cell highly demanding of energy, such is the neuron.

3.3. DHA and the activity of neuronal enzymes

Receptor functioning and the activation of membrane proteins involved in signaling transduction can be influenced by DHA, either as a free fatty acid and/or when it is incorporated into membrane phospholipids. DHA is concentrated in the phospholipids of neuronal tissues, including hippocampus and cerebellum, which are involved in learning as well as in memory storage [22]. Most recently we demonstrated that DHA supplementation to mother rats during the perinatal period, increases the DHA content of different brain segments of the pups, including hippocampus and cerebellum, and improves the learning and memory capacities of the pups when evaluated through the Skinner box test [23]. As part of the diacylglycerol molecule, DHA may enhance the diacylglycerol-dependent activation of the protein kinase C (PKC) [24]. It is interesting that PKC has an essential requirement for phosphatidylserine [25], which contains a high concentration of DHA. However, in vitro evidence is suggesting that unesterified DHA may competitively inhibit phosphatidylserine dependent PKC inhibition. Unesterified AA either stimulates or has no effect on PKC activity [26], showing that activation of the enzyme by omega-3 fatty acids may be specific to these fatty acids. Another example of an enzyme whose function is modified by DHA is Na+/K+ ATPase, also known as sodium pump, which is an integral protein of the neuronal membrane found in higher concentration at the axonal nodes (Ranvier nodes). The primary neuronal function of these ATPases is to generate and maintain Na+ and K+ gradients which are necessary to maintain the resting potential of the neuronal membrane. The activity of Na+/K+ ATPase is increased in the sciatic nerve of rats that are supplemented with DHA [27].

3.4. Inhibition of neuronal apoptosis by DHA

Neuronal cell survival is highly dependent on the presence of trophic nerve factors which influence downstream signalling pathways. Modifications in the concentration and/or number of these factors may lead to apoptotic cell death. Early signs of apoptosis include the loss of intracellular water, an increase in cytoplasmic calcium concentration, the releasing of cytochrome c from mitochondria and the translocation of phosphatidylserine to the outer leaflet of the plasma membrane [28]. The activation of the caspase-3 enzyme by self-cleavage results in the death of cells by apoptosis [29]. The prevention of apoptosis by DHA incorporation into phospholipids has been reported for rat retinal photoreceptors [30], HL-60 cells [31], and Neuro 2A cells [32]. Additionally, an increased dietary intake of DHA prevents apoptosis in mouse retinal photoreceptors when subjected to N-methyl-N-nitroso urea, a potent inducer of apoptosis [33]. DHA accumulation in phospholipids, mainly in phosphatidylserine, appears to promote neuronal survival under adverse conditions [32]. As discussed above, in the nervous system, DHA is incorporated primarily into anionic phospholipids such as phosphatidylserine and phosphatidylethanolamine [34]. Phosphatidylserine is synthesized from phosphatidylethanolamine or phosphatidylcholine by the serine replacement of ethanolamine or choline, respectively, in a base-exchange reaction. Phosphatidylserine is involved in a series of cell signaling events. The supplementation of cells with unesterified DHA promotes phosphatidylserine biosynthesis [35]. The enrichment of DHA in phosphatidylserine and its effect on phosphatidylserine biosynthesis are most likely due to the fact that phospholipid species containing DHA are the best substrates for phosphatidylserine synthesizing enzymes [36]. There is not a direct correlation between the level of phosphatidylserine and DHA content in different brain segments. The antiapoptotic effect of DHA in neurons occurs only when the fatty acid is added to cultured cells or when experimental animals have been treated previously with DHA, which may suggest that these effects are due to the incorporation of DHA into different phospholipids. It is interesting to note that in other non-neuronal cell types, DHA actually promotes apoptosis. For example, in CaCo-2 cells, a colon cancer cell line, DHA induces apoptosis by "down regulating" reducing the expression of antiapoptotic genes and increasing the expression of proapoptotic genes [37]. Therefore, the antiapoptotic effects of DHA-containing phosphatidylserine are probably specific to neuronal cells and critical for the long-term survival of these cells.

3.5. DHA and the regulation of gene expression in neurons

It has been demonstrated that polyunsaturated omega-3 fatty acids can modify gene expression by binding to specific receptors and transcription factors in the liver and adipose tissue. Receptors activated by DHA include retinoid X, peroxisome proliferator activated receptors (PPARs), hepatic nuclear receptor, and sterol regulatory element binding protein (SREBP) receptor [38]. The activation of each of these proteins modulates the expression of genes involved in the metabolism of glucose, fatty acids, triglycerides, and cholesterol. Of these proteins, the retinoid X receptor is present in significant levels in the brain, and DHA is an effective ligand and activator of the retinoid X receptor protein [39]. Activation of gene expression by DHA is not restricted to brain cells, the fatty acid activates several genes in other tissues, like liver or adipose tissue [40]. In rat brain cells, the stimulation of peroxisomal proliferator activated receptor β (PPAR β) resulted in the up regulation of the mRNA encoding a protein that converted DHA to the acyl-CoA derivative [41]. Upon alteration of the expression of genes involved in lipid metabolism, the optimal environment for neurite outgrowth can be achieved during neuronal differentiation and brain formation. For example, omega-6 and omega-3 PUFAs have been shown to decrease the expression and the activity of Δ-9 desaturase, the enzyme that converts stearic acid (18:0) to oleic acid (18:1, omega-9). This effect may be important to ensure that saturated fatty acids, whether newly synthesized or taken in from the diet, are available for the insertion of phospholipids into the sn-1 position as they are synthesized. Several studies have demonstrated that the DHA increasing effect on neurite outgrowth may be, in part, a consequence of the DHA stimulation of the expression of genes that promote phospholipids synthesis [42,43]. Using microarray gene expression methodology, it has been demonstrated that fish oil or DHA supplementation can modify the expression of many of the genes of the brain and retina involved in signal transduction, eicosanoid production, synaptic plasticity, and energy metabolism in rats [44].

4. DHA and alterations of neuronal functioning in mood disorders

Accelerated cognitive decline in middle age can make an individual more vulnerable to mood disorders in later life. Experts agree that once cognitive decline is accelerated and properly identify, it is advisable a prompt intervention [2]. During periods of nutritional deficiency of omega-3 fatty acids, DHA is retained to depletion from the phospholipids of neurons through two possible mechanisms: a) DHA released from membrane phospholipids is rapidly reacylated to specific phospholipids. b) It is produced a significant reduction in the rate of transfer of DHA out of the nervous system through the blood brain barrier. Many neurodegenerative conditions, such as Alzheimer's disease, retinal affections, and some peroxisomal disorders (Zellweger syndrome and adrenoleucodistrophy) are associated with reduced levels of omega-3 fatty acids. Mood disorders, such as depression, schizophrenia, and post-partum depression, have also been associated with modification of DHA metabolism. Epidemiological, experimental and clinical research support the hypothesis that DHA may play a role in the pathogenesis and eventually in the prevention and/or in treatment of these diseases [45,46].

4.1. Alzheimer's disease

Alzheimer's disease is a late-onset progressive, neurodegenerative disease of heterogeneous origin which is devastating both to the afflicted person and to the person's family. Before the dementia which characterizes the pathology is established, Alzheimer's disease may manifest through subtle cognitive decline greater than expected for an individual's age and education but with minimal impact on daily living. This transitory and still reversible stage is usually termed mild cognitive impairment [47]. However, once it is clinically diagnosed there is little prospect of improving the prognosis. The pathology is characterized by the formation of amyloid plaques, neurofibrillary tangles, and dystrophic neuritis. Data from numerous epidemiological studies suggest an inverse correlation between DHA intake and the likelihood of developing Alzheimer's disease. A reduction in the level of total phospholipids, as well as a decrease of DHA, has been described in various cerebral areas in Alzheimer's disease patients [48]. With aging, neural membrane fluidity is compromised due to the increased presence of cholesterol, and reduced activity of glial desaturase enzymes and blockages to phospholipids pathways of transduction signals and oxidative stress, all of which are inversely associated with omega-3 polyunsaturated fatty acids [49]. These processes are highly exacerbated in Alzheimer's patients. Brain autopsies of Alzheimer's disease patients have shown significantly higher saturated fatty acid and lower omega-3 polyunsaturated fatty acid content in the hippocampus and frontal lobes which govern memory and executive functions, respectively [50]. Studies have demonstrated that the levels of phosphatidylethanolamine, which is enriched in DHA, and phosphatidylinositol, which is enriched in AA, are significantly reduced in the brain of individuals affected by Alzheimer's disease. Specifically there is a significant reduction in the amount of DHA in the frontal cortex and hippocampus phospholipids of patients with Alzheimer's diseases. Alzheimer's disease is characterized by the accumulation of various β amyloid (Aβ) peptides resulting from the cleavage of the amyloid precursor protein, in particular peptides composed of 40 (Aβ 40) and 42 (Aβ 42) aminoacids. Aβ peptide is produced constitutively during cell metabolism but under normal conditions, the peptide does not accumulate in brain. It has been proposed that the central event in Alzheimer's disease pathogenesis is an imbalance between Aβ peptide production and clearance, with increased Aβ peptide production and/or decreased Aβ clearance during the onset of the pathology [51]. The pretreatment of rats with DHA protected the animals against the memory loss which typically occurs when animals are infused with Alzheimer's disease Aβ peptide, which triggers synapse destruction [52]. DHA inhibits the accumulation of insoluble Aβ peptide, partially by decreasing cholesterol levels in the detergent insoluble neuronal membrane domains (rafts) of the cerebral cortex [53] and this effect is strongly influenced by the age of animals [54]. It has been demonstrated that the effect of DHA in the reduction of insoluble Aβ peptide is attributable to a decrease in steady-state levels of presenilin 1 [55]. In cognitive test animals expressing high levels of a mutant amyloid precursor protein, showed low levels of DHA in brain phospholipids. Additionally, the activity of phospholipase A2, which is involved in the liberation of AA from brain phospholipids, increases in the brain of patients with Alzheimer´s disease, suggesting that an increased generation of AA-derived eicosanoids, which are antagonist of DHA-derived docosanoids, may contribute to the etiology of Alzheimer's disease. It has been proposed that DHA-derived neuroprotectin D1 induces an antiapoptotic and neuroprotective gene expression program that regulates the secretion of Aβ peptide, resulting in the modulation of inflammatory signaling, neuronal survival, and the preservation of brain function [7]. The typical Western diet provided < 30% of the 200-300 mg/day of DHA recommended by Expert Panels. Epidemiology show a risk reduction of 60% associated with a modest increase in DHA intake or plasma levels. DHA may works well in slowing down Alzheimer´s disease pathogenesis in mice with a human Alzheimer's disease gene [56]. DHA provided by supplementation (e.g. fish meals, fish oil capsules, or other forms of DHA supplementation), could restore DHA deficiency in membrane phospholipids in the cerebral cortex of patients with Alzheimer's disease [57]. DHA together with natural antioxidants, may exert general anti-Alzheimer's and anti-aging benefits [58]. Studies have indicated the apparently crucial role of DHA in preventing Alzheimer's disease in its very mild, precocious stages [46]. However, studies on the exact molecular mechanism underlying the beneficial effects of DHA are required to validate the hypothesis that changing dietary habits or promoting dietary supplementation with DHA can considerably improve human health and specially may prevent, or delay, the onset of cognitive impairment in mild cases of Alzheimer's disease.

4.2. Depression and postpartum depression

Depression is characterized by high levels of depressed or low mood, a lost in interest or pleasure in nearly all activities, changes in appetite, weight, sleep or activity, decreased energy, difficulties in thinking, concentration or making decisions, feeling or worthlessness or guilt, and recurrent thoughts of death or suicidal ideation, plans or attempts. Depression and major depressive disorder are serious affective illness with a high lifetime prevalence rate that particularly involves neurotransmission processes, especially serotonin receptors and membrane transporters [59]. The World Health Organization estimates that depressive disorder will become the second leading cause of disability worldwide by 2020, second to ischemic heart disease, and will be the leading cause in developing regions [60]. The etiology of the illness is multifactorial and is influenced by genetic, environmental and nutritional factors. Epidemiologic, neurobiologic, and clinical studies suggest that a relative deficiency in omega-3 polyunsaturated fatty acids contributes to depression. Support for a nutritional contribution to the disease derives from studies that report an inverse correlation between the level of omega-3 fatty acids as measured either in red blood cells phospholipids or adipose tissue, and symptoms of depression. An increasing ratio omega-6/omega-3 is frequently observed in patients with depression [61]. Numerous studies carry-out over the last few years are involving omega-3 long-chain fatty acid supplementation with the reduction of any of the symptoms of different forms of depression, including bipolar disorders, postpartum depression (included forward), agoraphobia, and anorexia nervosa. According to meta-analysis realized by Lin and Su [62], it is concluded that DHA supplementation may reduce the symptoms of depression. Depression and coronary artery disease often occurs in the same individuals who frequently have low plasma levels of DHA and high levels of AA. Omega-3 supplementation shows as effective for the treatment of these disorders. Reducing omega-6 polyunsaturated fatty acid intake as well as increasing omega-3 polyunsaturated fatty acids, specifically DHA, for a more balanced ratio may be beneficial [63]. However, the mechanism by which DHA may reduce depression is still unclear, and more research is needed. As discussed, increasing the nutritional level of omega-3 fatty acids may modify the activity of integral membranes proteins (receptors, ion channels, molecular pumps, etc.), and/or counteract the proinflammatory action of AA-derived eicosanoids. However, there is no consensus about the positive effect of omega-3 fatty acids in depression which is accompanied with other comorbid. Lespérance et al. [64] not observed significant differences of omega-3 supplementation over placebo in reducing depressive symptoms in patients with anxiety comorbid, but the same researchers observed a clear benefit of omega-3 supplementation in patients without comorbid anxiety disorders.

Depression during pregnancy and postpartum depression have negative impact on the development and health of the newborn. Maternal stress in humans is associated with fetal hypoxia, reduced gestational age, and low birth weight. Evans et al., in an study comprising different countries found that 13.5% of women (n= 14,451) experienced serious symptoms of depression during pregnancy and postpartum [65]. A cross-national analysis of seafood consumption, and the DHA content of breast milk, demonstrated an inverse correlation with the prevalence of pregnancy and postpartum depression. The prevalence varied from 0.5% in Singapore to 24.5% in South Africa, with a mean prevalence worldwide of 12.4%. Both, higher national seafood consumption and higher DHA content in the mother's breast milk predicted a lower prevalence of postpartum depression. The mean DHA intake of western women is estimated at 15-20 mg/day, whereas intake of countries with high fish consumption (e.g Japan, Korea and Norway) is approximately 1000 mg/day. During the third gestational trimester, the fetus accumulates an average of 67 mg/day of DHA, in excess of dietary intake of many mothers. Such transfer to the baby through the placenta and, subsequently through breast milk poses a risk to women to significant depletion of omega-3 fatty acids during lactation, contributing to the perinatal risk of depression. A review by Parker et al., about omega-3 fatty acids and postpartum depression, proposed that DHA supplementation in the perinatal period may have additional benefits to the infant's neurodevelopment. Women and their physicians prefer options to standard antidepressant medication during pregnancy and postpartum. DHA supplementation during these periods may be a plausible alternative. However, more clinical trials are needed to confirm the recommendation of omega-3 fatty acid supplementation to avoid or reduce symptoms of depression [3].

4.3. Schizophrenia

Schizophrenia is defined by a mixture of characteristics (positive and negative) signs and symptoms which have been present for a significant proportion of time during a one-month period with indications of the disorder persisting for at least six months. Positive symptoms reflect an extension or distortion of normal functions, for example, delusions, hallucinations, and disorganized speech or behavior. Negative symptoms reflect a diminution or loss of normal functions, for example, restrictions in the range or intensity of emotional expression, restriction in the fluency or productivity of thought or speech, and restrictions in the initiation of goal-directed behavior [66]. Schizophrenia is a psychiatric disease that affects 1-1.5% of the population with higher prevalence in males than in females. The predominant hypothesis regarding the pathophysiology of the disease is dysfunction of the dopaminergic system. However further finding concerning the disease suggests a close relationship with reduced tissue levels of omega-6 and omega-3 fatty acids specially AA and DHA [67]. A "phospholipid membrane hypothesis of schizophrenia" emerged in the late 1970's [68]. This hypothesis encompasses abnormalities of long-chain omega-6 (AA) and omega-3 (DHA) fatty acids. Fenton et al., list multiple analyses of red blood cell membranes (recognized markers for essential fatty acid status) that consistently document depletion of AA and DHA [68]. This depletion is also observed in plasma, thrombocytes and post-mortem brain tissue of schizophrenia patients. Several mechanism could explain these deficits, including an increased activity of phospholipase A2 thus producing the extraction of AA and DHA from cerebral membrane phospholipids [69]. Another argument in favor of a relationship between schizophrenia and omega-6/omega-3 fatty acids is that dietary supplementation of either AA and DHA or their precursors is able to alleviate the symptoms of the disease [70]. Tissue omega-3 and omega-6 levels are negatively and positively associated with the hostility and aggressive behavior in patients with schizophrenia [71]. It has been proposed that an alteration of DHA metabolism in the brain is involved in the pathophysiology of schizophrenia and that omega-3 fatty acid supplementation may be an important coadjutant in the treatment of the disease [72]. It seems therefore that schizophrenia might be an example of a disease in which omega-6 and omega-3 supplementation, presumably AA and DHA, associated with pharmacological treatment might be beneficial, although extended evaluation of such complementary treatment is still required [68].

4.4. Aggression, hostility and anti-social behavior

The role of diet in aggression, hostility and anti-social behavior has been extensity revised and a relationship with omega-3 fatty acid has been established [73]. Epidemiological studies have suggested a link between poor omega-3 fatty acid status and aggression, hostility and anti-social behavior. A negative correlation between seafood consumption and homicide mortality statistics has been observed in many countries [74]. The result of intervention studies with omega-3 fatty acids (DHA) plus other ingredients have been, however, equivocal. The study populations have been heterogeneous, sometimes with a small number of subjects. Despite this, there are some encouraging data emerging. Studies in prisoners in the USA have provided some support regarding micronutrients and omega-3 fatty acids as it was observed a 30% reduction in violence among a small population of young violent offenders in prison. However for more accurate results, the study needs to be replicated on a larger scale. The general conclusion is that high dietary intake of DHA may be related to lower likelihood of high hostility in young adulthood [75]. This is clearly an area where more research is required, particularly in defined populations with large number of subjects.

4.5. Retinal function and pathologies

Retinal pathologies are not directly involved with mood disorders. However, retinal tissue is derived from neuronal cells and DHA is essential for the proper development and functioning of this visual tissue. The fatty acid is particularly concentrated in the outer membrane segments of the photoreceptors cells, cones and rods. DHA is required for the survival of retinal photoreceptors and exerts a protective effect on apoptosis of these photoreceptors during visual development [36]. Retinitis pigmentosa is a visual disease with a worldwide prevalence of 1 in 4000 individuals [76]. Photoreceptor cell degeneration is a feature of the disease and the death of these cells in many instances seems to involve closely associated retinal pigment epithelial cells. Under normal circumstances, both cell types are subjected to potentially damaging stimuli (e.g. sunlight and high oxygen tension). However, the mechanism by which homeostasis is maintained in this part of the ye, which is crucial for sight, are an unsolved riddle. A correlation between retinitis pigmentosa and low retinal DHA levels has been observed, were evidence show that the synthesis of DHA is impaired in patients suffering from X-linked retinitis pigmentosa [32]. Supplementation with DHA (400 mg/day) for four years produces a significant reduction in the loss of functionality of rods in patients with retinitis pigmentosa, as assessed by an electroretinogram which measures the photoreceptor activity. For patients with retinitis pigmentosa beginning vitamin A therapy, together with DHA (1200 mg/day), slowed the evolution of the decline in visual field sensitivity [77]. It has been suggested that DHA upon its transformation in neuroprotectin D1 may inhibit oxidative stress-mediated proinflammatory gene induction and apoptosis, and consequently promotes retinal pigment epithelial cell survival [78]. Results suggest that early intervention with DHA, may be important in slowing down the progression of retinitis pigmentosa.

5. Possible mechanism for links between DHA and mood disorders

Several neurophysiological mechanisms have been proposed to explain the relationship between omega-3 polyunsaturated fatty acids and mood disorders [79]. DHA appears to decrease the production of inflammatory eicosanoids from AA by means two mechanisms:

First, DHA compete with AA for incorporation into membrane phospholipids, thus decreasing both cellular and plasma levels of AA. Second, DHA, compete with AA for cyclooxygenase enzyme system, inhibiting the production of proinflammatory eicosanoids derived from AA (e.g. prostaglandins, leukotrienes, thromboxanes). Prostagladin E2 and thromboxane B2 have linked to depression. DHA also inhibits the release of proinflammatory cytokines such as interleukin-1 beta, interleukin 2, interleukin 6, interferon gamma, and tumor necrosis factor alpha, which depends on eicosanoid release and are also associated with mood disorders, such as depression [80]. Another possible mechanism relates to the abundance of DHA in brain phospholipids were they play a vital role in maintaining the integrity and fluidity of neuronal membranes. By varying the lipid concentration in cell membranes, changes in fluidity can affect either the structure and/or functioning of proteins embedded in the membrane, including enzymes, receptors, ion channels, molecular pumps, leading to changes in cellular signaling [45]. Support for the involvement of DHA in receptor functioning, neurotransmitter levels and the metabolism of monoamines implicated in mood disorders has been provided by animal studies [81].

6. How to provide DHA supplementation

After the suggestion years ago of Expert Committees to include omega-3 long-chain polyunsaturated fatty acids from marine origin in infant formulas, efforts were made to identify suitable sources for these fatty acids, mainly DHA. Refined and deodorized fish oil was initially used because of it availability and relatively high content of DHA. However many concerns related to different levels of contamination of fish oil with heavy metals and organic compounds encouraged seeking others sources for DHA supplementation. Today the recommendation has been also extended to adults and especially to those going to elderly, due the possible beneficial effect of DHA supplementation to prevent mood and neurodegenerative diseases. At present, new other sources for DHA supplementation are available to provide the fatty acids in variable amounts and degrees of purity. The advantages/disadvantages of these DHA sources are discussed.

6.1. Free DHA and DHA-ethyl ester

Since fish oil contains a mixture of triacylglyerols with various fatty acids, the concentration of DHA may be relatively low (not higher than 18%, such as tuna or salmon oil). However, higher concentrations of DHA can be achieved from the hydrolysis of fish oil and further separation of selected fatty acids, such as DHA, by column chromatography or molecular distillation. Pure preparations of DHA as free fatty acid or as DHA-ethyl ester have been developed for supplementation. Pure DHA, as free fatty acid, may cause gastrointestinal complaints [82] and is very unstable to oxidation and difficult to be incorporated to food preparations (milk, dairy products, juices, etc.). Ethyl ester preparations have not side-effect and are less unstable than DHA free form. Although DHA-ethyl ester preparation has been used in several experimental protocols [83], the efficacy of these products is controversial due the low absorption efficiency observed in the intestinal tract [84]. Emulsions, soft capsules and beverages containing DHA ethyl ester are widely available in some western and oriental countries

6.2. Single cell algae DHA-rich oil

Some marine algae produce naturally large amounts of DHA that can be extracted from collected cells as a clear, odorless algae oil having concentrations up to 40% of DHA [85]. Antioxidants (tocopherols or some others natural antioxidants) are added to the oil to prevent oxidation. Algae oil rich in DHA has been considered a substance "Generally Recognized as Safe" (GRAS) by the US-FDA having good stability and biological availability. Algae oil can be added to a wide variety of food and nutraceutical products. The oil can also be microencapsulated allowing its incorporation to powdered foods to be reconstituted just when served.

6.3. DHA from egg yolk and marine phospholipids

Much evidence gleaned from animal studies (rodents and primates) indicates fatty acids are more available when provided in the form of phospholipids than triglycerides or ethyl esters [86]. Egg yolk is a complex oil/water emulsion containing 32% lipids. A substantial fraction of these lipids are phospholipids containing on average 0.4 – 0.6% of DHA. These concentrations can be increased by feeding laying hens with linseed oil, canola oil or directly with fish oil. Under these conditions DHA can be increased to 1.5 – 2.0% (150 – 170 mg DHA/yolk). Industrially, egg yolk powder is treated with solvents to isolate lipids and phospholipids and thereafter phospholipids are extracted by emulsifying with water followed by spray-drying. Egg yolk phospholipids can be safety incorporated to a wide variety of food products as has been used for many years to increase DHA content (and also AA content) of infant formulas and represent an interesting alternative for the development foods or supplements for the aged population.

Marine phospholipids are a more recently alternative to provide DHA. The main source for these phospholipids which have up to 20% DHA is krill (*Euphausia superba*), a small crustacean which is massively captured in the Antarctic sea. Krill is thought to be the largest single biomass on the planet and is life sustaining food for diverse marine animals [87]. The product obtained after processing krill is intense red colored oil, due its high concentration of carotenes (mainly astaxantin) which provided high stability to the oil. Due its coloration it is not suitable to be added to foods and is used mainly for the preparation of dark capsules. Also, dietary oils extracted from other crustacean (*Calanus finmarchicus*), have interesting features. Calanus oil is comprised of omega-3 fatty acids incorporated to phospholipids and to wax esters having a relatively high content of astaxantin [88]. Phospholipids containing DHA are also obtained from the enzymatic digestion of whole fatty fish, salmon or sardine by-products (viscera's) or salmon eggs [89].

6.4. sn-2 DHA monoacylglyceride

This is a new experimental source for providing DHA supplementation. It is a monoacylglyceride containing DHA at the sn-2 (central position) of the glycerol molecule, which is obtained from the controlled enzymatic hydrolysis of refined salmon oil [90]. The bioavailability of the product has been assayed in rats showing a high intestinal absorption and producing a high tissue accretion of DHA in animals [91]. The product, which contains added tocopherols as antioxidant, can be easily incorporated into water due its emulsifying properties that allow its incorporation into water-containing beverages, milk, milk-derived products, and also to baked products and sausages. The product is currently assayed by our group in the development of juices and soups for the elderly population which receive public nutritional support in Chile.

7. Conclusions and future prospects

The effectiveness of strategies involving DHA to reduce the risk of Alzheimer's disease or other cognitive and mood disorders depend on a good understanding of how the low intake or low tissue levels of DHA would increase the risk of these diseases. Solid basis now exist to believe that low DHA intake may contribute significantly to the early onset of cognitive and mood diseases, and that the supplementation with DHA may have substantial benefits. Epidemiological evidence suggest that a decrease in brain DHA levels, which normally occurs during elderly, and that it is exacerbated by reduced dietary intake of DHA, may increase the prevalence of several neurological diseases as such discussed in this chapter. However at present we do not understood at all the complex functions that DHA performs as either as free fatty acid and/or incorporated to neuronal phospholipids. The identification of several DHA-derived metabolites, probably involved in cell signaling, suggest that DHA is utilized to perform many functions beyond a structural role in phospholipids and membrane structure. Future research about food and/or additives that preferentially provide DHA and molecules that promote its internalization, transport and metabolism is clearly needed to understand the importance of DHA in the development, normal function and senescence of the brain and nervous system. Establishing the functions of DHA in the brain will be critical to evaluate the health implications of a reduced dietary intake of DHA as occurs in western populations, and the importance of DHA supplementation at the early stages of human life. The optimal duration of DHA supplementation, allowing a clinical benefit to be observed, still needs to be established. Basic, clinical and epidemiological research supports the importance of DHA in mood disorders. However, results are at present not fully convincing and in some case confounding and more research is definitively needed. Probably in the next years we will have more solid evidences about the function of DHA in the brain and nervous system and of its preventive or ameliorative effect in mood disorders.

Acknowledgements

The authors are grateful from FONDECYT, FONDEF and INNOVA-Chile the support of their research.

Author details

Alfonso Valenzuela[1] and Rodrigo Valenzuela[2*]

*Address all correspondence to: rvalenzuelab@med.uchile.cl

1 Lipid Center, Nutrition and Food Technology Institute, University of Chile. Faculty of Medicine. University of Los Andes, Chile

2 Nutrition and Dietetics School, Faculty of Medicine, University of Chile, Santiago, Chile

References

[1] Andlin-Sobocki, P., Jonsson, B., Wittchen, H., & Olesen, J. (2005). Cost of disorders of the brain in Europe. *Eur J Neurol*, 12, 1-27.

[2] Kidd, P. M. (2007). Omega-3 DHA and EPA for cognition, behavior, and mood: Clinical findings and structural-functional synergies with cell membrane phospholipids. *Altern Med Rev.*, 12, 207-227.

[3] Valenzuela, A., Sanhueza, J., & Nieto, S. (2006). Docosahexaenoic acid (DHA) essentiality and requirements: why and how to provide supplementation. *Grasas & Aceites*, 57, 229-237.

[4] Crawford, M., Bloom, M., Cunnane, S., Holmsen, H., et al. (2001). Docosahexaenoic acid and cerebral evolution. *World Rev Nutr Diet*, 8, 6-17.

[5] Simopoulos, A. (2002). The importance of the ratio omega-6/omega-3 essential fatty acids. *Biomed Phamacother*, 56, 365-379.

[6] Das, U. N. (2003). Long-chain polyunsaturated fatty acids in the growth and development of the brain and memory. *Nutrition*, 19, 62-65.

[7] Lukiw, W., Ciu, J., Marcheselli, V., Bodker, M., et al. (2005). A role of docosahexaenoic acid-derived neuroprotectin D1 in neural cell survival and Alzheimer disease. *J Clin Invest*, 115.

[8] Reinoso, M. A., Mukherjee, P., Marcheselli, V., et al. (2008). PEDF promotes biosynthesis of a novel anti-inflammatory and anti-apoptotic mediator NPD1 in retinal pigment epithelial cells. *Ochsner J*, 8, 39-43.

[9] Serham, C. N. (2005). Novel eicosanoid and docosanoid mediators: resolvins, docosatrienes and neuroprotectins. *Curr Opin Clin Nutr Medtab Care*, 8, 115-121.

[10] Breckenridge, W., Gombos, G., & Morgan, I. G. (1972). The lipid composition of adult rat brain synaptosomal plasma membranes. *Biochim Biophys Acta*, 266, 605-707.

[11] Salem, N., Litman, B., & Kim, H. Y. (2001). Mechanism of action of docosahexaenoic acid in the nervous system. *Lipids*, 36, 1-20.

[12] Martin, R. E., & Bazan, N. (1992). Changing fatty acids content of growth cone lipids prior to synaptogenesis. *J Neurochem*, 59, 318-325.

[13] Calderon, F., & Kim, H. Y. (2004). Docosahexaenoic acid promotes neurite growth in hippocampal neurons. *J Neurochem*, 90, 979-988.

[14] Ikemoto, A., Kobayashi, T., Watanabe, S., & Okuyama, H. (1997). Membrane fatty acid modifications of PC12 cells by arachinodate or docosahexaenoate affect neurite outgrowth but not epinephrine release. *Neurochem Res*, 22, 671-678.

[15] Holub, B. J. (1978). Differential utilization of 1-palmitoyl and 1-stearoyl homologues of various unsaturated 1,2-diacyl-sn-glycerols for phosphatidylcholine and phosphatidylethanolamine synthesis in rat liver microsomes. *J Biol Chem*, 253, 691-696.

[16] Mozzi, R., Buratta, S., & Goracci, G. (2003). Metabolism and function of phosphatidylserine in mammalian brain. *Neurochem Res*, 28, 195-214.

[17] Feller, S. E., Gawrisch, K., & Mac Kerell, A. D. (2002). Polyunsaturated fatty acids in lipid bilayers: intrinsic and environmental contributions to their unique physical properties. *J Am Chem Soc*, 124, 318-326.

[18] Teague, W. E., Fuller, N. L., Rand, R. P., & Gawrisch, K. (2002). Polyunsaturated lipids in membrane fusion events. *Cell Mol Biol Lett*, 7, 262-264.

[19] Niu, S. L., Mitchell, D. C., Lim, S. Y., et al. (2003). Reduced G protein-coupled signaling efficiency in retinal rod outer segments in response to n-3 fatty acid deficiency. *J Biol Chem*, 279, 1098-1104.

[20] Valentine, R. C., & Valentine, D. L. (2004). Omega-3 fatty acids in cellular membranes: a unified concept. *Prog Lipid Res*, 43, 383-402.

[21] Hulbert, A. J. (2003). Life, death and membrane bilayers. *J Exp Biol*, 206, 2303-2311.

[22] Ahmad, A., Moriguchi, T., & Salem, N. (2002). Decrease in neuron size in docosahexaenoic acid-deficient brain. *Pediatr Neurol*, 26, 210-218.

[23] Valenzuela, A., Nieto, S., Sanhueza, J., Morgado, N., & Zañartu, P. (2010). Supplementation of female rats with DHA-lysophosphatidylcholine increases DHA and acetylcholine content of the brain and improves the memory and learning capabilities of the pups. *Grasas & Aceites*, 61, 16-23.

[24] Chen, S. G., & Murakami, K. (1994). Effects of cis-fatty acids on protein kinase C activation and protein phosphorylation in the hippocampus. *J Pharm Sci Technol*, 48, 71-75.

[25] Nichizuka, Y. (1995). Protein kinase C and lipid signaling for sustained cellular responses. *FASEB J*, 9, 484-496.

[26] Seung Kim, H. F., Weeber, E. J., Sweatt, J. D., Stoll, A. L., & Marangell, L. B. (2001). Inhibitory effects of omega-3 fatty acids on protein kinase C activity in vitro. *Mol Psychiatry*, 6, 246-248.

[27] Gerbi, A., Maixent, J. M., Barbey, O., Jamme, I., & Pierlovisi, M. (1998). Alteration of Na, K-ATPase isoenzymes in the rat diabetic neuropathy: protective effect of dietary supplementation with n-3 fatty acids. *J Neurochem*, 71, 732-740.

[28] Sastry, P. S., & Rao, K. S. (2000). Apoptosis and the nervous system. *J Neurochem*, 74, 1-20.

[29] Nagata, S. (1997). Apoptosis by death factor. *Cell*, 88, 355-365.

[30] Rotstein, N. P., Aveldaño, M. I., Barrantes, F. J., Roccamo, A. M., & Politi, L. E. (1997). Apoptosis of retinalphotoreceptors during development in vitro: protective effect of docosahexaenoic acid. *J Neurochem*, 69, 504-513.

[31] Kishida, E., Yano, M., Kasahara, M., & Masuzawa, Y. (1998). Distinctive inhibitory activity of docosahexaenoic acid against sphingosine-induced apoptosis. *Biochim Biophys Acta*, 1391, 401-408.

[32] Kim, H. Y., Akbar, M., Lau, A., & Edsall, L. (2000). Inhibition of neuronal apoptosis by docosahexaenoic acid. J Biol Chem , 45, 35215-35223.

[33] Moriguchi, K., Yuri, T., Yoshizawa, K., Kiuchi, K., & Takada, H. (2003). Dietary docosahexaenoic acid protects against methyl-N-nitrosourea-induced retinal degeneration in rats. *Exp Eye Res*, 77, 167-173.

[34] Aid, S., Vancassel, S., Poumes-Ballihaut, C., Chalon, S., Guesnet, P., & Lavialle, M. (2003). Effect of a diet-induced n-3 PUFA depletion on cholinergic parameters in the rat hippocampus. *J Lipid Res*, 44, 1545-1551.

[35] Kim, H. Y., & Hamilton, J. (2000). Accumulation of docosahexaenoic acid in phosphatidylserine is selectively inhibited by chronic ethanol exposure in C-6 glioma cells. *Lipids*, 3, 187-195.

[36] Kim, H. Y., Bigelow, J., & Kevala, J. H. (2004). Substrate preference in phosphatidylserine biosynthesis for docosahexaenoic acid containing species. *Biochemistry*, 3, 1030-1036.

[37] Narayanan, B. A., Narayanan, K., & Eddy, B. S. (2001). Docosahexaenoic acid regulated genes and transcription factors inducing apoptosis in human colon cancer cells. *Int J Oncol*, 9, 1255-1262.

[38] Mata de Urquiza, A., Liu, S., Sjoberg, M., Zetterstrom, R., Griffiths, W., Sjovall, J., & Perlman, T. (2000). Docosahexaenoic acid, a ligand for the retinoid X receptor in mouse brain. *Science*, 290, 2140-2144.

[39] Lengqvist, J., Mata de Urquiza, A., Bergman, A. C., Willson, T. M., & Sjovall, J. (2004). Polyunsaturated fatty acids including docosahexaenoic acid and arachidonic acid

bind to retinoid X receptor alpha ligand-binding domain. *Mol Cell Proteomics*, 3, 692-703.

[40] Kitajka, K., Puskás, L., Zvara, A., Hackler, L., Barceló-Coblijn, G., Yeo, Y., & Farkas, T. (2002). The role of n-3 polyunsaturated fatty acids in brain: Modulation of brain gene expression by dietary n-3 fatty acids. *Proc Natl Acad Sci USA*, 99, 2619-2624.

[41] Marszalek, J. R., Kitidis, C., Dirusso, C. C., & Lodish, H. F. (2005). Long-chain acyl CoA synthetase 6 preferentially promotes DHA metabolism. *J Biol Chem*, 20, 10817-10826.

[42] Barcelo-Coblijn, G., Hogyes, E., Kitajka, K., Puskas, L. G., & Zvara, A. (2003). Modification by docosahexaenoic acid of age-induced alterations in gene expression and molecular composition of rat brain phospholipids. *Proc Natl Acad Sci USA*, 100, 11321-11326.

[43] Puskas, L. G., Kitajka, K., Nyakas, C., Barcelo-Coblijn, G., & Farkas, T. (2003). Short-term administration of omega-3 fatty acids from fish oil results in increased transthyretin transcription in old rat hippocampus. *Proc Natl Cad Sci USA*, 100, 1580-1585.

[44] Rojas, C. V., Martinez, J. I., Hoffman, D. R., & Uauy, R. (2003). Gene expression analysis in human fetal retinal explants treated with docosahexaenoic acid. *Invest Ophtalmol Vis Sci*, 4, 3170-3177.

[45] Stahl, L. A., Berg, D. P., Weisinger, R. S., & Sinclair, A. J. (2008). The role of omega-3 fatty acids in mood disorders. *Curr Opin Invest Drugs*, 9, 57-64.

[46] Hashimoto, M., & Hossain, S. (2011). Neuroprotective and ameliorative actions of polyunsaturated fatty acids against neuronal diseases: Beneficial effect of docosahexaenoic acid on cognitive decline in Alzheimer´s disease. *J Pharmacol Sci*, 116, 150-162.

[47] Gauthier, S., Reisberg, B., Zauding, M., et al. (2006). Mild cognitive impairment. *Lancet*, 367, 1262-1270.

[48] Prasad, M. R., Lowell, M. A., Yatin, M., et al. (1998). Regional membrane phospholipid alteration in Alzheimer's disease. *Neurochem Res*, 23, 81-88.

[49] Yehuda, S., Rabinovitz, S., Carasso, R., et al. (2002). The role of polyunsaturated fatty acids in restoring the aging neuronal membrane. *Neurobiol Aging*, 23, 843-853.

[50] Soderberg, M., Edlund, C., Kristensson, K., et al. (1991). Fatty acid composition of brain phospholipids in aging and in Alzheimer disease. *Lipids*, 26, 421-425.

[51] Blennow, K., de León, M., & Zetterberg, H. (2006). Alzheimer's disease. *Lancet*, 368, 387-403.

[52] Coleman, P. D., & Yao, P. J. (2003). Synaptic slaughter in Alzheimer's disease. *Neurobiol Aging*, 24, 1023-1027.

[53] Hashimoto, M., Hossain, S., Agdul, H., & Shido, O. (2005). Docosahexaenoic acid-induced amelioration on impairment of memory learning in amyloid β-infused rats re-

lates to decreases of amyloid β and cholesterol levels in detergent-insoluble membrane fractions. *Biochim Biophys Acta*, 1738, 91-98.

[54] Geula, C., Wu, C. K., Saroff, D., Lorenzo, A., Yuan, M., & Yankner, B. (1998). Aging renders the brain vulnerable to amyloid beta-protein neurotoxicity. *Nat Med*, 4, 827-831.

[55] Green, K. N., Martínez-Coria, H., Khashwji, H., et al. (2007). Dietary docosahexaenoic acid and docosapentaenoic acid ameliorate amyloid-β and tau pathology via a mechanism involving presenilin 1 levels. *J Neuroscien*, 27, 4385-4395.

[56] Calon, F., Lim, G. P., Yang, F., et al. (2004). Docosahexaenoic acid protects from dendritic pathology in an Alzheimer's disease mouse model. *Neuron*, 43, 47-55.

[57] Connor, W. E., & Connor, J. L. (2007). The importance of fish and docosahexaenoic acid in Alzheimer's disease. *Am J Clin Nutr*, 85, 929-930.

[58] Cole, G. M., Lim, G. P., Yang, F., et al. (2005). Prevention of Alzheimer's disease: omega-3 fatty acid and phenolic anti-oxidant interventions. *Neurobiol Aging*, 26S, S133-S136.

[59] Pao-Yen, L., Shih-Yi, H., & Kuan-Pin, S. (2010). A meta-analytic review of polyunsaturated fatty acids composition in patients with depression. *Biol Psychiatry*, 68, 140-147.

[60] Murray, C. J., & Lopez, A. D. (1997). Alternative projections of mortality and disability by cause 1990-2010: Global Burden of Disease Study. Lancet. , 349, 1498-1504.

[61] Appleton, K. M., Rogers, P. J., & Ness, A. R. (2008). Is there a role of n-3 long-chain polyunsaturated fatty acids in the regulation of mood and behavior? A review of the evidence to date from epidemiological studies, clinical studies and intervention trials. *Nutr Res Rev*, 21, 13-41.

[62] Lin, P. Y., Huang, S. Y., & Su, K. P. (2010). A metha-analytic review of polyunsaturated fatty acid composition in patients with depression. *Biol Psychiatry*, 68, 140-147.

[63] Sinn, N., Milte, C., Street, S., et al. (2012). Effects of n-3 fatty acids, EPA v. DHA, on depressive symptoms, quality of life, memory and executive function in older adults with mild cognitive impairment: a 6-moth randomized controlled trial. *Brit J Nutr*, 107, 1682-1693.

[64] Lespérance, F., Frasure-Smith, F., St-Andre, E., et al. (2011). The efficacy of omega-3 supplementation for major depression: A randomized controlled trial. *J Clin Psychiatry*, 72, 1054-1062.

[65] Evans, J., Heron, J., Francomb, H., Oke, S., & Golding, J. (2001). Cohort study of depressed mood during pregnancy and after childbirth. *Brit Med J*, 323, 257-260.

[66] American Psychiatric Association. (1994). Diagnostic and Statistical Manual for Psychiatric Disorders, 4th ed. *Washington, DC: American Psychiatric Association*.

[67] Yao, J. K., Leonard, S., & Reddy, R. D. (2000). Membrane phospholipid abnormalities in post-mortem brains from schizophrenic patients. *Schizophen Res*, 42, 7-17.

[68] Fenton, W. S., Hibbeln, J., & Knable, M. (2000). Essential fatty acid, lipid membrane abnormabilities, and the diagnosis and treatment of schizophrenia. *Biol Psychiatry*, 47, 8-21.

[69] Horrobin, D. F., Glen, A. L., & Vaddadi, K. (1994). The membrane hypothesis of schizophrenia. *Schizophr Res*, 13, 195-207.

[70] Arvindaskshan, M., Ghate, M., Ranjekar, P., Evans, D., & Mahadik, S. P. (2003). Supplementation with a combination of omega-3 fatty acids and antioxidants (vitamin E and C) improves the outcome of schizophrenia. *Schizophr Res*, 62, 195-204.

[71] Watari, M., Hamazaki, K., Hirata, T., et al. (2010). Hostility of drug-free patients with schizophrenia and n-3 polyunsaturated fatty acid levels in red blood cells. *Psychiatry Res*, 177, 22-26.

[72] Kale, A., Joshi, S., Naphade, N., Sapkale, S., Raju, M., Pillai, A., Nasrallah, H., & Mahadik, S. (2008). Opposite changes in predominantly docosahexaenoic acid (DHA) in cerebrospinal fluid and red blood cells from never-medicated first-episode psychotic patients. *Schizophr Res*, 98, 295-301.

[73] Benton, D. (2007). The impact of diet on anti-social, violent and criminal behavior. *Neuroscien. Biobehav Rev*, 31, 752-774.

[74] Hibbeln, J. R. (2001). Seafood consumption and homicide mortality. A cross-national ecological analysis. *World Rev Nutr Diet*, 88, 41-46.

[75] Iribarren, C., Markovitz, J., Jacobs, D., et al. (2004). Dietary intake of n-3, n-6 fatty acids and fish: Relationship with hostility in young adults-the CARDIA study. *Europ J Clin Nutr*, 58, 24-31.

[76] Bougham, J. A., Conneally, P. M., & Nance, W. E. (1980). Population genetic studies of retinitis pigmentosa. *Am J Hum Genet*, 32, 223-235.

[77] Berson, E. L., Rosner, B., Sandberg, M., et al. (2004). Further evaluation of docosahexaenoic acid in patients with retinitis pigmentosa receiving vitamin A treatment. *Arch Ophthalmol*, 122, 1306-1314.

[78] Bazan, N. (2006). Cell survival matters: Docosahexaenoic acid signaling, neuroprotection and photoreceptors. *Trends Neuroscien*, 29, 263-271.

[79] Mamalakis, G., Tornaritis, M., & Kafatos, A. (2002). Depression and adipose essential polyunsaturated fatty acids. *Prostaglandins Leukot Essent Fatty Acids*, 67.

[80] Logan, A. C. (2003). Neurobehavioral aspects of omega-3 fatty acids: possible mechanism and therapeutic value in major depression. *Altern Med Rev*, 8, 410-425.

[81] Hibbeln, J. R., & Salem, N. (1995). Dietary polyunsaturated fatty fats and depression: when cholesterol alone doesn't satisfy. *Am J Clin Nutr*, 62, 1-9.

[82] Beckermann, B., Beneke, M., & Seitz, I. (1990). Comparative bioavailability of eicosapentaenoic acid and docosahexaenoic acid from triacylglycerols, free fatty acids and ethyl esters in volunteers. *Arzneimittelforschung*, 40, 700-704.

[83] Zuijdgeewst-van, Leeuwen. S., Dagniele, P., Rietveld, T., et al. (1999). Incorporation and washout of orally administered n-3 fatty acid ethyl esters in different plasma lipid fractions. *Brit J Nutr*, 82, 481-488.

[84] Lawson, L., & Hughes, B. (1988). Human absorption of fish oil fatty acids as triacylglycerols, free fatty acids or ethyl esters. *Biochim Biophys Acta*, 152, 328-335.

[85] Becker, C., & Kyle, D. (1998). Developing functional foods containing algal docosahexaenoic acid. *Food Technol*, 52, 68-71.

[86] Wijendran, V., Huang, M. C., Diau, G. Y., et al. (2002). Efficacy of dietary arachidonic acid provided as triglyceride or phospholipid substrates for brain arachidonic accretion in baboon neonates. *Pediatr Res*, 51, 265-272.

[87] Mc Michael, A. J., & Butler, C. D. (2005). Fish health, and sustainability. *Am J Prev Med*, 29, 322-323.

[88] Larsen, R., Eilertsen, K. E., & Elvevoll, E. (2011). Health benefits of marine foods and ingredients. *Biotechnol Adv*, 29, 508-518.

[89] Kachaou, E. S., Dumay, J., Donnay-Moreno, C., et al. (2009). Enzymatic hydrolysis of cuttlefish (Sepia officinalis) and sardine (Sardina pilchardus) viscera using commercial proteases: Effects on lipid distribution and aminoacid composition. *J Bioscien Bioengineerig*, 107, 158-164.

[90] Nieto, S., Sanhueza, J., & Valenzuela, A. (1999). Preparation of sn-2 long-chain polyunsaturated monoacylglycerols from fish oil by hydrolysis with a stereo-specific lipase from Mucor Meihei. *Grasas & Aceites*, 50, 111-113.

[91] Valenzuela, A., Valenzuela, V., Sanhueza, J., et al. (2005). Tissue accretion and milk content of docosahexaenoic acid (DHA) in female rats after supplementation with different DHA sources. *Ann Nutr Metab*, 49, 325-332.

Chapter 11

Neuronal Insulin Receptor Signaling: A Potential Target for the Treatment of Cognitive and Mood Disorders

Toshihiko Yanagita, Takayuki Nemoto,
Shinya Satoh, Norie Yoshikawa, Toyoaki Maruta,
Seiji Shiraishi, Chihiro Sugita and
Manabu Murakami

Additional information is available at the end of the chapter

http://dx.doi.org/10.5772/54389

1. Introduction

Insulin is mainly known for its peripheral effects on the metabolism of glucose, fats, and proteins. Following the discovery of insulin by Banting and Best in 1921, major research works focused on the role of insulin in the peripheral tissues (liver, muscle and adipocytes) in regulating glucose homeostasis. During the last two decades, evidence has accumulated that insulin also exerts important actions within the central nervous system (CNS) and peripheral nervous system (PNS). Although neurons are not insulin-dependent, they are insulin-responsive (Benedict et al., 2004, 2011; de la Monte 2009, 2012; Laron 2009; Stockhorst et al., 2004; van der Heide et al., 2006).

Insulin acts as a neuropeptide in the brain to regulate food intake, body weight, mood, cognitive function, memory, neuronal survival and synaptic plasticity (Laron, 2009; Stockhorst et al., 2004). Conversely, dysregulated insulin receptor signaling (e.g. insulin deficiency and insulin resistance) in the brain is involved in the neurodegenerative disease, dementia and mood disorders (Craft and Watson, 2004; de la Monte. 2012; Rasgon & Kenna, 2005). Interestingly, intranasal insulin administration has an improving effect of learning and memory as well as mood stabilizing effect in the patients with Alzheimer's disease (AD) and healthy volunteers (Benedict et al., 2004, 2007; Reger et al., 2006, 2008). Based on these findings, novel hypothesis "Type 3 diabetes" has been proposed: insulin resistance in the brain causes AD (de la Monte & Wands, 2008; de la Monte 2012;

Steen et al., 2005). Thus, insulin receptor signaling attracts attention as the molecular target for the treatment of cognitive and mood disorders.

In the present review, we would like to summarize the novel biological and pathophysiological roles of neuronal insulin in health and disease. In addition, we also introduce several of our findings that modulation of neuronal insulin receptor signaling by therapeutic drugs and bioactive agents via multiple mechanisms in cultured bovine adrenal medullary chromaffin cells (embryologically derived from neural crest) ; 1) enhancement of insulin receptor signaling by nicotine (Sugano et al., 2006); 2) reduction of insulin receptor signaling by immunosuppressants (cyclosporine and tacrolimus) (Shiraishi et al., 2001: Satoh et al., 2008), ketone body acetoacetate (Yokoo et al., 2003), heat shock protein 90 (Hsp90) inhibitors (Saitoh et al., 2002; Yoshikawa et al., 2010); 3) negative-feedback regulation of insulin receptor signaling by insulin and glycogen synthase kinase-3 (GSK-3) inhibitors (lithium and valproic acid) (Yokoo et al., 2007; Nemoto et al., 2006, 2009) ; 4) neurite-like outgrowth induced by insulin (Nemoto et al., 2011), and up-regulation of cell surface voltage-dependent Na^+ channel induced by insulin, insulin-like growth factor-1 (IGF-1) and GSK-3 inhibitors (lithium and valproic acid) (Yamamoto et al., 1996, 1997; Yanagita et al., 2009, 2011).

2. Insulin and insulin receptor signaling in the brain

It is now generally thought that little or no insulin is produced in the brain itself (Woods, 2003; Banks, 2004; Laron 2009). Insulin crosses the blood-brain barrier (BBB) and enters the brain via a receptor-mediated active transport system (Baskin et al., 1987; Baura et al., 1993).

Insulin receptor is distributed in a widespread, but selective, pattern in the brain, including the olfactory bulb, hypothalamus, hippocampus, cerebellum, amygdale and cerebral cortex (Marks et al., 1990; Unger & Betz, 1998). The expression level of the insulin receptor is developmentally regulated, being higher at early stages and lower in the adult (Chiu & Cline 2010). Brain insulin receptors are present in particularly high concentrations in neurons, and in much lower levels in glia (Schwartz et al., 1992; Unger et al., 1989). Subcellularly, the insulin receptor is a component of synapses, where it concentrates at the postsynaptic density (Abbott et al., 1999; Marks et al., 1988). Cell surface insulin receptor, a member of receptor tyrosine kinase family, consists of two extracellular α- and two transmembrane β-subunits (~135 and ~95 kDa, respectively) that are encoded by the same gene and derived from the single-chain insulin receptor precursor molecule. The brain insulin receptor differs from its peripheral counterpart by having a lower molecular weight of both α- and β-subunits (Heidenreich et al., 1983). This is presumable the result of alternative mRNA splicing and differences in receptor glycosylation (Heidenreich et al., 1983; Goldstein & Dudley, 1992; Sugimoto et al., 2000). As shown in fig. 1, insulin receptor precursor undergoes translational glycosylation, intrachain disulfide-bond formation/isomerization (rearrangement), and disulfide-linked homodimerization at

http://dx.doi.org/10.5772/54389

the endoplasmic reticulum (ER). The homodimeric insulin receptor precursor is proteolytically processed at the *trans*-Golgi network into the disulfide-linked α2β2 complex, which is transported to plasma membrane (reviewed in Wada et al., 2005). Binding of insulin to the α-subunit causes autophosphorylation of the β-subunit tyrosine residues. Tyrosine phosphorylation of β-subunits induces specific recruitment of Src homology 2 (SH2) and phosphotyrosine-binding (PTB) domain containing proteins (SH2 and PTB domains are domains that recognize phosphorylated tyrosine residues). The most prominent scaffold proteins recruited to the insulin receptor are the insulin receptor substrate (IRS)-1/-2 and SHC (White, 1997, 1998). These scaffold proteins link the activated insulin receptor to downstream signal transduction pathways. Insulin binding to the insulin receptor activates two major parallel signal transduction cascades identified as the phosphoinositide 3-kinase (PI3K)/phosphoinositide-dependent kinase 1 (PDK-1)/Akt pathway and the Ras/extracellular signal-regulated kinase (ERK) pathway (van der Heide et al., 2006: Wada et al., 2005). Akt catalyzes inhibitory Ser^{21}/Ser^{9}-phosphorylation of GSK-3α/3β (Jope & Johnson, 2004; Jope et al., 2007).

3. Physiological roles of insulin in the brain

The neuronal specific insulin receptor knockout (NIRKO) mice study revealed that insulin receptor signaling in the CNS plays an important role in regulation of energy disposal, fuel metabolism, and reproduction: the inactivation of the insulin receptor had no impact on brain development or neuronal survival. However, female NIRKO mice showed increased food intake, and both male and female mice developed diet-sensitive obesity with increases in body fat and plasma leptin levels, mild insulin resistance, elevated plasma insulin levels, and hypertriglyceridemia. NIRKO mice exhibited impaired spermatogenesis and ovarian follicle maturation because of hypothalamic dysregulation of luteinizing hormone (Brüning et al., 2000). The NIRKO mice also had an impairment of the counter-regulatory response to hypoglycaemia (Fisher et al., 2005). The NIRKO mice exhibit a complete loss of insulin-mediated activation of PI3K and inhibition of neuronal apoptosis. In intact animals, this loss results in markedly reduced phosphorylation of Akt and GSK-3β, leading to substantially increased phosphorylation of the microtubule-associated protein Tau, a hallmark of neurodegenerative diseases. Nevertheless, these animals exhibit no alteration in neuronal proliferation/survival, memory (Schubert et al., 2003). Interestingly, the early postnatal inhibition of brain insulin receptor by using small interfering RNA causes structural and functional abnormalities (e.g. cerebellar hypofoliation and hypotrophy, impaired motor function, and altered expression of neurotrophins and neurotropin receptors) that resemble effects of fetal alcohol spectrum disorder (FASD). The findings suggest that major abnormalities in brains with FASD are mediated by impairments in insulin/IGF signaling. (de la Monte et al., 2011). Although there is little evidence to date from neuronal insulin receptor knockout and knockdown studies for a key role in learning and memory, there is evidence that insulin may play important roles in learning and memory (Williamson et al 2012). The deletion of IRS-2 (but not IRS-1) causes a similar phenotype; IRS-2 knockout mice displayed hypothalamic female infertility, and increased food intake and obesity (Burks et al., 2000). These findings implicate that neuronal insulin receptor ~ IRS-2 pathway plays crucial roles in the neuroendocrine regulation of reproduction and energy homeostasis. Furthermore, the disruption of the IRS-2 gene reduced neuronal proliferation during development by 50%, which dissociated brain growth from IRS-1-dependent body growth. In the old IRS-2 knockout mice, neurofibrillary tangles containing phosphorylated tau accumulated in the hippocampus, suggesting that IRS-2 signaling is neuroprotective. Thus, dysregulation of the IRS-2 branch of the insulin/IGF-1 signaling cascade reveals a molecular link between diabetes and neurodegenerative disease (Schubert et al., 2003). Indeed, intravenous and intranasal administrations of insulin improve cognitive performance in a humans and animals in a wide variety of settings, including healthy subjects, aged subjects, AD patients and in the various experimental models of insulin resistance (Reagan 2007; Stockhorst et al., 2004: Wada et al., 2005; Watson & Craft, 2004).

4. Insulin resistance and cognitive disorders

The intensively studied phenomenon of insulin resistance in peripheral tissues is tightly linked with overweight and a hallmark in the development of type 2 diabetes mellitus (T2DM). Insulin resistance and impaired glucose tolerance are considered early warning signs for the development of T2DM. Cognitive impairments are more common in diabetic patients than in non-diabetic subjects. In the Rotterdam study, of 6,370 elderly subjects studied for 2.1 years, 126 developed dementia; 89 of these were specifically diagnosed with AD. T2DM doubled the risk of a patient having dementia and patients on insulin had four times the risk (Ott et al., 1999). Hisayama Study in Japan also revealed that impaired glucose tolerance (an early warning sign of T2DM) increased risk of all-cause dementia (Ohara et al., 2011). This T2DM-associated dementia is in part due to ischemic events resulting from cerebral microvascular and/or macrovascular disease or to repeated episodes of severe hypoglycemia. These conditions have been referred to as secondary diabetic encephalopathy. However, there is accumulating evidence suggesting that cognitive dysfunction is also caused by diabetic dysmetabolism in the brain, so-called primary diabetic encephalopathy (Ott et al., 1999; Sima et al., 2004; Sima & Li. 2006).

Cerebral insulin resistance could be the result of various mechanisms at different levels. Acute elevations of plasma insulin levels have been found to correlate with cerebro-spinal-fluid (CSF) insulin concentrations in healthy, normal weight humans. However, in overweight humans, the ratio of CSF to plasma insulin seems altered – elevated plasma insulin levels due to peripheral insulin resistance are not accompanied by similar elevations in cerebral insulin levels (Ketterer et al., 2011).

The peripheral and CNS insulin abnormalities have been reported in AD patients. AD patients have an increased risk for hyperinsulinemia and hyperglycemia relative to healthy controls (Meneilly et al., 1993; Razay and Wilcock, 1994), and also have lower CSF insulin levels, higher plasma insulin levels, and reduced insulin-mediated glucose disposal, a pattern consistent with insulin resistance (Craft et al., 1999; Watson & Craft 2006). AD brains show reduced insulin receptor density and tyrosine kinase activity markers (Frölich et al., 1998). The expression of insulin receptor was increased in the hippocampal dentate gyrus and CA1 field following training of rodents on a spatial memory task, suggesting that neuronal insulin sensitivity could be enhanced during learning (Zhao et al., 1999). In addition, intravenous and intranasal administrations of insulin improve cognitive performance in AD patients and in the experimental models of insulin resistance (Wada et al., 2005; Watson & Craft, 2004). Taken together, these correlative findings suggest that insulin resistance in the brain may be associated with AD.

Moreover, de la Monte et al., proposed novel disease concept "Type 3 diabetes": AD is a brain DM (Steen et al., 2005; de la Monte and Wands, 2008). Postmortem brain studies demonstrated that the molecular, biochemical, and signal transduction abnormalities in AD are virtually identical to those that occur in T1DM and T2DM (see review de la Monte & Wands, 2008; de la Monte 2012). In addition, experimental brain diabetes produced by intracerebral administration of streptozotocin shares many features with AD, including cognitive impairment and disturbances in acetylcholine homeostasis. This experimental brain diabetes is treatable with insulin sensitizer agents, i.e., drugs currently used to treat T2DM (de la Monte & Wands, 2008).

5. Insulin resistance and mood disorders

Evidence has accumulated that obesity is associated with mood disorders. Obesity is associated with an approximately 25% increase in odds of mood and anxiety disorders and an approximately 25% decrease in odds of substance use disorders (Simon et al. 2006). The individuals meeting criteria for obesity are more likely to report a major depressive episode in the past 12 months when compared to healthy weight individuals (Chen et al. 2009). Prospective studies add further evidence that obesity is a significant risk factor for depression, although depression did not increase the risk of future obesity (Roberts et al. 2003).

Numerous studies describe the association between insulin resistance and depression. Low glucose utilization rates as well as abnormal glucose and insulin disposal rates have been reported in a significant proportion of patients with depressive disorders (Ramasubbu 2002; Rasgon & Kenna 2005). The evidence lending support to this association is the influence of therapeutic drugs for depression (e.g. selective serotonin-reuptake inhibitors (SSRIs) and tricyclic antidepressants) on insulin resistance. Improvement in insulin resistance has been reported with successful treatment of depression with SSRIs, but worsening of insulin resistance has been reported with tricyclic antidepressants (Rasgon & Kenna 2005; Sockynska et al., 2011). Furthermore, hyperinsulinemia, a feature of peripheral insulin resistance, may in part be responsible for decreased appetite and weight loss observed in depressive disorders (Licinio-Paixao, 1999).

Although precise mechanisms that insulin resistance induces mood disorder are not revealed, impairment of multi-neuroregulatory functions of insulin (e.g. CNS glucose metabolism, BBB transport and neuroprotective effect) caused by insulin resistance in the brain may contribute to evolution and progression of serious mental disorders including depression (Ramasubbu 2002).

6. Intranasal administration of insulin

Intranasal delivery is a noninvasive method of bypassing the BBB to deliver therapeutic agents to the brain and spinal cord. The use of intranasal administration to target therapeutics to the CNS has many benefits (safety, cost, and easy handling) in the treatment of neurologic disorders, and has been used to target a wide variety of therapeutics to the CNS [e.g. Nerve growth factor (Chen X-Q et al., 1998), IGF-1 (Thorne RG et al., 2004), glucagon-like peptide-1 antagonist, exendin9–39 (Banks WA et al., 2004) and carbamazepine (Barakat NS et al., 2006)]. Intranasal administration of insulin provides direct access of the hormone to the CSF within 30 min without substantial uptake into the bloodstream (Born et al., 2002). Direct delivery of therapeutics from the nose to the brain was initially attributed to the olfactory pathway (Thorne et al., 1995). More recently, the contribution made by the trigeminal pathway to intranasal delivery to the CNS has also been recognized (Thorne RG et al., 2004). Because intraneuronal transport of neuropeptides from the nasal cavity to the olfactory bulb takes several hours (Thorne et al., 1995), extra-neuronal passage through intercellular clefts of the olfactory epithelium is assumed to be the preferential pathway of peptide transport into the CNS compartment (Ott et al., 2012).

Intranasal insulin improves memory function both in healthy humans and AD patients. Chronic (8 weeks) administration of intranasal insulin in cognitively normal young adults is associated with increased memory performance (Benedict et al., 2004, 2007). Intranasal insulin has also been studied in cognitively impaired patients. Intranasal insulin treatment produced significant memory improvement in memory-impaired subjects (early stage AD or amnestic mild cognitive impairment) (Reger et al., 2006, 2008). Interestingly, memory-improving effects of intranasal insulin were found only in non-carriers of the APOE4 gene allele that is linked to an increased risk of developing AD (Cummings and Cole, 2002), whereas the APOE4-postive subjects showed no benefits or even a decline in memory function (Reger et al., 2006). In addition, intranasal insulin administration to obese males over 8 weeks caused improvement of declarative memory and mood without reduction in body weight and fat (Hallschmid et al., 2008). Thus, the enhancement of insulin signaling in the CNS by intranasal insulin administration may be a useful approach in the treatment and/or prevention of cognitive and mood dysfunction.

http://dx.doi.org/10.5772/54389

7. Modulation of neuronal insulin receptor signaling by therapeutic drugs and bioactive agents.

There are two major approaches to improve insulin signal impairment: 1) stimulation of insulin receptor signaling by insulin such as intranasal administration of insulin, and 2) adjustment of insulin receptor signaling via modulation of expression and function of insulin receptor signaling molecules. We have previously reported that several therapeutic drugs and bioactive agents affect cell surface density of insulin receptor and protein levels of IRS-1, IRS-2 and other various downstream signaling molecules via multiple intracellular mechanisms in cultured bovine adrenal medullary chromaffin cells. In this part, we would like to introduce several of our findings that the modulation of neuronal insulin receptor signaling by therapeutic drugs and bioactive agents (Fig. 1).

7.1. Nicotine and protein kinase C-α (PKC-α) activation: enhancement of insulin receptor signaling via increase in IRS-1, IRS-2, and cell surface insulin receptor (Fig.1 ① and ①').

Activation of neuronal nicotinic acetylcholine receptors (nAChRs) enters Na^+ into the cells and rapidly evokes excitatory postsynaptic potentials and Ca^{2+}-dependent exocytosis of neurotransmitters, while generating longer-lasting multiple effects (e.g. synaptic plasticity, learning and memory, and cell survival) (Dajas-Bailador & Wonnacott 2004; Sugano et al., 2006). The aberrant down-regulation of nAChRs accounts for cognitive deficits in normal aging and age-related neurodegenerative diseases, such as AD (Picciotto & Zoli 2002), with impairment of acetylcholine synthesis in AD brain (Hoshi et al. 1997). Enhancement of nAChRs signaling caused by choline esterase inhibitors is the major therapeutic strategy against these cognitive impairments, but the therapeutic mechanisms have not been fully identified at the cellular level (Newhouse et al. 2001; Nordberg 2001; Picciotto and Zoli 2002).

In cultured bovine adrenal chromaffin cells treated with nicotine (10 μ M for 24 h), insulin (100 nM for 10 min)-induced phosphorylation of Akt, GSK-3β and ERK1/2 was enhanced by ~62%, without altering levels of these protein kinases. Treatment with nicotine produced time (≧ 12 h)- and concentration (EC_{50} = 3.6 and 13 μ M)-dependent increases in IRS-1 and IRS-2 levels by ~125 and 105%, without altering cell surface density of insulin receptor. Nicotine also increased IRS-1 and IRS-2 mRNA levels by ~57 and ~50%. Nicotine-induced increase in IRS-1 and IRS-2 was prevented by nAChR antagonists (d-tubocurarine and mecamylamine), cell membrane-permeable Ca^{2+} chelator (BAPTA-AM), protein synthesis inhibitor (cycloheximide), transcription inhibitor (actinomycin D), conventional protein kinase C (cPKC) inhibitor (Gö6976), or ERK kinase inhibitor (PD98059 and U0126). Nicotine phosphorylated cPKC-α, thereby increasing phosphorylation of ERK1/ERK2, as demonstrated by using Gö6976, PD98059 or U0126. Selective activation of cPKC-α by thymeleatoxin mimicked these effects of nicotine. Interestingly, activation of PKC-α by thymeleatoxin or other phorbol esters up-regulated cell surface insulin receptor via transcriptional/translational events (Yamamoto et al., 2000), although nicotine did not affect cell surface insulin receptor. Thus, stimulation of nAChRs up-regulates expression of IRS-1/IRS-2 via Ca^{2+} -dependent sequential activation of cPKC-α and ERK, and enhances insulin-induced PI3K/Akt/GSK-3β and ERK signaling pathways (Sugano et al., 2006). This nicotine-induced enhancement of insulin receptor signaling may contribute to the neuroprotective effects of nicotine.

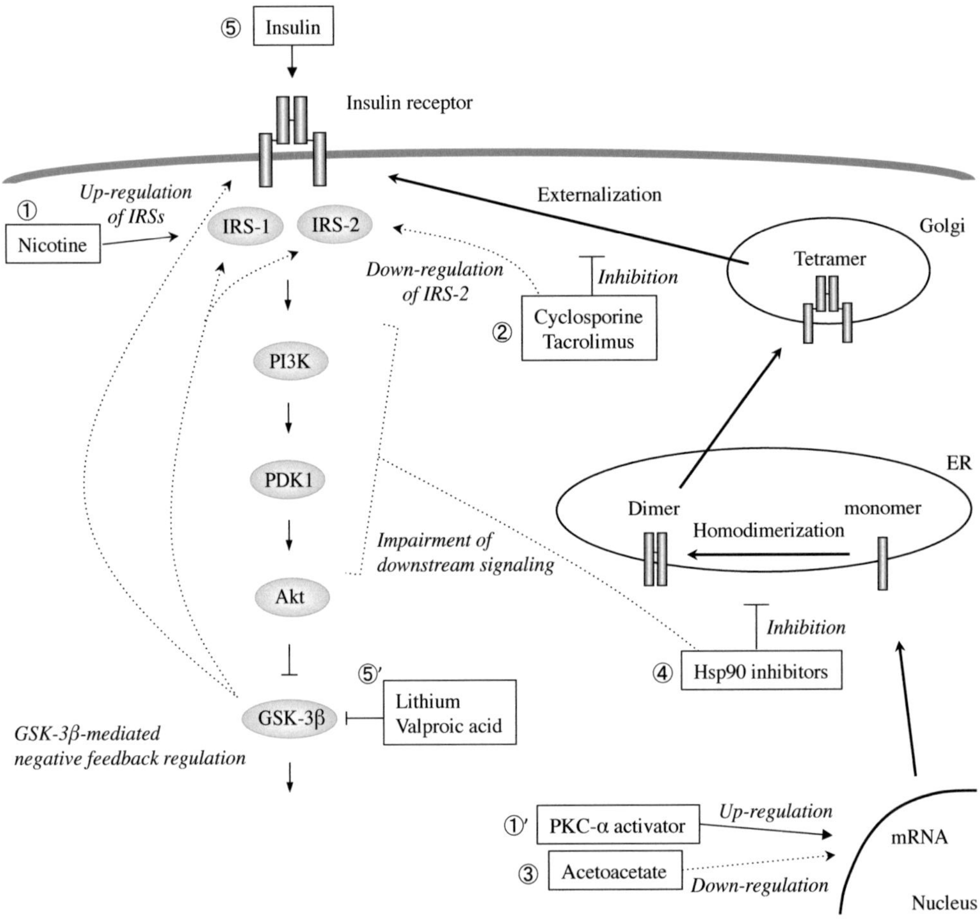

Figure 1. Modulation of insulin receptor signaling by therapeutic drugs and bioactive agents via multiple intracellular mechanisms in adrenal chromaffin cells. ① and ①′: Nicotine-induced up-regulation of IRS-1 and IRS-2, and PKC-α activation-induced up-regulation of insulin receptor (see 7-1).②: Immunosuppressants (cyclosporine and tacrolimus)-induced down-regulation of cell surface insulin receptor and IRS-2 (see 7-2).③: Acetoacetate-induced down-regulation of insulin receptor.④: Hsp90 inhibition-induced impairment of insulin receptor signaling via down-regulation of cell surface insulin receptor and various downstream signaling molecules (e.g. IRS-1, PI3K, PDK-1, Akt, GSK-3β, and Raf-1) (see 7-4). ⑤ and ⑤′: GSK-3β-mediated negative feedback regulation of insulin receptor signaling caused by chronic treatment with insulin and GSK-3 inhibitors (lithium and valproic acid) (see 7-5).

http://dx.doi.org/10.5772/54389

7.2. Immunosuppressants, cyclosporine and tacrolimus: reduction of insulin receptor signaling via down-regulation of cell surface insulin receptor and IRS-2. (Fig.1②)

Cyclosporine (Cyclosporin A) and tacrolimus (FK506) are clinically important immunosuppressive drugs that are widely used to prevent organ rejection after transplantation. In addition, an increasing number of autoimmune diseases are treated with these drugs (Oetjen et al., 2003). Both structurally distinct drugs bind to their respective intracellular receptors, the immunophilins, and the drug-immunophilin complexes then bind to and inhibit calcineurin phosphatase; this inhibition of calcineurin is well known as the mechanism of immunosuppressive effect (Ho et al., 1996). In addition, cyclosporine and tacrolimus directly inhibit peptidyl prolyl *cis-trans* isomerase (PPIase) activity of immunophilin (Shiraishi et al., 2000). Among the most serious adverse effects of cyclosporine and tacrolimus are the impaired glucose tolerance leading to hyperglycemia and DM (Kahan, 1989, 1994; Jindal et al., 1997; Saltiel, 2001; Oetjen et al., 2003) as well as neurotoxicity (Bechstein 2000; Gijtenbeek et al., 1999). The incidence of glucose tolerance has been estimated to be 10 to 30% (Kahan, 1989; Jindal et al., 1997; Oetjen et al., 2003). Between 10~28 % of patients who receive cyclosporine experience some form of neurotoxic adverse event. Mild symptoms are common and include tremor, neuralgia, and peripheral neuropathy. Severe symptoms affect up to 5 % of patients and include psychoses, hallucinations, blindness, seizures, cerebellar ataxia, motoric weakness, or leukoencephalopathy. The mechanisms of neurotoxicity associated with cyclosporine and tacrolimus are less well-understood (Bechstein 2000; Gijtenbeek et al., 1999).

Chronic (≧ 3 h) treatment of cultured bovine adrenal chromaffin cells with cyclosporin A or FK506 selectively decreased IRS-2 protein level by w50% (IC_{50} = 200 or 10 nM), without changing IRS-2 mRNA level, and protein levels of insulin receptor, IGF-1 receptor, IRS-1, PI3K / PDK-1 / Akt / GSK-3β and ERK1 / ERK2 via inhibition of calcineurin activity (IC_{50} = 500 or 40 nM, in vitro assay). Cyclosporin A and FK506 accelerated IRS-2 degradation rate ($t_{1/2}$) from >24 to ~4.2 h, without altering IRS-2 protein synthesis. IRS-2 reduction induced by cyclosporin A or FK506 was prevented by lactacystin (proteasome inhibitor), but not by calpeptin (calpain inhibitor) or leupeptin (lysosome inhibitor). Cyclosporin A or FK506 increased serine-phosphorylation and ubiquitination of IRS-2. These results suggest that calcineurin inhibition by cyclosporin A or FK506 decreased IRS-2 protein level via proteasomal IRS-2 degradation (Satoh et al., 2008). Interestingly, inhibition of PPIase activity of immunophilin by cyclosporin A or FK506 inhibits externalization of insulin receptor (but not IGF-1 receptor), and down-regulates cell surface expression of insulin receptor (Shiraishi et al., 2000). Cell surface density of IGF-1 receptor was not changed in cyclosporin A- or FK506-treated cells; however, IGF-1-induced phosphorylations of GSK-3β and ERK1/ERK2 were attenuated by ~50%. Therefore, cyclosporin A and FK506 reduced insulin receptor signaling via two mechanisms; (1) down-regulation of cell surface expression of insulin receptor via inhibition of PPIase activity of immunophilin, and (2) selective reduction of IRS-2 protein via inhibition of calcineurin. As mentioned above, knockout mice of insulin receptor, IRS-1 or IRS-2 study revealed that neuronal insulin receptor ~ IRS-2 pathway plays crucial roles in the regulation of reproduction, energy homeostasis, cognitive performance, and neuroprotection. In addition, forebrain-specific calcineurin knockout mice exhibit impairment of bidirectional synaptic plasticity, working/episodic-like memory, and multiple abnormal behaviors related to schizophrenia (miyagawa et al., 2003; Zeng et al., 2001). Thus, this reduction of insulin receptor signaling might be involved in the neuronal disorders caused by immunosuppressants. Our findings raise a possibility that intranasal insulin administration might be effective in the treatment for immunosuppressants-induced neuronal disorders.

7.3. Ketone body acetoacetate: reduction of insulin receptor signaling via down-regulation of cell surface insulin receptor. (Fig.1③)

It has been widely accepted that glucose is the main energy source in the brain. However, in some circumstances, such as diabetes, starvation, during the suckling period and the ketogenic diet, brain uses the ketone bodies, acetoacetate and β-hydroxybutyrate, as energy sources (Massieu et al., 2003; Nehlig & Pereira de Vasconcelos, 1993). Ketone body utilization in brain depends mainly on its blood concentration, which is normally very low, but increases substantially during the conditions mentioned above (Massieu et al., 2003), although astrocyte can produce ketone body (Guzmán & Blázquez 2004). Under normal conditions, blood levels of ketone bodies are maintained below 0.5 mM (Sokoloff, 1973), but, during fasting or a high-fat, low-protein, and low-carbohydrate diet, blood levels of ketone bodies become elevated (referred to as ketosis) (Massieu et al., 2003; Noh 2006). Previous studies have demonstrated that, during starvation or administration of ketone bodies, the ketone bodies have neuroprotective effects against hypoxia / ischemia- and glutamate-induced neuronal damage toxicity, AD, and Parkinson's disease (Maalouf et al., 2009; Massieu et al., 2003; Noh 2006). Ketone bodies are converted from free fatty acid (FFA) when there is not enough insulin. The increased level of FFA is linked to the insulin-resistance in DM and obesity because FFA interferes with insulin's intracellular signaling (Boden et al., 2001; Patti, 1999). Diabetic ketoacidosis is a severe and life threatening metabolic disease caused by an absolute or relative deficiency of insulin (Wolfsdorf et al, 2009; Yokoo et al., 2003). Cerebral edema is the most important neuronal complication of diabetic ketoacidosis as it is associated with a high mortality rate of 20 to 90 %. Of the survivors, 20 to 40 % suffer from serious and permanent neurologic disability including motor deficits, visual impairment, seizure disorder, learning disability and speech disturbance. Clinically, apparent cerebral edema occurs in approximately 1% of episodes of diabetic ketoacidosis, and the pathogenesis of diabetic ketoacidosis-related cerebral edema is unclear and incompletely understood (Glaser 2009; Shastry & Bhatia 2006; Wolfsdorf et al, 2009).

Chronic (≧ 24 h) treatment of cultured bovine adrenal chromaffin cells with ketoacidosis-related concentrations (≧3 mM) of acetoacetate (but not β-hydroxybutyrate, acetone, and acidic medium) caused a time- and concentration-dependent reduction of cell surface insulin receptor by ~38%. Acetoacetate decreased protein and mRNA levels of insulin receptor via shortening insulin receptor mRNA half-life (stability). In cells treated with

http://dx.doi.org/10.5772/54389

acetoacetate (10 mM, 24 h), insulin-induced (100 nM for 10 min) tyrosine-phosphorylation of IRS-1 was attenuated by 56% in acetoacetate-treated cells, with no change in IRS-1 level. These results suggest that chronic treatment with ketoacidosis-related concentrations of acetoacetate (but not β-hydroxybutyrate and acetone) down-regulated the density of cell surface insulin receptor, thereby reducing insulin receptor signaling (Yokoo et al., 2003). Further in vivo and in vitro investigations are required to elucidate the relationship between the acetoacetate-induced impairment of neuronal insulin receptor signaling and the diabetic ketoacidosis-related neuronal damages.

7.4. Hsp90 inhibitors: impairment of insulin receptor signaling via down-regulation of cell surface insulin receptor and various downstream signaling molecules. (Fig.1④)

Hsp90 is the most abundant molecular chaperone in eukaryotic cells (Welch and Feramisco, 1982). It has been increasingly recognized that Hsp90 plays a important role in the regulating signal transduction pathways that control cell proliferation and cell death, since its chaperone function is restricted to a subset of proteins including nuclear hormone receptors, tyrosine kinases, serine/threonine kinases, and transcription factors (Kamal et al., 2004; Richter and Buchner, 2001; Zhang and Burrows 2004). These findings were evidenced by using selective Hsp90 inhibitors [geldanamycin (GA), 17-allylamino-17-demethoxy-geldanamycin (17-AAG), Herbimycin A (HA) or radicicol] (Saitoh et al., 2002; Whitesell et al., 1994; Yoshikawa et al., 2010). GA binds to the adenosine nucleotide binding site of N-terminal domain of Hsp90 with affinity higher than that of ATP, inhibiting the ATPase activity/chaperone function of Hsp90 (Whitesell et al., 1994; Young et al., 2001).

In adrenal chromaffin cells, inhibition of Hsp90 by GA or HA decreased cell surface ^{125}I- insulin binding in a concentration- and time-dependent manner. GA (1 μM for 24 h) lowered the B_{max} value of ^{125}I-insulin binding by 80%, without changing the K_d value. Western blot analysis showed that GA (1 μM for 24 h) lowered α2β2 tetramer-form of insulin receptor level by 83%, while raising insulin receptor precursor level by 100%. [^{35}S]methionine/cysteine pulse-chase study of insulin receptor revealed that monomeric insulin receptor precursor (~190 kDa) developed into the homodimeric insulin receptor precursor (~380 kDa) and the mature α2β2 insulin receptor (~410 kDa) in nontreated cells. In contrast, in GA-treated cells, the homodimerization of monomeric insulin receptor precursor was completely blocked. GA had no effect on insulin receptor mRNA levels and internalization rate of cell surface insulin receptor. Thus, inhibition of chaperone activity of Hsp90 by GA completely blocked homodimerization of monomeric insulin receptor precursor in the ER; the dimeric insulin receptor precursor and the tetrameric mature-form of insulin receptor were significantly decreased, whereas the monomeric insulin receptor precursor was accumulated in the ER. Chaperone activity of Hsp90 is indispensable to the homodimerization of monomeric insulin receptor precursor (Saitoh et al., 2002).

GA also affects the protein levels of downstream signaling molecules of insulin receptor. GA treatment significantly decreased protein levels of IRS-1, PI3K, PDK-1, Akt, GSK-3β, and Raf-1, without altering protein levels of ERK and ERK kinase. Interestingly, GA increased protein level of IRS-2. Chronic (≧12 h) treatment with 0.1–10 μM Hsp90 inhibitor (GA, 17-AAG, HA, and radicicol) decreased IRS-1 level by ~66%, while increasing IRS-2 level by ~160%. These effects of GA (IC_{50} = 155 nM, EC_{50} = 177 nM) and 17-AAG (IC_{50} = 310 nM, EC_{50} = 260 nM) were time- and concentration- dependent. GA-induced decrease of IRS-1 was attenuated by proteasome inhibitors (lactacystin, β-lactone or MG132), but not by calpain inhibitor (calpastatin) or lysosome inhibitor (leupeptin). GA-induced increase of IRS-2 was prevented by cycloheximide or actinomycin D. GA lowered IRS-1 mRNA level by ~39%, while raising IRS-2 mRNA level by ~109%, without changing the stability of IRS-1 and IRS-2 mRNA. Nuclear run-on assay revealed that GA retarded IRS-1 gene transcription by 42%, while accelerating IRS-2 gene transcription by 41%. Hsp90 inhibitors oppositely altered IRS-1 and IRS-2 levels via proteasomal degradation and gene transcription (Yoshikawa et al., 2010).

Increasing evidence has accumulated over the past 2 decades that anti-Hsp90 autoantibodies in CSF may be involved in the various neuropsychological diseases. Aberrant increase in anti-Hsp90 antibodies in CSF or blood were found in the patient with Schizophrenia (Kim et al., 2001), autism (Evers et al., 2002), acute bipolar mania (Shen et al., 2006), and multiple sclerosis (Cid et al., 2007). The autoantibodies to Hsp90 in CSF from multiple sclerosis induced cell death of cultured oligodendrocyte precursor cells (Cid et al 2005). Moreover, it has been reported that schizophrenia associated with abnormalities in glucose metabolism that may lead to insulin resistance and a 3-fold higher incidence of T2DM (Zhao et al 2006). In postmortem brain tissue from schizophrenic patients, protein level of insulin receptor β-subunit and Akt activity were drastically decreased (Zhao et al 2006). These correlative findings imply that chaperone activity of Hsp90 plays crucial roles in the regulation of various neuropsychological functions in brain via maintenance the expression and function of insulin receptor and downstream signaling molecules.

A derivative of GA, 17-AAG, has similar cellular effects of GA but lower hepatotoxicity than GA. 17-AAG exerts a potent antitumor activity in preclinical models and is currently in clinical trials (Neckers 2002). Aberrant expression of IRS-1 has been associated with pathogenesis and progression of breast cancer and prostatic cancer (Morelli et al., 2003; Reiss et al., 2000; Koda 2006). In breast cancer, IRS-1 overexpression has been associated with tumor development, hormone independence, and anti-estrogen resistance (Surmacz 2000). In hormone dependent breast cancer cell lines, the expression of IRS-1 has been correlated with estrogen receptorα (ERα, and numerous studies have demonstrated that IRS-1 is one of the central elements of ERα-IGF-1 crosstalk (Surmacz 2000). In patients with primary breast cancer, IRS-1 expression is correlated with poorly differentiation and with lymph node metastasis (Koda et al 2006). Human prostatic cancer LNCaP cells are characterized by having a frame-shift mutation of the tumor suppressor gene piedmont triad entrepreneurial network, low levels of IGF-I receptor and no IRS-1. Reiss et al. reported that ectopic expression of IRS-1 in LNCaP cells increases cell adhesion and decreases cell motility; over-expression of IGF-1 receptor, in the absence of IRS-1, causes growth arrest and a combination of IGF-1 receptor and IRS-1 restores the transformed phenotype of LNCaP cells. These correlative findings indicated that IRS-1 expression is involved in the growth regulation of breast and prostatic cancer. Thus, the decreasing effect of 17-AAG on the IRS-1 could be contributed to the anti-tumor effect against these cancers, although our results were obtained from primary cultured bovine chromaffin cells. In addition, previous studies with IRS-1 knockout mice or the cells derived from these mice have suggested that IRS-2 could compensate for IRS-1 deficiency more effectively in liver and pancreatic cells than in skeletal muscle, fibroblasts, or adipocytes (Tanemoto et al. 1994; Bruning et al 1997; Sesti et al. 2001). It has been shown that IRS-2 has a major role in regulating hepatic glucose production and in controlling pancreatic cell development and survival (Sesti et al. 2001). Indeed, IRS-2 knockout mice exhibit insulin resistance with abnormal glucose tolerance at birth and progressively develop fasting hyperglycemia as a result of inadequate compensatory insulin secretion because of pancreatic β-cell apoptosis (Kubota et al. 2000; Withers et al. 1998). Thus, the increasing effect of 17-AAG on the IRS-2 expression would be convenient for avoiding side effects such as hyperglycemia, insulin resistance, and pancreatic β-cell damage, during anti-cancer therapy by 17-AAG. Therefore, it is interesting to investigate precisely the down- and up-regulation of IRS-1 / IRS-2 by 17-AAG in the animal model, *in vivo* study.

7.5. Insulin, IGF-1 and potent GSK-3 inhibitors (lithium and valproic acid): negative feedback regulation of insulin receptor signaling. (Fig.1 ⑤ and ⑤')

Control over insulin signaling can be achieved by autoregulation, whereby insulin-stimulated downstream components (e.g. Akt, GSK-3β, mTOR, and ERK1/2) inhibit upstream elements (negative feedback control; autologous regulation). The insulin receptor and the IRS proteins are targets for these feedback control mechanisms, with phosphorylation of IRS proteins on Ser / Thr residues being a key step in these feedback control processes. For example, Ser / Thr-phosphorylation of IRS-1 caused by downstream signals of the PI3K pathway (e.g., mTOR) results in the self-attenuation of IRS-1 activity. Additionally, signals from apparently unrelated (heterologous) pathways also inhibit insulin signaling. The agents inducing insulin resistance (e.g., tumor necrosis factor-α) increase Ser / Thr-phosphorylation of IRS-1 via activating protein kinases (e.g., c-Jun N-terminal kinase) and caused negative feedback regulation of insulin receptor signaling (Boura-Halfon & Zick 2009; Copps & White.2012; Zick 2001).

GSK-3, a serine/threonine protein kinase, is constitutively active in nonstimulated cells, causing phosphorylation and inactivation/degradation of various signaling molecules (e.g., glycogen synthase), transcription factors (e.g., β-catenin), translation initiation factor eIF2B, and structural proteins (e.g., tau) (Jope & Johnson, 2004; Jope et al., 2007; Meijer et al., 2004; Nemoto et al., 2006). Insulin- or IGF-I-induced activation of Akt increases Ser^{21}/Ser^{9} phosphorylation of GSK-3α/-3β and inhibits catalytic activity of GSK-3α/-3β.

In adrenal chromaffin cells, insulin activated insulin receptor but not IGF-1 receptor, whereas IGF-1 activated both insulin receptor and IGF-1 receptor (Yanagita et al., 2011). Insulin treatment increased Ser^9-phosphorylated GSK-3β level by 47% within 1 min, with peaking to 104% increase at 1 h and declining to 57% increase at 24 h (Nemoto et al., 2006). IGF-1 (100 nM) also increased Ser^9-phosphorylated GSK-3β level within 1 min, and inhibited GSK-3β activity. The maximum inhibition of GSK-3β activity (~50%) was observed at 1 min after treatment with 100 nM IGF-1, and inhibition of GSK-3β activity was continued for up to 24 h (Yanagita et al., 2011). Inhibition of GSK-3β by chronic treatment with insulin, IGF-1, lithium or valproic acid up-regulated cell surface $Na_V1.7$ Na^+ channel via acceleration of Na^+ channel α-subunit gene transcription, thereby resulting in the enhancement of Na^+ influx, Ca^{2+} channel gating and catecholamine secretion (Yamamoto et al., 1996, 1997; Yanagita et al., 2009, 2011). Chronic insulin treatment also up-regulated tau protein via acceleration of protein synthesis, and induced neurite-like process outgrowth (Nemoto et al., 2011).

In addition to these physiological effects of insulin, chronic insulin treatment down-regulated cell surface density of insulin receptor via reduction of insulin receptor mRNA stability (Yokoo et al., 2007), and protein levels of IRS-1 and IRS-2 via regulating proteasomal degradation and/or synthesis of IRS-1 and IRS-2 (Nemoto et al., 2006). These insulin-induced negative feedback regulations of insulin receptor and IRS-1/-2 were mimicked by treatment with potent GSK-3 inhibitors (lithium, valproic acid, or SB216763) (Nemoto et al., 2006, 2009; Yokoo et al., 2007). LiCl (20 mM) decreased cell surface ^{125}I-insulin binding and insulin receptor protein levels by ~48% in a time-dependent manner. LiCl destabilized insulin receptor mRNA ($t_{1/2}$ = 9.3 vs. 6.5 h), decreasing insulin receptor mRNA level by ~47%, without altering insulin receptor gene transcription (Yokoo et al., 2007). LiCl also decreased protein levels of IRS-1 and IRS-2 by ~38 and ~48% in a concentration- and time-dependent manner. Proteasome inhibitors (β-lactone or lactacystin) completely blocked LiCl-induced reduction of IRS-1, and partially blocked LiCl-induced reduction of IRS-2. LiCl lowered IRS-2 mRNA level, with no effect on IRS-1 mRNA level (Nemoto et al., 2006). These findings suggest that long-term treatment with insulin, lithium or valproic acid causes negative feedback regulation of insulin receptor signaling via inhibition of GSK-3, thereby withdrawal of these therapeutic drugs after long-term treatment may occurs severe depletion of insulin signaling.

8. Conclusion and future perspectives

Multiple lines of experiments in the last two decades have accumulated compelling evidence that brain insulin receptor signaling plays pivotal roles in regulating brain region-specific pleiotropic function, including cognitive and mood stabilizing function. Aberrant decrease in brain insulin receptor signaling (e.g. insulin resistance) may be involved in the various cognitive and mood disorder. There are two major approaches to improve insulin signal impairment: 1) stimulation of insulin receptor signaling by insulin such as intranasal administration of insulin and 2) adjustment of insulin receptor signaling via modulation of expression and function of insulin receptor signaling molecules. The information of up- and down-regulation of insulin receptor signaling by various therapeutic drugs may provide a new avenue for the prevention and treatment of neurodegenerative disease, dementia and mood disorders.

Acknowledgements

This study was supported in part by a Grant-in-Aid for The Scientific Research (C) (to TY 60295227), Young Scientists (A) (to TY 60295227), and Young Scientists (B) (to TN 90506833), from the Ministry of Education, Culture, Sports, Science and Technology, Japan.

Author details

Toshihiko Yanagita[1], Takayuki Nemoto[1], Shinya Satoh[2], Norie Yoshikawa[3], Toyoaki Maruta[4], Seiji Shiraishi[5], Chihiro Sugita[1] and Manabu Murakami[1]

1 Department of Pharmacology, Miyazaki Medical College, University of Miyazaki, Japan

2 Department of Otorhinolaryngology, Miyazaki Medical College, University of Miyazaki, Japan

3 Department of Orthopaedic Surgery, Miyazaki Medical College, University of Miyazaki, Japan

4 Department of Anesthesiology, Miyazaki Medical College, University of Miyazaki, Japan

5 Cancer Pathophysiology Division, National Cancer Center Research Institute, Tokyo, Japan

References

[1] Abbott, M.A.; Wells, D.G., & Fallon, J.R. (1999). The insulin receptor tyrosine kinase substrate p58/53 and the insulin receptor are components of CNS synapses. *J Neurosci*;19:7300-7308.

[2] Banks, W.A. (2004). The source of cerebral insulin. *Eur J Pharmacol*; 490: 5–12.

[3] Banks, W.A.; During, M.J., & Niehoff, M.L. (2004). Brain uptake of the glucagon-like peptide-1 antagonist exendin(9–39) after intranasal administration. *J Pharmacol Exp Ther;* 309: 469-475.

[4] Barakat, N.S.; Omar, S.A., & Ahmed, A.A. (2006). Carbamazepine uptake into rat brain following intra-olfactory transport. *J Pharm Pharmacol;* 58:63-72.

[5] Baskin, D.G.; Figlewicz, D.P.; Woods, S.C.; Porte, D., & Dorsa, D.M. (1987). Insulin in the brain. *Ann Rev Physiol;* 49: 335–347.

[6] Baura, G.D.; Foster, D.M.; Porte, D. Jr.; Kahn, S.E.; Bergman, R.N.; Cobelli, C., & Schwartz, M.W. (1993). Saturable transport of insulin from plasma into the central nervous system of dogs in vivo. A mechanism for regulated insulin delivery to the brain. *J Clin Invest;* 92: 1824–1830.

[7] Bechstein, W.O. (2000). Neurotoxicity of calcineurin inhibitors: impact and clinical management. *Transpl Int;* 13: 313-326.

[8] Benedict. C.; Frey, W.H. 2nd.; Schiöth, H.B.; Schultes, B.; Born, J., & Hallschmid, M. (2011). Intranasal insulin as a therapeutic option in the treatment of cognitive impairments. *Exp Gerontol;* 46: 112-115.

[9] Benedict, C.; Hallschmid, M.; Hatke, A.; Schultes, B.; Fehm, H.L.; Born, J., & Kern, W. (2004). Intranasal insulin improves memory in humans. *Psychoneuroendocrinology;* 29: 1326-1334.

[10] Benedict, C.; Hallschmid, M.; Schmitz, K.; Schultes, B.; Ratter, F.; Fehm, H.L.; Born, J., & Kern, W. (2007). Intranasal insulin improves memory in humans: superiority of insulin aspart. *Neuropsychopharmacology;* 32: 239–243.

[11] Boden, G.; Lebed, B.; Schatz, M.; Homko, C., & Lemieux, S. (2001). Effects of acute changes of plasma free fatty acids on intramyocellular fat content and insulin resistance in healthy subjects. *Diabetes;* 50: 1612–1617.

[12] Born, J.; Lange, T.; Kern, W.; McGregor, G.P.; Bickel, U., & Fehm, H.L. (2002). Sniffing neuropeptides: a transnasal approach to the human brain. *Nat. Neurosci;* 5: 514–516.

[13] Boura-Halfon, S., & Zick, Y. (2009). Phosphorylation of IRS proteins, insulin action, and insulin resistance. *Am J Physiol Endocrinol Metab;* 296: E581-591.

[14] Brüning, J.C.; Gautam, D.; Burks, D.J.; Gillette, J.; Schubert, M.; Orban, P.C.; Klein, R.; Krone, W.; Müller-Wieland, D., & Kahn, C.R. (2000). Role of brain insulin receptor in control of body weight and reproduction. *Science;* 289: 2122–2125.

[15] Bruning, J. C.; Winna, J.; Cheatham, B., & Kahn, C. R. (1997). Differential signaling by insulin receptor substrate 1 (IRS-1) and IRS-2 in IRS-1-deficient cells. *Mol. Cell. Biol;* 17: 1513–1521.

[16] Burks, D.J.; de Mora, J.F.; Schubert, M.; Withers, D.J.; Myers, M.G.; Towery, H.H.; Altamuro, S.L.; Flint, C.L., & White, M.F. (2000). IRS-2 pathways integrate female reproduction and energy homeostasis. *Nature;* 407: 377–382.

[17] Chen, X-Q.; Fawcett, J.R.; Rahman, Y-E.; Ala, T.A., & Frey, W.H. 2nd. (1998). Delivery of nerve growth factor to the brain via the olfactory pathway. *J Alzheimer's Dis;* 1: 35-44.

[18] Chen, Y., Jiang, Y., & Mao, Y. (2009). Association between obesity and depression in Canadians. *J Womens Health (Larchmt);* 18: 1687–1692.

[19] Chiu, S.L., & Cline, H.T. (2010). Insulin receptor signaling in the development of neuronal structure and function. *Neural Dev;* 15: 5-7.

[20] Cid, C.; Alvarez-Cermeño, J.C.; Salinas, M., & Alcázar, A. (2005). Anti-heat shock protein 90β antibodies decrease pre-oligodendrocyte population in perinatal and adult cell cultures. Implications for remyelination in multiple sclerosis. *J Neurochem;* 95: 349-360.

[21] Cid, C.; Regidor, I. & Alcázar, A. J. (2007). Anti-heat shock protein 90β antibodies are detected in patients with multiple sclerosis during remission. *Neuroimmunol;* 184: 223-226.

[22] Copps, K.D., & White, M.F. (2012). Regulation of insulin sensitivity by serine/threonine phosphorylation of insulin receptor substrate proteins IRS1 and IRS2. *Diabetologia;* Aug 8. [Epub ahead of print]

[23] Craft, S.; Asthana, S.; Schellenberg, G.; Cherrier, M.; Baker, L.D.; Newcomer, J.; Plymate, S.; Latendresse, S.; Petrova, A.; Raskind, M.; Peskind, E.; Lofgreen, C., & Grimwood, K. (1999). Insulin metabolism in Alzheimer's disease differs according to apolipoprotein E genotype and gender. *Neuroendocrinology;* 70: 146-152.

[24] Craft, S., & Watson, G.S. (2004). Insulin and neurodegenerative disease: shared and specific mechanisms. *Lancet Neurol;* 3: 169-178.

[25] Cummings, J.L., & Cole, G. (2002). Alzheimer disease. *JAMA;*287:2335–2338.

[26] Dajas-Bailador, F., & Wonnacott, S. (2004). Nicotinic acetylcholine receptors and the regulation of neuronal signalling. *Trends Pharmacol Sci;* 25: 317–324.

[27] de la Monte, S.M. (2009). Insulin resistance and Alzheimer's disease. *BMB reports;* 42: 475- 481.

[28] de la Monte, S.M. (2012). Brain insulin resistance and deficiency as therapeutic targets in Alzheimer's disease. *Curr Alzheimer Res;* 9: 35-66.

[29] de la Monte, S.M.; Tong, M.; Bowling, N., & Moskal, P. (2011). si-RNA inhibition of brain insulin or insulin-like growth factor receptors causes developmental cerebellar abnormalities: relevance to fetal alcohol spectrum disorder. *Mol Brain;* 28: 4-13.

[30] de la Monte, S.M., & Wands, J.R. (2008). Alzheimer's disease is type 3 diabetes-evidence reviewed. *J Diabetes Sci Technol;* 2: 1101–1113.

[31] Evers, M.,; Cunningham-Rundles, C., & Hollander, E. (2002). Heat shock protein 90 antibodies in autism. *Mol Psychiatry;* 7 Suppl 2: S26-28.

[32] Fisher, S.J.; Bruning, J.C.; Lannon, S., & Kahn, C.R. (2005). Insulin signaling in the central nervous system is critical for the normal sympathoadrenal response to hypoglycemia. *Diabetes;* 54: 1447–1451.

[33] Frölich, L.; Blum-Degen, D.; Bernstein, H.G.; Engelsberger, S.; Humrich, J.; Laufer, S.; Muschner, D.; Thalheimer, A.; Türk, A.; Hoyer, S.; Zöchling, R.; Boissl, K.W.; Jellinger, K., & Riederer, P. (1998). Brain insulin and insulin receptors in aging and sporadic Alzheimer's disease. *J Neural Transm;* 105: 423-438.

[34] Gijtenbeek, J.M.; van den Bent, M.J., & Vecht, C.J. (1999). Cyclosporine neurotoxicity: a review. *J Neurol;* 246: 339-346.

[35] Glaser, N. (2009). Cerebral injury and cerebral edema in children with diabetic ketoacidosis: could cerebral ischemia and reperfusion injury be involved? *Pediatr Diabetes;* 10: 534-541.

[36] Goldstein, B.J., & Dudley, A.L. (1992). Heterogeneity of messenger RNA that encodes the rat insulin receptor is limited to the domain of exon 11. Analysis by RNA heteroduplex mapping, amplification of cDNA, and in vitro translation. *Diabetes;* 41: 1293–1300.

[37] Guzmán, M., & Blázquez, C. (2004). Ketone body synthesis in the brain: possible neuroprotective effects. *Prostaglandins Leukot Essent Fatty Acids;* 70: 287-292.

[38] Hallschmid, M.; Benedict, C.; Schultes, B.; Born, J., & Kern, W. (2008). Obese men respond to cognitive but not to catabolic brain insulin signaling. *Int J Obes;* 32: 275–282.

[39] Hanson, L.R., & Frey, W.H. 2nd. (2008). Intranasal delivery bypasses the blood-brain barrier to target therapeutic agents to the central nervous system and treat neurodegenerative disease. BMC Neurosci; 9 Suppl 3: S5.

[40] Heidenreich, K.A.; Zahniser, N.R.; Berhanu, P.; Brandenburg, D., & Olefsky, J.M. (1983). Structural differences between insulin receptors in the brain and peripheral target tissues. *J Biol Chem;* 258: 8527–8530.

[41] Ho, S.; Clipstone, N.; Timmerman, L.; Northrop, J.; Graef, I.; Fiorentino, D.; Nourse, J., & Crabtree, G.R. (1996). The mechanism of action of cyclosporin A and FK560. *Clin Immunol Immunopathol;* 80: S40-45.

[42] Hoshi, M.; Takashima, A.; Murayama, M.; Yasutake, K.; Yoshida, N.; Ishiguro, K.; Hoshino, T., & Imahori, K. (1997). Nontoxic amyloid β peptide1-42 suppresses acetylcholine synthesis. Possible role in cholinergic dysfunction in Alzheimer's disease. *J Biol Chem;* 272: 2038–2041.

[43] Huang, C.C.; Lee, C.C., & Hsu, K.S. (2010). The role of insulin receptor signaling in synaptic plasticity and cognitive function. *Chang Gung Med J;* 33:115-125.

[44] Jindal, R.M.; Sidner, R.A., & Milgrom, M.L. (1997). Post-transplant diabetes mellitus. *Drug Saf;* 16: 242–257.

[45] Jope, R.S., & Johnson, G.V.W. (2004). The glamour and gloom of glycogen synthase kinase-3. *Trends Biochem. Sci.* ; 29: 95–102.

[46] Jope, R.S.; Yuskaitis, C.J., & Beurel, E. (2007). Glycogen synthase kinase-3 (GSK3): inflammation, diseases, and therapeutics. *Neurochem. Res.* ; 32: 577–595.

[47] Kahan, B.D. (1989). Cyclosporine. *N Engl J Med;* 321: 1725–1738.

[48] Kahn, C.R. (1994). Insulin action, diabetogenes and the cause of type II diabetes. *Diabetes;* 43: 1066–1084.

[49] Kamal, A.; Boehm, M.F., & Burrows, F.J. (2004). Therapeutic and diagnostic implications of Hsp90 activation. *Trends Mol Med.;* 10: 283-290.

[50] Kroner, Z. (2009). The relationship between Alzheimer's disease and diabetes: Type 3 diabetes? *Altern Med Rev.;* 14: 373-379.

[51] Ketterer, C.; Tschritter, O.; Preissl, H.; Heni, M.; Häring, H.U., & Fritsche, A. (2011). Insulin sensitivity of the human brain. *Diabetes Res Clin Pract.;* 93 Suppl 1: S47-51.

[52] Koda, M.; Sulkowska, M.; Kanczuga-Koda, L., & Sulkowski, S. (2005). Expression of insulin receptor substrate 1 in primary breast cancer and lymph node metastases. *J Clin Pathol.;* 58:645-649.

[53] Kubota, N.; Tobe, K.; Terauchi, Y.; Eto, K.; Yamauchi, T.; Suzuki, R.; Tsubamoto, Y.; Komeda, K.; Nakano, R.; Miki, H.; Satoh, S.; Sekihara, H.; Sciacchitano, S.; Lesniak, M.; Aizawa, S.; Nagai, R.; Kimura, S.; Akanuma, Y.; Taylor, S.I., & Kadowaki, T. (2000). Disruption of insulin receptor substrate 2 causes type 2 diabetes because of liver insulin resistance and lack of compensatory β-cell hyperplasia. *Diabetes;* 49: 1880-1889.

[54] Laron, Z. (2009). Insulin and the brain. *Arch Physiol Biochem;* 115: 112-116.

[55] Licinio-Paixao, J. (1989). Hyperinsulinemia; a mediator of decreased food intake and weight loss in anorexia nervosa and major depression. *Med Hypotheses;* 28: 125–130.

[56] Maalouf, M.; Rho, J.M., & Mattson, M.P. (2009). The neuroprotective properties of calorie restriction, the ketogenic diet, and ketone bodies. *Brain Res Rev.;* 59: 293-315.

[57] Marks, J.L.; Maddison, J., & Eastman, C.J. (1988). Subcellular localization of rat brain insulin binding sites. *J Neurochem;* 50: 774-781.

[58] Massieu, L.; Haces, M.L.; Montiel, T., & Hernández-Fonseca, K. (2003). Acetoacetate protects hippocampal neurons against glutamate-mediated neuronal damage during glycolysis inhibition. *Neuroscience;* 120: 365-378.

[59] Meijer, L.; Flajolet, M., & Greengard, P. (2004). Pharmacological inhibitors of glycogen synthase kinase 3. *Trends Pharmacol.Sci.;* 25: 471–480.

[60] Meneilly, G.S.; Cheung, E.; Tessier, D.; Yakura, C., & Tuokko, H. (1993). The effect of improved glycemic control on cognitive functions in the elderly patient with diabetes. *J Gerontol;* 48: M117-121.

[61] Miyakawa, T.; Leiter, L.M.; Gerber, D.J.; Gainetdinov, R.R., Sotnikova, T.D.; Zeng, H.; Caron, M.G., & Tonegawa, S. (2003). Conditional calcineurin knockout mice exhibit multiple abnormal behaviors related to schizophrenia. *Proc Natl Acad Sci U S A.*; 100: 8987-8992.

[62] Morelli, C.; Garofalo, C.; Bartucci, M., & Surmacz, E. (2003). Estrogen receptor-α regulates the degradation of insulin receptor substrates 1 and 2 in breast cancer cells. *Oncogene*; 22: 4007–4016.

[63] Morris, J.K., & Burns, J.M. (2012). Insulin: An Emerging Treatment for Alzheimer's Disease Dementia? Curr Neurol Neurosci Rep. Jul 13. [Epub ahead of print].

[64] Neckers, L. (2002). Hsp90 inhibitors as novel cancer chemotherapeutic agents. *Trends Mol Med.*; 8: S55-S61.

[65] Nehlig, A., & Pereira de Vasconcelos, A. (1993). Glucose and ketone body utilization by the brain of neonatal rats. *Prog Neurobiol*; 40: 163–221.

[66] Nemoto, T.; Yanagita, T.; Kanai, T., & Wada, A. (2009). Drug development targeting the glycogen synthase kinase-3β (GSK-3β)-mediated signal transduction pathway: the role of GSK-3β in the maintenance of steady-state levels of insulin receptor signaling molecules and Nav1.7 sodium channel in adrenal chromaffin cells. *J Pharmacol Sci*; 109: 157-161.

[67] Nemoto, T.; Yanagita, T.; Satoh, S.; Maruta, T.; Kanai, T.; Murakami, M., & Wada A. (2011). Insulin-induced neurite-like process outgrowth: Acceleration of tau protein synthesis via a phosphoinositide 3-kinase~mammalian target of rapamycin pathway. *Neurochem Int*; 59: 880-888.

[68] Nemoto, T.; Yokoo, H.; Satoh. S.; Yanagita, T.; Sugano, T.; Yoshikawa, N.; Maruta, T.; Kobayashi, H., & Wada A. (2006). Constitutive activity of glycogen synthase kinase-3β: positive regulation of steady-state levels of insulin receptor substrates-1 and -2 in adrenal chromaffin cells. Brain Res; 1110: 1-12.

[69] Newhouse, P. A.; Potter, A.; Kelton, M., & Corwin, J. (2001). Nicotinic treatment of Alzheimer's disease. *Biol. Psychiatry*; 49: 268–278.

[70] Noh, H.S.; Hah, Y.S.; Nilufar, R.; Han, J.; Bong, J.H.; Kang, S.S.; Cho, G.J., & Choi, W.S. (2006). Acetoacetate protects neuronal cells from oxidative glutamate toxicity. *J Neurosci Res*; 83:702-709.

[71] Nordberg, A. (2001). Nicotinic receptor abnormalities of Alzheimer's disease: therapeutic implications. *Biol. Psychiatry*; 49: 200–210.

[72] Oetjen, E.; Baun, D.; Beimesche, S.; Krause, D.; Cierny, I.; Blume, R.; Dickel, C.; Wehner, S., & Knepel, W. (2003). Inhibition of human insulin gene transcription by the immunosuppressive drugs cyclosporin A and tacrolimus in primary, mature islets of transgenic mice. *Mol. Pharmacol.*; 63: 1289–1295.

[73] Ohara, T.; Doi, Y.; Ninomiya, T.; Hirakawa, Y.; Hata, J.; Iwaki, T.; Kanba, S., & Kiyohara, Y. (2011). Glucose tolerance status and risk of dementia in the community: the Hisayama Study. *Neurology;* 77: 1126–1134.

[74] Ott, A.; Stolk, R.P.; van Harskamp, F.; Pols, H.A.; Hofman, A., & Breteler, M.M. (1999). Diabetes mellitus and the risk of dementia: the Rotterdam study. *Neurology;* 58: 1937-1941.

[75] Ott, V.; Benedict, C.; Schultes, B.; Born, J., & Hallschmid, M. (2012). Intranasal administration of insulin to the brain impacts cognitive function and peripheral metabolism. *Diabetes Obes Metab.;* 14: 214-221.

[76] Patti, M-E. (1999). Nutrient modulation of cellular insulin action. *Ann NY Acad Sci;* 892: 187–203.

[77] Picciotto M. R. and Zoli M. (2002). Nicotinic receptors in aging and dementia. J. Neurobiol. 53, 641–655.

[78] Ramasubbu, R. (2002). Insulin resistance: a metabolic link between depressive disorder and atherosclerotic vascular diseases. *Med Hypotheses;* 59: 537-551.

[79] Rasgon, N.L., & Kenna, H.A. (2005). Insulin resistance in depressive disorders and Alzheimer's disease: revisiting the missing link hypothesis. *Neurobiol Aging;* 26 Suppl 1:103-107.

[80] Razay, G., & Wilcock G.K. (1994). Hyperinsulinaemia and Alzheimer's disease. *Age Ageing;* 23: 396-399.

[81] Reagan, L.P. (2007). Insulin signaling effects on memory and mood. *Curr Opin Pharmacol.;* 7:633-637.

[82] Reger, M.A.; Watson, G.S.; Frey, W.H.; Baker, L.D.; Cholerton, B.; Keeling, M.L.; Belongia, D.A.; Fishel, M.A.; Plymate, S.R.; Schellenberg, G.D.; Cherrier, M.M., & Craft, S. (2006). Effects of intranasal insulin on cognition in memory-impaired older adults: modulation by APOE genotype. *Neurobiol. Aging;* 27: 451-458.

[83] Reger, M.A.; Watson, G.S.; Green, P.S.; Baker, L.D.; Cholerton, B.; Fishel, M.A.; Plymate, S.R.; Cherrier, M.M.; Schellenberg, G.D.; Frey, W.H., & Craft, S. (2008). Intranasal insulin administration dose-dependently modulates verbal memory and plasma amyloid-β in memory-impaired older adults. *J. Alzheimers Dis;* 13: 323–331.

[84] Reiss, K.; Wang, J.Y.; Romano, G.; Furnari, F.B.; Cavenee, W.K.; Morrione, A.; Tu, X., & Baserga, R. (2000). IGF-I receptor signaling in a prostatic cancer cell line with a PTEN mutation. *Oncogene;* 19: 2687–2694.

[85] Richter, K., & Buchner, J. (2001). Hsp90: Chaperoning signal transduction. *J Cell Physiol;* 188: 281-290.

[86] Roberts, R. E.; Deleger, S.; Strawbridge, W. J., & Kaplan, G. A. (2003). Prospective association between obesity and depression: Evidence from the Alameda County Study. *Int J Obes Relat Metab Disord;* 27: 514-521.

[87] Saltiel, A.R. (2001). New perspective into molecular pathogenesis and treatment of type 2 diabetes. *Cell;* 104: 517–529.

[88] Saitoh, T.; Yanagita, T.; Shiraishi, S.; Yokoo, H.; Kobayashi, H.; Minami, S.; Onitsuka, T., & Wada, A. (2002). Down-regulation of cell surface insulin receptor and insulin receptor substrate-1 phosphorylation by inhibitor of 90-kDa heat-shock protein family: endoplasmic reticulum retention of monomeric insulin receptor precursor with calnexin in adrenal chromaffin cells. *Mol Pharmacol;* 62: 847-855.

[89] Satoh, S.; Yanagita, T.; Maruta, T.; Nemoto, T.; Yoshikawa, N.; Kobayashi, H.; Tono, T., & Wada, A. (2008). Proteasomal degradation of IRS-2, but not IRS-1 by calcineurin inhibition: attenuation of insulin-like growth factor-I-induced GSK-3β and ERK pathways in adrenal chromaffin cells. *Neuropharmacology;* 55: 71-79.

[90] Schwartz, M.W.; Figlewicz, D.P.; Baskin, D.G.; Woods, S.C., & Porte, D. Jr. (1992). Insulin in the brain: a hormonal regulator of energy balance. *Endocr Rev;* 13: 387-414.

[91] Schubert, M.; Brazil, D.P.; Burks, D.J.; Kushner, J.A.; Ye, J.; Flint, C.L.; Farhang-Fallah, J.; Dikkes, P.; Warot, X.M.; Rio, C.; Corfas, G., & White, M.F. (2003). Insulin receptor substrate-2 deficiency impairs brain growth and promotes tau phosphorylation. *J Neurosci;* 23: 7084-7092.

[92] Schubert, M.; Gautam, D.; Surjo, D.; Ueki, K.; Baudler, S.; Schubert, D.; Kondo, T.; Alber, J.; Galldiks, N.; Küstermann, E.; Arndt, S.; Jacobs, A.H.; Krone, W.; Kahn, C.R., & Brüning, J.C. (2004). Role for neuronal insulin resistance in neurodegenerative diseases. *Proc Natl Acad Sci U S A;* 101: 3100–3105.

[93] Sesti, G.; Federici, M.; Hribal, M.L.; Lauro, D.; Sbraccia, P., & Lauro, R. (2001). Defects of the insulin receptor substrate (IRS) system in human metabolic disorders. *FASEB J;* 15: 2099-2111.

[94] Shastry, R.M., & Bhatia, V. (2006). Cerebral edema in diabetic ketoacidosis. *Indian Pediatr;* 43: 701-708.

[95] Shen, W.W.; Liu, H.C.; Yang, Y.Y.; Lin, C.Y.; Chen, K.P.; Yeh, T.S., & Leu, S.J. (2006). Anti-heat shock protein 90 is increased in acute mania. *Aust N Z J Psychiatry;* 40: 712-716.

[96] Shiraishi, S.; Yokoo, H.; Kobayashi, H.; Yanagita, T.; Uezono, Y.; Minami, S.; Takasaki, M., & Wada, A. (2000). Post-translational reduction of cell surface expression of insulin receptors by cyclosporin A, FK506 and rapamycin in bovine adrenal chromaffin cells. *Neurosci Lett;* 293: 211-215.

[97] Sima, A.A.; Kamiya, H., & Li, Z.G. (2004). Insulin, C-peptide hyperglycemia and central nervous system complications in diabetes. *Eur J Pharmacology;* 490: 187-197.

[98] Sima, A.A., & Li, Z.G. (2006). Diabetes and Alzheimer's disease - is there a connection? *Rev Diabet Stud;* 3: 161-168.

[99] Simon, G. E.; Von Korff, M.; Saunders, K.; Miglioretti, D. L.; Crane, P. K.; van Belle, G., & Kessler, R.C. (2006). Association between obesity and psychiatric disorders in the US adult population. *Arch Gen Psychiatry;* 63, 824–830.

[100] Soczynska, J.K.; Kennedy, S.H.; Woldeyohannes, H.O.; Liauw, S.S.; Alsuwaidan, M.; Yim, C.Y., & McIntyre, R.S. (2011). Mood disorders and obesity: understanding inflammation as a pathophysiological nexus. *Neuromolecular Med;* 13: 93-116.

[101] Steen, E.; Terry, B.M.; Rivera, E.J.; Cannon, J.L.; Neely, T.R.; Tavares, R.; Xu, X.J.; Wands, J.R., & de la Monte, S.M. (2005). Impaired insulin and insulin-like growth factor expression and signaling mechanisms in Alzheimer's disease-is this type 3 diabetes? *J Alzheimers Dis;* 7: 63–80

[102] Stockhorst, U., de Fries, D., Steingrueber, H.J., & Scherbaum, W.A. (2004). Insulin and the CNS: effects on food intake, memory, and endocrine parameters and the role of intranasal insulin administration in humans. *Physiol Behav;* 83: 47-54.

[103] Sugano, T.; Yanagita, T.; Yokoo, H.; Satoh, S.; Kobayashi, H., & Wada, A. (2006). Enhancement of insulin-induced PI3K/Akt/GSK-3βand ERK signaling by neuronal nicotinic receptor/PKC-α/ERK pathway: up-regulation of IRS-1/-2 mRNA and protein in adrenal chromaffin cells. *J Neurochem;* 98: 20-33.

[104] Sugimoto, K.; Murakawa, Y.; Zhang, W.; Xu, G., & Sima, A.A. (2000). Insulin receptor in rat peripheral nerve: its localization and alternatively spliced isoforms. *Diab. Metab. Res. Rev.;* 16: 354-363.

[105] Surmacz, E. (2000) Function of the IGF-I receptor in breast cancer. *J Mammary Gland Biol Neoplasia;* 5: 95-105.

[106] Tanemoto, H.; Kadowaki, T.; Tobe, K.; Yagi, T.; Sakura, H.; Hayakawa, T.; Terauchi, Y.; Ueki, K.; Kaburagi, Y., & Satoh, S. (1994). Insulin resistance and growth retardation in mice lacking insulin receptor substrate-1. *Nature;* 372, 182–186.

[107] Thorne, R.G.; Emory, C.R.; Ala, T.A., & Frey, W.H. (1995). Quantitative analysis of the olfactory pathway for drug delivery to the brain. *Brain Res;* 692: 278 – 282.

[108] Thorne, R.G.; Pronk, G.J.; Padmanabhan, V., & Frey, W.H. 2nd. (2004). Delivery of insulin-like growth factor-I to the rat brain and spinal cord along olfactory and trigeminal pathways following intranasal administration. *Neuroscience;* 127: 481-496.

[109] Unger, J.; McNeill, T.H.; Moxley, R.T.; White, M.; Moss, A., & Livingston, J.N. (1989). Distribution of insulin receptor-like immunoreactivity in the rat forebrain. *Neuroscience;* 31: 143-157.

[110] van der Heide, L.P.; Ramakers, G.M., & Smidt, M.P. (2006). Insulin signaling in the central nervous system: learning to survive. *Prog Neurobiol;* 79: 205-221.

[111] Wada, A.; Yokoo, H.; Yanagita, T., & Kobayashi, H. (2005). New twist on neuronal insulin receptor signaling in health, disease, and therapeutics. *J Pharmacol Sci;* 99: 128-143.

[112] Watson, G.S., & Craft, S. (2004). Modulation of memory by insulin and glucose: neuropsychological observations in Alzheimer's disease. *Eur J Pharmacol;* 490: 97-113.

[113] Watson, G.S., & Craft, S. (2006). Insulin resistance, inflammation, and cognition in Alzheimer's Disease: lessons for multiple sclerosis. *J Neurol Sci;* 245: 21-33.

[114] Welch, W.J., & Feramisco, J.R. (1982). Purification of the major mammalian heat shock proteins. *J Biol Chem;* 257: 14949 -14959.

[115] White, M.F. (1997). The insulin signalling system and the IRS proteins. *Diabetologia;* 40 (Suppl. 2): S2–17.

[116] White, M.F. (1998). The IRS-signalling system: a network of docking proteins that mediate insulin action. *Mol Cell Biochem;* 182: 3–11.

[117] Whitesell, L.; Mimnaugh, E.G.; De Costa, B.; Myers, C.E., & Neckers, L.M. (1994) Inhibition of heat shock protein HSP90-pp60v-src heteroprotein complex formation by benzoquinone ansamycins: essential role for stress proteins in oncogenic transformation. *Proc Natl Acad Sci USA;* 91: 8324-8328.

[118] Williamson, R.; McNeilly, A., & Sutherland, C. (2012). Insulin resistance in the brain: An old-age or new-age problem? *Biochem Pharmacol;* 84:737-745.

[119] Withers, D.J.; Gutierrez, J.S.; Towery, H.; Burks, D.J.; Ren, J.M.; Previs, S.; Zhang, Y.; Bernal, D.; Pons, S.; Shulman, G.I.; Bonner-Weir, S., & White, M.F. (1998). Disruption of IRS-2 causes type 2 diabetes in mice. *Nature;* 391: 900-904.

[120] Wolfsdorf, J.; Craig, M.E.; Daneman, D.; Dunger, D.; Edge, J.; Lee, W.; Rosenbloom, A.; Sperling, M., & Hanas, R. (2009). Diabetic ketoacidosis in children and adolescents with diabetes. *Pediatr Diabetes;* 10 Suppl 12: 118-133.

[121] Woods, S.C.; Seeley, R.J.; Baskin, D.G., & Schwartz, M.W. (2003). Insulin and the blood–brain barrier. *Curr Pharm Res;* 9: 795–800.

[122] Yamamoto, R.; Kobayashi, H.; Yanagita, T.; Yokoo, H.; Kurose, T.; Shiraishi, S.; Minami, S.; Matsukura, S., & Wada, A. (2000). Up-regulation of cell surface insulin receptor by protein kinase C-α in adrenal chromaffin cells: involvement of transcriptional and translational events. *J Neurochem;* 75: 672-682.

[123] Yamamoto, R.; Yanagita, T.; Kobayashi, H.; Yokoo, H., & Wada, A. (1997). Up-regulation of sodium channel subunit mRNAs and their cell surface expression by antiepileptic valproic acid: activation of calcium channel and catecholamine secretion in adrenal chromaffin cells. *J Neurochem;* 68: 1655-1662.

[124] Yamamoto, R.; Yanagita, T.; Kobayashi, H.; Yuhi, T.; Yokoo, H., & Wada, A. (1996). Up-regulation of functional voltage-dependent sodium channels by insulin in cultured bovine adrenal chromaffin cells. *J Neurochem;* 67:1401-1408.

[125] Yanagita, T.; Maruta, T.; Nemoto, T.; Uezono, Y.; Matsuo, K.; Satoh, S.; Yoshikawa, N.; Kanai, T.; Kobayashi, H., & Wada, A. (2009). Chronic lithium treatment up-regu-

http://dx.doi.org/10.5772/54389

lates cell surface $Na_V1.7$ sodium channels via inhibition of glycogen synthase kinase-3 in adrenal chromaffin cells: enhancement of Na^+ influx, Ca^{2+} influx and catecholamine secretion after lithium withdrawal. *Neuropharmacology;* 57: 311-321.

[126] Yanagita, T.; Satoh, S.; Uezono, Y.; Matsuo, K.; Nemoto, T.; Maruta, T.; Yoshikawa, N.; Iwakiri, T.; Minami, K., & Murakami, M. (2011). Transcriptional up-regulation of cell surface Na_V 1.7 sodium channels by insulin-like growth factor-1 via inhibition of glycogen synthase kinase-3β in adrenal chromaffin cells: enhancement of $^{22}Na^+$ influx, $^{45}Ca^{2+}$ influx and catecholamine secretion. *Neuropharmacology;* 61: 1265-1274.

[127] Yokoo, H.; Saitoh, T.; Shiraishi, S.; Yanagita, T.; Sugano, T.; Minami, S.; Kobayashi, H., & Wada, A. (2003). Distinct effects of ketone bodies on down-regulation of cell surface insulin receptor and insulin receptor substrate-1 phosphorylation in adrenal chromaffin cells. *J Pharmacol Exp Ther;* 304: 994-1002.

[128] Yoshikawa, N.; Nemoto, T.; Satoh, S.; Maruta, T.; Yanagita, T.; Chosa, E., & Wada, A. (2010). Distinct regulation of insulin receptor substrate-1 and -2 by 90-kDa heat-shock protein in adrenal chromaffin cells. *Neurochem Int;* 56: 42-50.

[129] Young, J.C.; Moarefi, I., & Hartl, F.U. (2001). Hsp90: a specialized but essential protein folding tool. *J Cell Biol;* 154: 267-273.

[130] Zhang, H., & Burrows, F. (2004). Targeting multiple signal transduction pathways through inhibition of Hsp90. *J Mol Med (Berl);* 82:488-499.

[131] Zhao, W.; Chen, H.; Moore, E.; Meiri, N.; Quon, M.J., & Alkon, D.L. (1999). Brain insulin receptors and spatial memory. *J Biol Chem;* 274: 34893–34902.

[132] Zhao, Z.; Ksiezak-Reding, H.; Riggio, S.; Haroutunian, V., & Pasinetti, G.M. (2006). Insulin receptor deficits in schizophrenia and in cellular and animal models of insulin receptor dysfunction. *Schizophr Res;* 84: 1-14.

[133] Zeng, H.; Chattarji, S.; Barbarosie, M.; Rondi-Reig, L.; Philpot, B.D.; Miyakawa, T.; Bear, M.F., & Tonegawa, S. (2001). Forebrain-specific calcineurin knockout selectively impairs bidirectional synaptic plasticity and working memory. *Cell;* 107: 617-629.